Nutrition and Heart Disease: An Integrated Approach

Nutrition and Heart Disease: An Integrated Approach

Editor: Brooke Dowson

AMERICAN
MEDICAL PUBLISHERS
www.americanmedicalpublishers.com

AMERICAN
MEDICAL PUBLISHERS
www.americanmedicalpublishers.com

Cataloging-in-Publication Data

Nutrition and heart disease : an integrated approach / edited by Brooke Dowson.
p. cm.
Includes bibliographical references and index.
ISBN 978-1-63927-759-9
1. Heart--Diseases--Nutritional aspects. 2. Heart--Diseases--Diet therapy.
3. Reducing diets. 4. Diet therapy. I. Dowson, Brooke.
RC682 .N88 2023
616.12--dc23

American Medical Publishers,
41 Flatbush Avenue,
1st Floor, New York,
NY 11217, USA

ISBN 978-1-63927-759-9 (Hardback)

Contents

Preface

This book was inspired by the evolution of our times; to answer the curiosity of inquisitive minds. Many developments have occurred across the globe in the recent past which has transformed the progress in the field.

Heart disease refers to a variety of disorders that affect the heart in the human body. It includes heart valve disease, coronary artery disease, infections of the heart, heart rhythm issues, etc. There are several symptoms of heart disease, such as shortness of breath, chest pain and neck pain. The risk factors of heart disease include a poor diet, aging, high blood pressure, elevated cholesterol levels, a family history of heart disease, etc. Plant-based foods and diets rich in low-saturated fat and fiber can significantly lower the risk of developing heart disease. Potassium and sodium are two interconnected minerals that are crucial for maintaining a healthy heart and controlling blood pressure. The consumption of potassium-rich foods and less salty foods may considerably reduce the risk of heart disease. Furthermore, foods that are beneficial to heart health include vegetables and fruits, oily fish, whole grains, foods containing vitamin E, etc. This book covers in detail some existent theories and innovative concepts revolving around nutrition and heart disease. It is appropriate for students seeking detailed information in this area as well as for experts.

This book was developed from a mere concept to drafts to chapters and finally compiled together as a complete text to benefit the readers across all nations. To ensure the quality of the content we instilled two significant steps in our procedure. The first was to appoint an editorial team that would verify the data and statistics provided in the book and also select the most appropriate and valuable contributions from the plentiful contributions we received from authors worldwide. The next step was to appoint an expert of the topic as the Editor-in-Chief, who would head the project and finally make the necessary amendments and modifications to make the text reader-friendly. I was then commissioned to examine all the material to present the topics in the most comprehensible and productive format.

I would like to take this opportunity to thank all the contributing authors who were supportive enough to contribute their time and knowledge to this project. I also wish to convey my regards to my family who have been extremely supportive during the entire project.

Editor

1

Nutrients, Genetic Factors and their Interaction in Non-Alcoholic Fatty Liver Disease and Cardiovascular Disease

Rosa Lombardi [1,2], Federica Iuculano [1], Giada Pallini [1], Silvia Fargion [1] and Anna Ludovica Fracanzani [1,2,*]

1 Department of Pathophysiology and Transplantation, University of Milan, 20122 Milan, Italy; rosa.lombardi@unimi.it (R.L.); federica.iuculano@unimi.it (F.I.); giada.pallini@unimi.it (G.P.); silvia.fargion@unimi.it (S.F.)

2 Ca' Granda IRCCS Foundation, Policlinico Hospital of Milan, 20122 Milan, Italy

* Correspondence: anna.fracanzani@unimi.it

Abstract: Non-alcoholic fatty liver disease (NAFLD) is the most common chronic liver disease in Western countries and expose patients to increased risk of hepatic and cardiovascular (CV) morbidity and mortality. Both environmental factors and genetic predisposition contribute to the risk. An inappropriate diet, rich in refined carbohydrates, especially fructose, and saturated fats, and poor in fibers, polyunsaturated fats, and vitamins is one of the main key factors, as well as the polymorphism of patatin-like phospholipase domain containing 3 (PNPLA3 gene) for NAFLD and the apolipoproteins and the peroxisome proliferator-activated receptor (PPAR) family for the cardiovascular damage. Beyond genetic influence, also epigenetics modifications are responsible for various clinical manifestations of both hepatic and CV disease. Interestingly, data are accumulating on the interplay between diet and genetic and epigenetic modifications, modulating pathogenetic pathways in NAFLD and CV disease. We report the main evidence from literature on the influence of both macro and micronutrients in NAFLD and CV damage and the role of genetics either alone or combined with diet in increasing the risk of developing both diseases. Understanding the interaction between metabolic alterations, genetics and diet are essential to treat the diseases and tailoring nutritional therapy to control NAFLD and CV risk.

Keywords: nutrigenomic; fructose; PUFA; micronutrients; cardiovascular disease; NAFLD; diet; epigenetic; PNPLA3; genetic influence

1. Introduction

Non-alcoholic fatty liver disease is defined by the presence of fat in more than 5% of hepatocytes without excessive alcohol consumption and after exclusion of all other causes of liver disease. It is the most common chronic liver disease in Western countries [1] and includes a group of hepatic disorders ranging from simple steatosis to more progressive forms such as non-alcoholic steatohepatitis (NASH), characterized by hepatic inflammation, and hepatic fibrosis, possibly leading to NAFLD-related cirrhosis and hepatocellular carcinoma.

NAFLD is characterized by metabolic alterations, mostly overweight and central obesity, dyslipidemia, hypertension, insulin-resistance, and type 2 diabetes mellitus so that the acronym NAFLD has been substituted with the term MAFLD (i.e., metabolic associated fatty liver disease) [2]. However, given the really recent coin of MAFLD term and the almost totality of literature data on fatty liver disease referred as NAFLD, in the present review, we'll keep using the acronym NAFLD.

This metabolic imbalance exposes NAFLD patients to increased cardiovascular (CV) risk, so that the leading cause of mortality in patients with NAFLD is cardiovascular disease (CVD) [3]. Besides coronary artery disease, patients with NAFLD present also higher rate of atrial fibrillation, heart failure, atherosclerosis, altered arterial stiffness, and myocardial remodeling [4].

Actually, NAFLD and CVD share common pathogenetic risk factors. Insulin resistance is one of the key factors in the development of both diseases, prompting increased circulation of free fatty acids (FFAs) to the liver and imbalance in lipid metabolism, with consequent hepatic and vessels fat accumulation [5]. Increased lipid accumulation fosters mitochondrial dysfunction by lipo-toxicity and activation of oxidative stress, both in the liver and in peripheral arteries. Moreover, impairment in lipid metabolism enhances hepatic production of adipokines and inflammatory cytokines, as well as of procoagulant factors. In addition, diet may alter gut microbiota, which is involved in bile acid metabolism and systemic and hepatic inflammation [1].

Both environmental factors and genetic predisposition play a central role in sustaining the above-mentioned pathogenetic mechanisms. Among environmental factors, an inappropriate diet, rich in refined carbohydrates, especially fructose, and saturated fats, and physical inactivity are the key factors. As for the genetic substratum, the polymorphism of I148M PNPLA3 gene (patatin-like phospholipase domain containing 3) is the major determinant of NAFLD, whilst the transmembrane 6 superfamily member 2 gene (TM6SF2), the membrane bound O-acyltransferase domain-containing 7 gene (MBOAT7), and the glucokinase regulatory protein (GCKR) variants play a minor role [6]. Conversely, TM6SF2 mutation seems to reduce CV risk [7]. Along with genetic alterations, epigenetics modifications are also responsible for various clinical manifestations of both hepatic and CVD.

Nowadays, no established pharmacological treatment is available for NAFLD, so that modification in lifestyle, especially diet and regular physical exercise, are standard of care. Similarly, the same approach is advisable to prevent and manage CVD. Many dietary approaches have been proposed and the Mediterranean diet has recently been shown to have a role in improving risk factors associated with metabolic syndrome and NAFLD [8], as well as in reducing CV events [9].

Given the complexity of NAFLD and cardiovascular disease, understanding the interaction between metabolic alterations, genetics, and diet, is essential to treat the diseases and tailoring nutritional therapy to control NAFLD and CV risk.

The aim of our review is to explore the impact of macro and micro-nutrients on development and progression of NAFLD and to assess their influence on CV risk, as well as the interplay between micro/macro-nutrients and genetic substrate in the etiopathogenetic pathway. Finally, we will also report our preliminary data of an observational study conducted at the Outpatient Hepatology Service of Policlinico Hospital of Milan evaluating the impact of macro and micronutrients on liver disease and cardiovascular damage in patients with NAFLD.

2. Role of Carbohydrates in NAFLD and Cardiovascular Disease

2.1. *Carbohydrates and NAFLD*

The Mediterranean diet is one of the mostly suggested dietetic regimen for patients with NAFLD and is characterized by reduced carbohydrate intake (40% of the calories vs. 50–60% in a typical low-fat diet), with particular decrease of sugars and refined carbohydrates [9].

Carbohydrates are classified into monosaccharides (fructose, glucose, and galactose) and disaccharides. Fructose is naturally present in fruits; however, it is often present in the form of added sugar, as a sweetener to other products such as soft drinks, biscuits, and bakery products in the form of sucrose (made of 50% of glucose and 50% of fructose) and high fructose corn syrup (HFCS) (with up to 55% of fructose).

Fructose has been demonstrated as the main carbohydrate determinant in hepatic fat accumulation. In fact, Schwarz et al. [10] demonstrated a higher fat accumulation in patients exposed to a high-fructose diet compared to those with a diet poor in fructose and rich in complex carbohydrates like cereals, bread, pasta, rice, and potatoes.

Indeed, fructose exerts a negative metabolic effect promoting de novo lipogenesis (DNL) and hepatic fat accumulation [11] either directly, being a substrate of DNL, or leading to a hyperproduction of Acetyl-Co-A from citrate, another substrate for DNL as well as a powerful activator of key enzymes in the DNL itself [12]. In addition, the higher intake of fructose fosters oxidative stress and hepatic insulin resistance [13], which, along with intrahepatic fat accumulation, promote the development of hepatic steatosis and cardiometabolic events [14,15]. Moreover, fructose inhibits the production of insulin and leptin, hormones which modulate the feeling of satiety, fostering increased energy intake and weight gain. Finally, fructose ingestion alters gut microbiota, with a reduced capacity to degrade carbohydrates to short-chain fatty acids, and increases gut permeability promoting metabolic dysfunction [16].

Population studies revealed a close association between overconsumption of added sugar (e.g., sucrose and high-fructose corn syrup) and the presence of NAFLD in both adults and children [17–19]. In particular, the Framingham Heart Study, involving more than 2600 subjects examined by abdomen computer tomography for the presence of NAFLD, showed a dose–response association between soft drinks consumption and fatty liver disease [20]. In addition, soft-drinks' usual consumers with NAFLD have a higher rate of inflammation and fibrosis [21] compared to non-consumers, and an improvement of liver histology consequent to fructose restriction has been demonstrated [22]. In contrast, Cortez-Pinto et al. [23] reported in a cohort of 45 biopsy proven NAFLD patients a higher consumption of fat and less carbohydrate in NASH subjects compared to non-NASH ones, with only a slight increase in the consumption of fructose in those with more severe histological features.

Besides observational data, a large number of interventional studies explored the role of carbohydrates in patients with NAFLD.

Solid data demonstrated that consumption of a high-fructose diet even for a short term (i.e., 1–2 weeks) significantly favor hepatic fat deposition [24–26], possibly because of the stimulation of DNL by fructose, especially when combined with glucose ingestion. The role of fructose in DNL has been confirmed by a Sevastianova et al. [27] who demonstrated that a 3-week hypercaloric (+1000 kcal/day) diet enriched with sugars (i.e., candy, fruit juice, and sugar-sweetened beverages) led to an increase in fatty liver and was associated with an increase in the secretion of very low density lipoprotein and an increase in the lipogenic index, (i.e., the ratio of palmitate to linoleate acid), an indirect measure of DNL.

Another study demonstrated the specific steatogenic role of fructose showing that a highly hypercaloric diet, containing a low amount of fructose, did not elicit an increase in liver fat content [24].

Consistently with these results, Maersk et al. [14] compared the effects of ingesting 1 L/day of a sugar-sweetened beverage with a calorie-matched milk for six months and showed that sugar-sweetened beverage significantly increased liver fat by approximately 1.5 fold, despite similar calorie intake and weight gain.

While the causative role of fructose in hypercaloric diet has a consistent evidence, data on the impact of carbohydrates on liver fat accumulation in the setting of hypo or isocaloric diet are scarce and with contrasting results. One study involving NAFLD patients exposed to hypocaloric diet reported a more evident reduction in liver fat content obtained by reducing carbohydrate intake compared to the reduction of total calories without changing the macronutrient composition of the diet [28]. In contrast, Haufe et al. and Volynets et al. [29,30] suggested that total calorie deficit is the mediating factor for decreasing liver fat and that the carbohydrate intake has little influence. Likewise, also data from isocaloric diets enriched with added sugars did not show an influence on liver fat content which vice-versa was highlighted in subjects assuming hypercaloric high-fructose diets, possibly because of increased substrate availability for DNL.

Along with its specific effect, fructose pathogenetic action is modulated by co-ingestion of other macronutrients. Sobrecases et al. showed in a study comparing a 7-day hypercaloric diet enriched with fructose or saturated fatty acids (SFA) that the latter increased liver fat to a greater extent than fructose (~86% vs. ~16% change in hepatic fat content), and that SFA also had an additive effect on hepatic fat accumulation exerted by sugars [26]. On the other hand, supplementation of high-fructose diet with small amount of proteins (6.6 g of essential amino acids/day) leads to an attenuation of hepatic fat accumulation [31]. The beneficial effect of proteins may rely on the augmented fatty acid oxidation due to the increased energy required by the metabolism of amino acids (i.e., gluconeogenesis and cycle of urea) [32].

Finally, the timing of food intake also affects hepatic fat deposition, being more dangerous when consumed between rather than alongside meals [33].

2.2. Carbohydrates and Cardiovascular Disease

As for the impact in the development of NAFLD, fructose has been demonstrated to exert a negative effect on CV risk. Interestingly, the amount of added sugar, consumed mainly as HFCS, dramatically increased during the last few decades in Europe and the USA [34] paralleling the augmented prevalence of coronary artery disease (CAD) [35], as supported by a prospective study involving a large female cohort [36]. The association between HCFC and CVD has been confirmed by consistent data. A prospective study involving a cohort of adults in the USA showed that added sugar intake was a risk factor for CV mortality even when adjusted for conventional cardiovascular risk factors such hypertension and dyslipidemia [37]. Another prospective study involving more than 2600 Iranian subjects, without a history of CV events followed-up for approximately seven years, demonstrated that consumption of food with added fructose, but not natural sugars, was associated with an increased risk of CV events, either myocardial infarction or stroke, and cardiovascular mortality. This result points out that only industrial sweetened products expose to cardiovascular risk, whilst consumption of natural fructose food, like fresh fruit, is safe. In another population-based cohort study of nearly 40,000 adults, daily soft drink consumption increased the risk of CV events by 21% [38] and in the UK, The National Health Service (NHS) showed that sugar-sweetened beverages significantly increased the risk of stroke by 16% per one serving per day and coronary heart disease by 20% [39].

As a consequence, European guidelines for the management of CVD strongly discourage the intake of added sugars in diet, especially sweetened beverages, allowing no more than 25 g per day [40].

One underlying mechanism which may explain the adverse cardiometabolic outcome of fructose intake is the induction of hepatic lipogenesis and increased circulatory triglycerides levels, as well as the promotion of insulin resistance and oxidative stress [41], as already mentioned in the previous paragraph.

As a confirmation of the deleterious effect of added sugars on cardiovascular risk, in a 4-week prospective randomized study, 24 Hispanic overweight adolescents with hepatic steatosis, all usual high fructose containing beverages drinkers, were randomized to fructose-drinks vs. glucose only beverages. After the intervention period, patients randomized to glucose beverage presented a significant improvement in the cardiometabolic profile (plasma C-reactive protein, insulin-resistance indexes, plasma free fatty acids, and circulating oxydated low-density lipoprotein levels) compared to baseline and to those in the fructose-beverage arm of the study [42].

Conversely to fructose, whole grains seem to have a protective role on cardiovascular risk, mainly due to the high concentration of fibers. Fibers reduce inflammation and reactive oxidation and improve lipid profiles and blood pressure [43]. Ultimately, they inhibit absorption of fats and simple carbohydrates, with improvement of the cardiometabolic profile.

A small randomized clinical trial including a cohort of 300 participants explored the impact of a diet enriched with whole grain on surrogate markers of cardiovascular disease such as blood pressure, cholesterol, and markers of inflammation, and demonstrated a significant improvement of all of them [44]. In addition, a meta-analysis of seven prospective studies showed that an increased consumption of whole grain prompted a 21% reduction in cardiovascular disease events and mortality [45].

3. Role of Lipids in NAFLD and Cardiovascular Disease

3.1. Lipids and NAFLD

Fatty acids are long hydrocarbon chains and are divided in four categories: saturated fatty acids (SFAs), without double bound between carbon atoms, monounsaturated fatty acids (MUFAs), with only one double bound, polyunsaturated fatty acids (PUFAs), with more than one double bound, and trans fatty acids (TFAs), when the two hydrogen atoms are on opposite sides of the double bond [46]. Among PUFAs, n-3 PUFAs and n-6 PUFAs are essential because humans cannot synthesize them and their precursors (linoleic (18:2 n-6) acid and linolenic acid (18:3 n-3) need to be introduced in the diet, to build longer carbon chains [46]. Indeed, if on one hand a great supply of linolenic acid is beneficial, on the other hand, evidence is rising on the need of reducing that of linoleic acid which may favor inflammation and metabolic diseases [47].

In the last century, fatty acids consumption in the daily life has dramatically changed from a diet rich in MUFAs, principally found in olive oil, and, in PUFAs, contained in fish and shellfish, vegetable oils, seeds, and nuts, to a Westernized dietary, where SFAs and TFAs, present in meat and dairy products, prevail [48].

Regarding the consumption of fatty acids, Donnelly et al. demonstrated that 15% of hepatic fat derived from diet and that this percentage could increase if dietary fat consumption was higher than 30% of daily energy requirements [49]. Moreover, two epidemiological studies by Toshimitsu at al. and Musso at al. illustrated that NASH patients had a diet richer in saturated fat and cholesterol and poorer in PUFAs compared to the diet of age, gender, and BMI matched controls without NASH [50,51]. Analyzing PUFA intake, a lower consumption of n-3 PUFA and a higher n-6/n-3 ratio were observed in NAFLD and NASH patients compared to controls [23]. Moreover, patients with NAFLD had a depletion in blood and tissue PUFAs content, especially those of marine origin, the n-3 PUFAs (eicosapentaenoic acid (EPA) and docosahexaenoic acid (DHA)) [52,53].

A diet enriched in PUFAs or SFAs has a distinct effect on liver metabolism and visceral fat accumulation because SFAs result in a significant increase in liver and visceral fat compared to PUFAs. Preclinical studies illustrated that a diet rich in n-3 PUFAs, like docosahexaenoic acid (DHA), suppresses diet-induced steatosis, inflammation, and fibrosis [54], along with a positive effect on insulin resistance and serum triglycerides [55,56]. Furthermore, a preclinical study highlighted that, among 3-PUFAs, DHA is superior to eicosapentaenoic acid (EPA) to reduce NASH related inflammation and fibrosis, as well as hepatic fat content [57,58].

The harmful role of SFAs compared to PUFAs has also been confirmed by Bjermo et al. who analyzed two hypercaloric diets, one enriched in n-6 PUFA and the other in SFAs, and showed that, after seven weeks, a similar weight gain was observed, with a dramatically increment in hepatic fat and a two-fold increase in visceral fat only in patients assigned to the SFAs diet compared to the PUFAs diet [59]. In addition, a 10-week randomized clinical trial comparing two isocaloric diets containing n-6 PUFA or SFAs showed an improvement in metabolic status and a decrease in hepatic fat using n-6 PUFAs diet, despite no weight modification [60].

Besides PUFAs, a protective role in fat accumulation has been demonstrated also for MUFAs. In fact, an energy balanced diet with a high proportion of MUFAs was associated with a reduction in hepatic fat in patients with prediabetes [61], type 2 diabetes [62], and NAFLD [63], differently from an energy balanced diet with a very high proportion of SFAs. Indeed, the EASL–EASD–EASO Clinical Practice Guidelines recommended the Mediterranean diet for NAFLD patients in consideration of its high content of MUFAs, present in olive oil and nuts, and the large amount of fruits, legumes, vegetables, and fish and low in red and processed meats and sweets [64].

Multiple checkpoints are influenced by the high-fat diet and oxidative stress is directly associated with an excess of n-6 PUFAs and a low amount of n-3 PUFAs, generating lipid oxidation and NAFLD progression [65]. Firstly, diet modulates gut microbiota, whose metabolic products are delivered to the liver by the portal vein. The alterations of intestinal microbiota, characterized by overgrowth of some bacteria phyla and alteration of epithelial barrier permeability, contribute to inflammation, insulin resistance, and fat accumulation. Consequently, these modifications lead to obesity and NAFLD, dysregulating liver functions [66]. Secondly, SFAs promote mitochondrial dysfunction, altering respiratory chain activity and ATP homeostasis, increasing formation of reactive oxygen species (ROS) and inducing apoptosis, consequently impairing phospholipid metabolism and increasing insulin resistance [67]. Lastly, high-fat diet enriched with SFAs was hypothesized to trigger de novo lipogenesis through activation of the peroxisome proliferator-activated receptor (PPARγ)-coactivator-1beta (PGC-1) and the enhancement of transcription in genes involved in lipid metabolism, like the stearoyl-CoA desaturase-1, fatty acid synthase, and diacylglycerol acyltransferase compared to a PUFA diet [68]. On the contrary, n-3 PUFAs control the activity of transcription factors regulating the expression of gene encoding for de novo lipogenesis, fatty acid oxidation, fat uptake from the circulation and VLDL assembly and secretion [54]. Moreover, n-3 PUFAs have also been hypothesized to attenuate fibrosis, possibly by reducing the expression of a broad array of proteins involved in fibrosis [58]. Moreover, DHA has been supposed to act directly on human stellate cells suppressing the expression of Col1A1, the major collagen subtype induced in rodent and human NASH [69]. However, future studies are needed to clarify the role of DHA in hepatic fibrosis.

3.2. *Lipids and Cardiovascular Disease*

Cardiovascular disease (CVD) is the first cause of death and disability worldwide, and diet is one of the most important modifiable risk factors [70].

As described in the previous paragraph, in the last few decades, the daily diet is dramatically changed increasing the proportion of fatty acids, which nowadays represent 28–42% of total energy consumed by European populations [71], whereas in the past was approximately 20–30% of total energy [72]. Moreover, the kind of fatty acids in the diet is mutated, n-3 PUFAs intake is reduced, and the ratio between n-6 and n-3, which was 1:1, nowadays is dramatically increased to a range between 10:1 and 20:1 [72]. Several studies illustrate that a low ratio between n-6 and n-3 PUFAs has been considered protective for the development of many diseases, such as cardiovascular disease, cancer, and metabolic disease [73]. The cardioprotective action of the eicosanoids derived from n-3 PUFAs is justified by their anti-inflammatory, antiatherogenic, antiarrhythmic, antithrombotic/antiplatelet, antioxidant, hypotensive effects, and the positive action on lipid metabolism [74].

Regarding the food rich in n-3 PUFAs, the consumption of tree nuts, for example, almonds, reduces LDL cholesterol levels by 3 to 19% [75], while fish consumption has beneficial effects on insulin sensitivity, type 2 diabetes mellitus (T2DM), and lipid profile [76]. In addition, 3-PUFA contained in fish have been associated with a reduced risk for death from coronary heart diseases in healthy individuals [74,77], and in particular the α-linolenic acid with a reduced risk of myocardial infarction [78].

According to the literature consensus, healthy adults should have a daily intake of at least 0.5–1 g/d n-3PUFAs, equivalent to 2–4 servings per week of fish or a half serving of oily fish, in order to reduce the risk of CVD and improve the features of metabolic syndrome [79]. Indeed, conversely to the past when the total intake of n-3PUFAs exceeded 5–6 g/d [80], nowadays only the traditional Japanese diet contains that level [81].

Moreover, many epidemiological studies demonstrated a low cardiovascular risk associated with Mediterranean diet. In particular, the most important factor is the daily consumption of olive oil, the greatest source of dietary MUFA (about 90% of all MUFA). In fact, the PREDIMED trial (Primary Prevention of Cardiovascular Disease with a Mediterranean Diet) demonstrated that extra-virgin olive oil or nuts in supplementation to Mediterranean diet reduced the incidence of major cardiovascular events [9].

The protective role of an adequate consumption of olive oil (23 g/day) in the CV risk has already been recognized at the end of the last century by the Food and Drug Administration, addressing olive oil as a qualified dressing able to decrease the risk of coronary heart disease [82]. Indeed, olive oil has several beneficial effects on the cardiovascular system: decreases oxidative stress, inhibits oxidation of LDL-cholesterol, cuts-down serum level of triglycerides [83], modulates inflammation [84], reduces blood pressure, delays gastric emptying, decreasing postprandial hyperglycaemia, and improves glycaemic control in diabetic patients [85].

If on one hand MUFAs reduce CV risk, on the other hand, SFAs are associated with an unfavorable metabolic and CV profile, especially because of the increase in low density lipoprotein (LDL) cholesterol. In consideration of that, International Guidelines strongly recommended to reduce the daily consumption of SFAs to a maximum of 5–6% of the total lipid intake [86].

4. Role of Proteins in NAFLD and Cardiovascular Disease

4.1. Proteins and NAFLD

Data on the effects of dietary protein in patients with NAFLD are limited and controversial, while, in animal models, results suggest that dietary proteins have a beneficial effect on glucose metabolism, are essential for the regeneration of hepatocytes and could counteract the development of steatosis providing the amino acids needed for the inclusion of fat in lipoproteins and favoring its export from the liver. In addition, the energy requirement for amino acid catabolism could lead to oxidation of hepatic lipids with a consequent increase in fat depletion from the liver [87,88]. On the contrary, in population studies, diets enriched in animal proteins, especially in overweight patients, are associated with an increased risk of NAFLD development [89]. However, in the few available controlled trials, diets enriched in proteins were often also low-caloric diets, thus it is not possible to draw any firm conclusions.

Recent studies have highlighted sarcopenia as a risk factor for disease severity in NAFLD. In sarcopenic obesity, defined by the concomitant presence of sarcopenia and obesity, the coexistence of muscle loss and fat accumulation accelerates insulin resistance and inflammation, which lead to atherosclerotic damage and a more severe liver disease (NASH and advanced fibrosis) [90,91].

Very recently, nutritional and behavioral models have been proposed to contrast the increased risk of frailty in the obese, diabetic, and elderly patients (>75 years old) in whom quantities and qualities of various nutrients, including proteins, have been modified compared to younger subjects. These categories of patients should undergo anthropometric measurements and muscle function tests to allow targeted early nutrition interventions (i.e., 1.5 g/kg/day of protein intake, 2–3 hourly food intake with kidney function monitoring) and promotion of physical exercise [92].

4.2. Proteins and Cardiovascular Disease

Several large cohort observational and intervention studies in both Western and Asian populations have evaluated whether plant and animal proteins differ in the reduction/promotion of CV risk [93,94]. However, evidence is not definitive because it is difficult to isolate the independent effects of specific proteins from the contribution of other non-protein components in both plant and animal food source, the content of particular amino acids and the interaction with the intestinal microbiome. Red meat, for example, is rich in proteins but also in cholesterol and heme-iron, nutrients associated with the development of CVD through different mechanisms (increase of free fatty acids, oxidative stress, free radical production) [95,96]. In addition, as reported above, sarcopenia also, consequent to protein deficiency, is a risk factor for atherosclerosis, thus increasing CV risk [90].

5. Role of Fibers in the Setting of NAFLD and Cardiovascular Disease

5.1. Fibers and NAFLD

The role of fibers in NAFLD has been studied in animal models and in patients. However, results do not allow for understanding whether the impact of fibers is a direct consequence of the modulation of gut microbiome or if fibers, by themselves, reduce inflammation and thus counteract the development of NASH. Fibers can be distinguished into soluble and insoluble, and both can be non-fermentable and fermentable.

Cellulose, a type of insoluble non-fermentable fiber, exhibits protective anti-inflammatory effects through alteration of microbiota [97]. In mice, low-cellulose diets alter the intestinal mucosa by inducing crypt atrophy and reduction of goblet cells, resulting in development of inflammation. Conversely, diets rich in cellulose reduce IL-1β and TNF-α, both mediators of inflammation. Furthermore, it has been shown in mouse models of endotoxemia that a diet rich in cellulose acts by reducing the macrophage activity of the spleen and by attenuating the activity of hepatic NF-κB [98]. In addition, most soluble fibers are fermented by gut microbiota to produce metabolites that impact metabolic processes.

For example, inulin is a type of soluble fiber, the activity of which depends on its chemical structure and the presence of inulin in the diet of overweight, non-diabetic patients, induces a reduction in insulin resistance, coinciding with a change in the gut bacterial population [99]. In addition, β-glucan supplementation, derived from plant or fungal cell walls, and considered a soluble fiber, reduces insulin resistance, dyslipidemia, and hepatic steatosis jointly with alterations of gut microbiome [100].

5.2. Fiber and Cardiovascular Disease

The benefic effect of fibers is documented by the evidence that vegetarian diets reduce atherosclerotic cardiovascular damage with a significant decrease in coronary artery calcifications [101]. In a meta-analysis of nine cohort studies including 222,081 men and women, the overall reduction in coronary heart disease risk was 7% for each additional portion of vegetable intake per day [102]. Dark green leafy vegetables had the highest reduction in coronary heart disease risk, but it has to be stressed that vegetarian diets are often deficient in many nutrients that have to be supplemented.

6. Role of Micronutrients in NAFLD and Cardiovascular Disease

The potential role of micronutrients in both NAFLD and CVD has been debated for years and, although hundreds of papers have been published, sound results are still not available as proven by the fact that very rarely do these compounds reach clinical practice.

The main results reported in literature on bioactive compounds will be described below. The best results on the micronutrients utilization derive from cellular or animal models, while those obtained in patients often are conflicting. In many studies, multiple compounds are combined to enhance the antioxidant, anti-inflammatory, and anti-fibrogenic properties of individual compounds making even more difficult to understand the effect of the individual compounds.

Vitamin E is a fat-soluble vitamin that works as an antioxidant. It was evaluated alone or in combination with other antioxidants such as Sylimarin. The steatohepatitis study (PIVENS) showed that supplementation of 800 IU vitamin E (α-tocopherol) per day (in people without diabetes) improved steatosis and inflammation and induced resolution of NASH [103]. However, a long-term risk of increased mortality has been demonstrated at these dosages. A recent meta-analysis of 16 controlled studies showed that low doses of vitamin E alone would reduce the risk of myocardial infarction (RR 0.82; 95% CI, 0.70–0.96; $p = 0.01$) [104]. Furthermore, supplementation with Vitamin E is associated with a 2.5% increase in flow-mediated vasodilation and consequently a reduction in CV risk [105].

Silymarin, one of the most studied nutraceutical of plant origin, has been shown in numerous studies to have several positive effects on the liver and on the cardiovascular system: anti-oxidant (direct scavenger activity, optimization of mitochondrial function), anti-inflammatory (inhibition of NF-kB activity, reduction of the synthesis of proinflammatory cytokines IL-1, IL6, TNFa, TNFb), anti-apoptotic activity (modulation of caspase release) antifibrotic (inhibition of the conversion of stellate cells to fibroblasts, downregulation of target genes) and choleretic (upregulation of the bile salts export pump). Finally, it also exerts a favorable metabolic action by fostering the PPAR-agonist activation and increasing the expression of Glucose transporter-4 (GLUT4) on the cell surface, inhibition of Hydroxyl-Methyl-Glutaryl-Coenzyme-A reductase).

The studies that have documented the effect of silymarin (or its isoforms) in vivo have used this compound in monotherapy or in association with Vitamin E, and have demonstrated normalization of transaminases, reduction of GGT, and of the degree of steatosis (evaluated by ultrasound), improvement of fasting blood glucose and insulin resistance. However, these positive effects disappear upon discontinuation of the drug [106].

The combined use of vitamin E and Sylibin, the main active compound of sylimarin, in addition to a low-calorie diet is associated with a reduction of transaminases (ALT and AST), GGT and hepatic steatosis index, while results on HOMA, BMI, and lipids are conflicting. A mixture of vitamin E and C (600 IU/day and 500 mg/day, respectively) given to patients with elevated levels of ALT and biopsy-proven NAFLD that followed a weight-reducing diet showed a significative reduction of transaminases and of fibrosis [107]. It has also been reported that addition of atorvastatin to vitamin C and E would reduce the risk of fatty liver development [108].

7. Vitamin D

Vitamin D is a fat soluble secosteroid hormone, about 10% derived from the diet, while 90% from the cutaneous conversion of 7-dehydrocholesterol to cholecalciferol due to exposure to ultraviolet B rays.

Animal and cellular studies showed that vitamin D plays a fundamental role in the metabolism of minerals, but also in inflammation, regulation of the immune response and cell differentiation, with impact on the liver and on the cardiovascular system [109].

An interaction between vitamin D and NAFLD has been described. Recently, some literature data showed a higher prevalence of vitamin D deficiency in NAFLD, with vitamin D playing a role in NAFLD and cardiovascular disease through increasing insulin sensitivity, reducing inflammation of the adipose tissue, reducing liver inflammation and fibrosis [110]. However, it is still debated whether patients with NAFLD have a higher prevalence of vitamin D deficiency than people without steatosis and the effectiveness of adding vitamin D on NAFLD histological damage [111].

The decrease in sun exposure and the modern lifestyle, besides the reduction of the hepatic and renal hydroxylation capacity with aging, causes vitamin D deficiency in a large part of the population. Vitamin D deficiency has been reported in chronic liver diseases of different etiology, and it has even been associated with hepatic decompensation in liver cirrhosis. However, the most reliable data demonstrate effectiveness of vitamin D supplementation when associated with diet, thus it is not clear which is the real impact of vitamin D by itself.

8. Vitamin K

The role of vitamin K on CV alterations is documented in cohorts of patients with CVD, hypertension, and in the general population. The Multi-Ethnic Study of Atherosclerosis (MESA) demonstrated an increased prevalence of CAC in patients with a low intake of vitamin K1 with diet, especially in patients on antihypertensive drugs. A population-based study of 4807 participants found that the incident risk for chronic heart disease was reduced by Vitamin K [112,113].

9. Curcumin

Curcumin is an insulin sensitizing agent extracted from *Curcuma longa*, whose effect on NAFLD is reported in few preclinical and clinical studies. Curcumin would reduce some altered parameters of NAFLD including transaminases, abdominal circumference, and especially ultrasound steatosis. However, given the high dosage needed to obtain the effect, the only recent availability of pharmaceutical preparations with a known dose of the drug and finally the presence of a few randomized controlled trials with adequate numbers of patients, make these data still preliminary [114,115].

Curcumin displays a role also in CVD. In fact, in mice models, it significantly attenuates collagen deposition and inhibits cardiac fibroblast proliferation and migration after coronary damage [116]. In a study of 121 patients, curcumin reduced myocardial infarction after coronary artery bypass graft from 30% to 13% [117].

The potential effect on NAFLD of the administration of the mixed extracts obtained from natural sources was also evaluated. In general, these mixtures are very rich in phenolic compounds, carotenoids, vitamins, and minerals. Among them, some preparations were used more rigorously. Most of the beneficial effects of curcumin or its bioactive agents are still limited to preclinical studies in animal models [118], while randomized, controlled studies in humans have not reported conclusive results even for the small sample size [119].

10. Polyphenols

Polyphenols derive from plant metabolism and are divided into flavonoids and non-flavonoids and are contained in many natural compounds, as vegetables, cereals and fruits), as well as in tea, coffee, red wine, and beer. Normally, the daily diet intake is around 800–1300 mg [120] and their supplementation is essential because of their antioxidant, anti-inflammatory, anti-mutagenic and immunomodulatory action. As a consequence, a diet rich in polyphenols would reduce dyslipidemia and oxidative stress [121]. There are numerous studies in animal models: polyphenols can decrease the transcription of SREBP-1c and determine an increase in the transcription of PPAR-a, reducing insulin resistance and inflammation. However, clinical data on patients are conflicting. Some clinical studies which evaluated the effect of anthocyanins, phenolic acids, and catechins in NAFLD, found a reduction in biomarkers of hepatocyte apoptosis, ALT levels and liver fat content, evaluated by CT [122]. Resveratrol is currently one of the most evaluated polyphenols and some studies have been conducted in NAFLD with opposite results, showing a transient reduction in ALT and AST and CK18, but not of fibrosis [123].

It is therefore possible to hypothesize, on the basis of the data reported in the literature, that catechins and anthocyanins could have some effect on steatosis; however, data need to be confirmed in further research.

11. Caffeine

Several studies have evaluated the efficacy of caffeine, an alkaloid derivative of xanthine, which is the main compound in coffee, and of coffee consumption itself, in NAFLD. A reduction in the risk of developing NAFLD of approximately 30% has been described. In addition, a reduction in fibrosis has also been reported, the mechanism of which could be linked to inhibition of adhesion and activation of hepatic stellate cells. However, the definition of regular coffee consumption varies widely between studies and this may represent a limitation of the results presented in different meta-analyses [124,125]. It is also unclear whether the beneficial effect of caffeine/coffee is due to an association rather than a real causal mechanism. Finally, it is possible that other compounds present in coffee, including polyphenols and melanoidins, are the real culprits.

12. Genetics and Diet in NAFLD and Cardiovascular Disease

As already said, NAFLD is characterized by metabolic alterations, an incorrect diet, mainly rich in SFA and sugars, and physical inactivity. In addition, patients with NAFLD and metabolic alterations are exposed to high cardiovascular risk and a high rate of CV events. However, not all patients with a risky metabolic profile or unhealthy lifestyle develop hepatic steatosis or a cardiovascular disease.

12.1. Genetic Bases of NAFLD and CV Risk

The role of genetic predisposition is well established in the pathogenesis of NAFLD, and the strong heritability component is sustained by epidemiological, familial, and twin studies [126]. Several single nucleotide polymorphisms (SNPs) in genes involved in lipid metabolism play a role in the onset of NAFLD and progression towards advanced forms of liver damage. The patatin-like phospholipase domain-containing 3 (PNPLA3) is the major determinant of hepatic fat content and of its progression [127,128] and leads to accumulation of a mutated protein, with an impaired function in lipase activity on hepatocellular lipid droplets, thus favoring triglycerides accumulation within the liver. Another genetic determinant in NAFLD is the variant in a transmembrane 6 superfamily member 2 gene (TM6SF2) which predisposes to an increased hepatic fat content because of retention of lipids and impairment in very low-density lipoprotein (VLDL) release by the liver [129]. In addition, mutations in the membrane bound O-acyltransferase domain-containing 7 gene (MBOAT7) foster liver fat accumulation and inflammation. In fact, this gene encodes for an enzyme localized on the mitochondria-associated membrane, where lipid droplets formation occurs, thus regulating the desaturation of membranes phospholipids and the production of arachidonic acid, which is involved in inflammatory processes [130]. Finally, the glucokinase regulatory protein (GCKR) gene, which modulates the glucose influx into the hepatocytes and the de novo lipogenesis, is involved in NAFLD development [131]. However, less than 10% of inherited variability is explained by these common variants.

Likewise, a large number of genes and their variants may influence the CV risk by different routes. Among them, the 5–10-Methylene tetrahydrofolate reductase (MTHFR) and the Methionine synthase (MTR), both regulating homocysteine metabolism, an atherogenic and prothrombotic protein, have been related with an increased risk of coronary artery disease (CAD) [132,133]. Similarly, the LDL receptors gene which is involved in low-density lipoprotein (LDL) and triglyceride metabolism and the LIPC gene (hepatic lipase C), the major determinant of plasma HDL concentration, are linked to increased prevalence of myocardial infarction and CAD in the general population [134,135]. Finally, the apolipoprotein APO-A and APO-E family gene, encoding key regulators of plasma lipids, have a significant impact on CAD [136]. The possible mechanisms and interactions between liver, cardiovascular, and nutrient damage are shown in Figure 1.

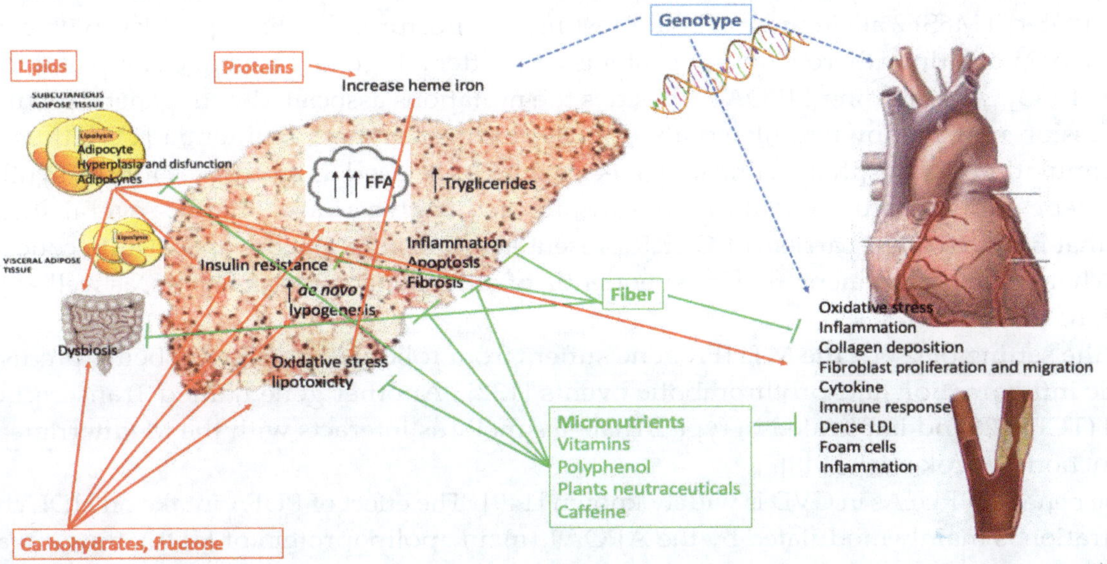

Figure 1. Potential multiple distinct and interrelated mechanisms by which nutrients promote (red line) or prevent (green line) liver and cardiovascular damage. Influence of genetics on NAFLD and cardiovascular damage (blue line).

12.2. Nutritional Genomics or Nutrigenomics

Besides pure genetic bases of diseases, in the last few years, evidence is accumulating on the complex interplay between genetic predisposition and environmental influences, particularly diet, in the development of NAFLD as well as in the increase in cardiovascular risk, possibly suggesting common etiopathogenetic pathways linking both hepatic and CVD.

Therefore, since 2013, the term nutritional genomics or "nutrigenomics" has been coined, defining the interaction between cellular, genetic processes, and nutritional environment [137]. Nutrigenomic has the aim of exploring the effect of diet on disease development by modulating the expression of an individual's genetic pattern.

Three main fields of study cover this interaction: (1) the genetic variability response towards nutrition, named nutrigenetics; (2) the effect of nutrients on DNA metabolism; and (3) the effect of nutrients on genetic expression.

12.2.1. Nutrigenetic: Genetic Variability Response towards Nutrition

The most widely studied gene which interacts with the environment in NAFLD is represented by PNPLA3. In fact, accumulation of the protein encoded by the mutated gene is triggered by acquired factors, like obesity [138], alcohol consumption [139], and diet, especially with a high content in carbohydrates [140]. A nutrigenetic analysis in a cohort of Italian adolescents showed that hepatic triglycerides accumulation was related to carbohydrate and sugar intake in the homozygous mutated group but not in the wild type group [141]. The rationale of this influence relies on carbohydrate-mediated upregulation of PNPLA3, which in turn favors the accumulation of the pathological protein on the surface of lipid droplets.

Indeed, PNPLA3 is influenced also by fatty acids in the diet, particularly n-6/n-3 PUFA [142]. In 127 Caucasian adolescents with steatosis evaluated by MRI, increased transaminases and free fatty acids were associated with a diet with a high n-6/n-3 PUFA ratio, but only in patients homozygous for the mutated PNPLA3 variable. This result is possibly related to the impaired hydrolyzing function of PNPLA3, with accumulation of hepatic triglycerides and metabolites of omega 6 PUFA with pro-inflammatory action (Santoro, 2012) [142]. In addition, patients with NAFLD and mutated PNPLA3 seem to have no response in terms of reduction of the novo lipogenesis and improvement in transaminases by n-3 PUFA supplementation in the diet [143].

In addition, mutated patients for the TM6SF2 and MBOAT7 genes are affected by diet. Carriers of the mutated TM6SF2 allele present better fasting and postprandial lipid profiles, with consequent reduction of circulating atherogenic lipoproteins even after a high fat challenge compared to the wild types [144,145]. As regarding MBOAT7, besides the mutations associated with genetic predisposition, its expression may be downregulated also by diet-induced hyperinsulinemia [146], thus fostering the accumulation of phosphatidylinositol species which are used as substrates for the synthesis and hepatic deposition of saturated and mono-unsaturated triglycerides. Finally, several studies have shown that mutated allele carriers of GCKR present lower fasting glucose and insulin concentrations after a whole-grain supplementation independently of other metabolic risk factors, as well as to dietary restrictions [147].

In the setting of CVD, the MTHFR gene suffers from folic acid deficiency, being predisposed to systemic inflammation and prothrombotic events [132]. Another gene named Transcription factor 7-like-2 (TCF7L2) and implicated in type 2 diabetes mellitus interacts with the Mediterranean diet in the reduction of stroke risk [148].

The benefit of PUFAs in CVD is widely known [149]. The effect of PUFA intake on HDL cholesterol concentration is mainly modulated by the APOA1 (main apolipoprotein of HDL), thus it was shown that PUFAs consumption was associated with higher HDL cholesterol concentration depending on APOA1 polymorphism [150]. In addition, the APO-E4 polymorphism has been associated with the development of CAD. A study examining the effect of a quercetin supplementation (flavonoid glycosides) in a cohort of overweight-obese individuals with metabolic syndrome showed a significant reduction in HDL in the subgroup of patients carrying the APO-E4 polymorphism, differently from the APO-E3 carriers [151]. In another population-based study involving nearly 2000 subjects, the APO-E3 and APO-E4 genotypes were significantly associated with a high risk of acute myocardial infarction in patients treated with high saturated fatty acids (>10%) diet compared with APO-E2 carriers [152].

12.2.2. Effect of Nutrients on DNA Metabolism

Studies of the effect of micronutrients on DNA metabolism have shown that several micronutrients (especially calcium, folate, nicotinic acid, vitamin E, retinol) are necessary for DNA homeostasis, being cofactors of a several enzymes essential to DNA synthesis and repair [153], whereas others, as the TFAs, favor DNA damage [154]. Their depletion may prompt unfavorable DNA modifications.

In addition, telomeres shortening is typical of aging and of many chronic diseases, including NAFLD [155] and cardiovascular disease [156]. Diet has an impact on telomeres homeostasis, with vegetables, fibers, and omega-3 fatty acids preventing telomeres shortening, whereas saturated fatty acids, processed meat, or carbohydrates with a high glycemic index favoring it [157,158].

12.2.3. Effect of Nutrients on Genetic Expression

The study of the effect of nutrients on gene expression primary identifies the transcription factors that are sensitive to a specific nutrient and their target genes, then the signaling pathways activated by these transcription factors and the possible proteins and metabolites created, detected by "omics" techniques, and finally the organ-specific response to nutrients [159].

Many transcription factors are susceptible to diet influences. In particular, the peroxisome proliferator-activated receptor (PPAR) family, which is involved in glucose and lipid metabolism, adipocyte differentiation, and inflammatory response, is one of the most widely studied. In fact, each PPAR family member α, δ, and γ is responsive to specific dietary fatty acids (PUFAs, monounsaturated fatty acids, and SFAs) [160,161]. Interestingly, PPARγ expression induced by omega 3 PUFA can increase the lipid storage capacity of adipose tissue along with hepatic fatty acid oxidation and reduce systemic inflammation, with consequent improvement in insulin sensitivity, hepatic steatosis, and CV risk. Polymorphisms in PPAR-γ2, the most important form associated with CVD, have been analyzed in a 2-year nutritional intervention with a Mediterranean-style diet vs. conventional low-fat diet in 774 patients at high-cardiovascular risk [162]. The results showed that only carriers of the mutated allele allocated in the low-fat diet and not in the Mediterranean diet arm significantly increased waist circumference compared with non-mutated participants. Therefore, it could be speculated that the Mediterranean diet could mitigate the adverse metabolic effects of mutation in PPAR-g2 gene in a high-cardiovascular risk population.

12.3. Epigenetic, Diet, NAFLD, and CVD

Along with genetic predisposition to NAFLD and CVD, disease development and natural history are also modulated by epigenetic mechanisms, heritable but reversible phenomena that modify gene transcription without altering DNA sequence [163].

The epigenetic modulation of gene expression includes (a) DNA methylation; (b) chromatin remodeling (histone modifications); and (c) microRNAs formation (small particles of non-coding RNA with specific functionality). Epigenetic modifications affect hepatic lipid metabolism, insulin resistance, mitochondrial function, and oxidative stress and diet may modulate all these [164,165].

(a) Some nutrients, such as choline, methionine, folate and vitamin B12 are considered "methyl-donor" promoting methylation of DNA and histones. Actually, DNA methylation, considered a key factor in the progression from simple steatosis to NASH and in triglycerides metabolism, may be increased by dietary deficiency of choline, betaine, B12, and folate. In fact, their supplementation is associated with an increase in the hepatic efflux of triglycerides [166]; conversely, their deficiency promotes hepatic triglycerides accumulation by fostering over-expression of genes involved in fatty acids synthesis [167]. In addition, in a rodent model, supplementation of methyl-donor micronutrients to a high-fat-sucrose diet mitigated the effect on triglycerides accumulation within the liver through a hypermethylation of a key enzyme involved in fatty acids synthesis [168]. In vivo studies showed the epigenetic effect of these nutrients, altering endothelial cell function, and inflammation processing, with consequent plaque formation and increased CV risk [169].

(b) Post-translational modification of histones is essential to define chromatin architecture and thus gene accessibility. In response to caloric restriction, Sirt1, a key enzyme involved in DNA repair, induces histone and non-histone deacetylation of genes involved in insulin-resistance and inflammation of the adipose tissue, promoting gluconeogenesis and fatty acid oxidation in the liver [170]. A histone acetyltransferase inhibitor, the tannic acid, a plant-derived polyphenol, has been demonstrated to block the hyperacetylation of histones of the promoter of DNL, thus reducing its activity and hepatic fat accumulation [171]. Likewise, SFAs, produced by fermentation of polysaccharide by gut microbiota, also inhibit histone deacetylases with consequent impairment in metabolic and inflammatory processes [172].

(c) Alteration of mRNA stability may arise through formation of small RNA molecules called microRNAs which bind to transcriptional mRNA turning into post-transcriptional repression of targeted protein-coding genes. Unhealthy diets may foster NAFLD development by altering miRNAs. One of the most represented in liver and hallmark of fat accumulation and steatosis severity, the miR-122 has been shown to be responsive to diet either in vitro or in vivo models and in humans. In particular, a high-fat-diet upregulated miR-122 with consequent promotion of lipogenesis within the liver [173]. However, non-conclusive data were reported on plant-derived dietary microRNAs which may potentially cross the intestinal and once in the bloodstream regulate host gene expression involved in cardiometabolic risk [174]. On the other hand, host derived small RNAs regulating processes of relevance to cardiometabolic risk are altered by dietary intervention [175].

Interestingly, epigenetic mechanisms may arise during the gestational period, as the fetus liver may be "primed" with unhealthy metabolic pattern by mother over-nutrition, as well as in post-natal period and over time with aging. For example, in pregnant women with a diet rich in fat, a state of chronic-low grade inflammatory arises in the placenta as well in the fetal organs, including the liver, contributing to steatosis development [176].

Based on this background, the role of gene–diet interaction in patients with NAFLD is crucial because, by modifying dietary pattern in genetically predisposed individuals, it could be possible to modulate specific clinical outcome. The long-term hypothetical objective could be the tailored therapy based also on a personalized nutritional approach.

13. Preliminary Data

In order to evaluate the role of diet on clinical presentation and cardiovascular alterations in patients with NAFLD, we enrolled 154 newly diagnosed, consecutive, untreated NAFLD patients (M/F 112/42 mean age 49 ± 12 years), who were administered a semi-quantitative food-frequency questionnaire (dietary record including 118 food items covering seven days) to calculate energy and nutrients intake. Steatosis, carotid intima-media thickness (IMT), and plaques were evaluated by ultrasonography; diastolic dysfunction ($E/A < 1$), left ventricular mass, and epicardial adipose thickness (EAT) by echocardiography. Twenty-three (15%) patients had "lean" NAFLD ($BMI < 25\ kg/m^2$). Moderate to severe steatosis was present in 61%, IMT above normal value in 13%, carotid plaques in 28%, and $E/A < 1$ in 39%; mean EAT was 5.8 ± 4 mm. Total calories and macro-nutrient intake (g/day) were: 1705 ± 5 750 kcal; proteins 98 ± 46, fat 65 ± 32 (saturated 23 ± 14; PUFA 10 ± 5; monounsaturated 25 ± 12), carbohydrates 164 ± 75 (simple sugar 64 ± 35), fibers 23 ± 14. Interestingly, no difference in daily dietary composition of nutrients and total Kcal between lean and overweight patients was observed, despite a higher prevalence of metabolic comorbidities and moderate-severe steatosis in the latter. Among nutrients, fructose intake was significantly higher in patients with plaques ($p = 0.03$) and vitamin E lower in those with $E/A < 1$ ($p = 0.01$). At multivariate analysis adjusted for age, sex, and BMI, diet fat content was significantly associated with dyslipidemia (OR 1.2, 95%CI 1–1.4, $p = 0.04$), fat, and carbohydrate with moderate-severe US steatosis (OR 1.2, 95%CI 1.03–1.5, $p = 0.01$).

14. Conclusions

In conclusion, both diet and genetic factors strongly impact on both NAFLD and cardiovascular damage, either alone or when interacting.

In particular, solid data in literature highly stress the potentially negative role of an incorrect diet, rich in fructose and added sugars, as well as in n-6 PUFAs and SFAs, in the development of both hepatic and cardiovascular diseases. Therefore, the elimination of soft drinks and sweetened bakery products, along with dairy and animal fat, from daily consumption, preferring complex carbohydrates, possibly whole grain, fibers, olives, and vegetable oils, fish, seeds, and nuts rich in MUFAs, and n-3 PUFAs is highly advisable. Indeed, one of the most recommended diet for patients with NAFLD is the Mediterranean diet, which has also been demonstrated to dramatically reduce cardiovascular events. If the role of carbohydrates and fat is well established, that of proteins and micronutrients (especially vitamins) is not completely elucidated, despite a protective role mediated by antioxidant and anti-inflammatory actions having been suggested.

Along with the diet, some genetic bases, either congenital or caused by environmental actions (i.e., epigenetic), have been implicated in the pathogenesis and progression of hepatic and cardiovascular disease. Even more interestingly, in the last few years, evidence is accumulating on the interplay between genetic predisposition and environmental influences, particularly diet, in the setting of NAFLD and cardiovascular disease, coining the new concept of nutritional genomics or nutrigenomics.

Based on this evidence, an accurate correction of patients' diet along with the understanding of the gene-diet interaction become crucial because modification of dietary pattern in genetically predisposed individuals could modulate specific clinical outcomes, either the metabolic, hepatological, or cardiovascular ones, so that a personalized nutritional therapy should be speculated on in the future.

Author Contributions: R.L. revised the literature, focusing on the full text regarding diet and genetic influence on NAFLD development and increased cardiovascular risk; R.L., F.I., and G.P. wrote the draft of the manuscript; S.F. and A.L.F. were involved in the critical revision of the manuscript into its final form and contributed to the review for important intellectual content. All authors have read and agreed to the published version of the manuscript.

Abbreviations

NAFLD	non-alcoholic fatty liver disease
NASH	non-alcoholic steatohepatitis
CVD	cardiovascular disease
FFAs	free fatty acids
TFA	trans fatty acids
PNPLA3	patatin-like phospholipase domain containing 3
TM6SF2	transmembrane 6 superfamily member 2
MBOAT7	membrane bound O-acyltransferase domain-containing 7
HFCS	high fructose corn syrup
DNL	de novo lipogenesis
CAD	coronary artery disease
APO	apolipoprotein
SFAs	saturated fatty acids
MUFA	monounsaturated fatty acids
PUFA	unsaturated fatty acids
MTHFR	methylene tetrahydrofolate reductase
DHA	docosahexaenoic acid
EPA	eicosapentaenoic acid
PPAR	peroxisome proliferator activated receptor
HFCS	high fructose corn syrup
GLUT4	glucose transporter-4

References

1. Byrne, C.D.; Targher, G. NAFLD: A multisystem disease. *J. Hepatol.* **2015** *62*, S47–S64. [CrossRef] [PubMed]

2. Eslam, M.; Sanyal, A.J.; George, J.; International Consensus Panel. MAFLD: A Consensus-Driven Proposed Nomenclature for Metabolic Associated Fatty Liver Disease. *Gastroenterology* **2020**, *158*, 1999–2014.e1. [CrossRef] [PubMed]
3. Ekstedt, M.; Hagstrom, H.; Nasr, P.; Fredrikson, M.; Stal, P.; Kechagias, S.; Hultcrantz, R. Fibrosis stage is the strongest predictor for disease-specific mortality in NAFLD after up to 33 years of follow-up. *Hepatology* **2015**, *61*, 1547–1554. [CrossRef] [PubMed]
4. Valbusa, F.; Bonapace, S.; Agnoletti, D.; Scala, L.; Grillo, C.; Arduini, P.; Turcato, E.; Mantovani, A.; Zoppini, G.; Arcaro, G.; et al. Nonalcoholic fatty liver disease and increased risk of 1-year all-cause and cardiac hospital readmissions in elderly patients admitted for acute heart failure. *PLoS ONE* **2017**, *12*, e0173398. [CrossRef]
5. Bugianesi, E.; Moscatiello, S.; Ciaravella, M.F.; Marchesini, G. Insulin resistance in nonalcoholic fatty liver disease. *Curr. Pharm. Des.* **2010**, *16*, 1941–1951. [CrossRef]
6. Eslam, M.; Valenti, L.; Romeo, S. Genetics and epigenetics of NAFLD and NASH: Clinical impact. *J. Hepatol.* **2018**, *68*, 268–279. [CrossRef]
7. Dongiovanni, P.; Petta, S.; Maglio, C.; Fracanzani, A.L.; Pipitone, R.; Mozzi, E.; Motta, B.M.; Kaminska, D.; Rametta, R.; Grimaudo, S.; et al. Transmembrane 6 superfamily member 2 gene variant disentangles nonalcoholic steatohepatitis from cardiovascular disease. *Hepatology* **2015**, *61*, 506–514. [CrossRef]
8. Godos, J.; Federico, A.; Dallio, M.; Scazzina, F. Mediterranean diet and nonalcoholic fatty liver disease: Molecular mechanisms of protection. *Int. J. Food. Sci. Nutr.* **2017**, *68*, 18–27. [CrossRef]
9. Estruch, R.; Ros, E.; Salas-Salvado, J.; Covas, M.I.; Corella, D.; Aros, F.; Gómez-Gracia, E.; Ruiz-Gutiérrez, V.; Fiol, M.; Lapetra, J.; et al. Primary Prevention of Cardiovascular Disease with a Mediterranean Diet Supplemented with Extra-Virgin Olive Oil or Nuts. *N. Engl. J. Med.* **2018**, *378*, e34. [CrossRef]
10. Schwarz, J.M.; Noworolski, S.M.; Wen, M.J.; Dyachenko, A.; Prior, J.L.; Weinberg, M.E.; Herraiz, L.A.; Tai, V.W.; Bergeron, N.; Bersot, T.P.; et al. Effect of a High-Fructose Weight-Maintaining Diet on Lipogenesis and Liver Fat. *J. Clin. Endocrinol. Metab.* **2015**, *100*, 2434–2442. [CrossRef]
11. Strable, M.S.; Ntambi, J.M. Genetic control of de novo lipogenesis: Role in diet-induced obesity. *Crit. Rev. Biochem. Mol. Biol.* **2010**, *45*, 199–214. [CrossRef] [PubMed]
12. Softic, S.; Cohen, D.E.; Kahn, C.R. Role of Dietary Fructose and Hepatic De Novo Lipogenesis in Fatty Liver Disease. *Dig. Dis. Sci.* **2016**, *61*, 1282–1293. [CrossRef] [PubMed]
13. Jornayvaz, F.R.; Shulman, G.I. Diacylglycerol activation of protein kinase Cepsilon and hepatic insulin resistance. *Cell Metab.* **2012**, *15*, 574–584. [CrossRef] [PubMed]
14. Maersk, M.; Belza, A.; Stodkilde-Jorgensen, H.; Ringgaard, S.; Chabanova, E.; Thomsen, H.; Pedersen, S.B.; Astrup, A.; Richelsen, B. Sucrose-sweetened beverages increase fat storage in the liver, muscle, and visceral fat depot: A 6-mo randomized intervention study. *Am. J. Clin. Nutr.* **2012**, *95*, 283–289. [CrossRef] [PubMed]
15. Rosset, R.; Surowska, A.; Tappy, L. Pathogenesis of Cardiovascular and Metabolic Diseases: Are Fructose-Containing Sugars More Involved Than Other Dietary Calories? *Curr. Hypertens. Rep.* **2016**, *18*, 44. [CrossRef]
16. Santos-Marcos, J.A.; Perez-Jimenez, F.; Camargo, A. The role of diet and intestinal microbiota in the development of metabolic syndrome. *J. Nutr. Biochem.* **2019**, *70*, 1–27. [CrossRef]
17. Jia, Q.; Xia, Y.; Zhang, Q.; Wu, H.; Du, H.; Liu, L.; Wang, C.; Shi, H.; Guo, X.; Liu, X.; et al. Dietary patterns are associated with prevalence of fatty liver disease in adults. *Eur. J. Clin. Nutr.* **2015**, *69*, 914–921. [CrossRef]
18. Lim, J.S.; Mietus-Snyder, M.; Valente, A.; Schwarz, J.M.; Lustig, R.H. The role of fructose in the pathogenesis of NAFLD and the metabolic syndrome. *Nat. Rev. Gastroenterol. Hepatol.* **2010**, *7*, 251–264. [CrossRef]
19. Papandreou, D.; Karabouta, Z.; Pantoleon, A.; Rousso, I. Investigation of anthropometric, biochemical and dietary parameters of obese children with and without non-alcoholic fatty liver disease. *Appetite* **2012**, *59*, 939–944. [CrossRef]
20. Ma, J.; Fox, C.S.; Jacques, P.F.; Speliotes, E.K.; Hoffmann, U.; Smith, C.E.; Saltzman, E.; McKeown, N.M. Sugar-sweetened beverage, diet soda, and fatty liver disease in the Framingham Heart Study cohorts. *J. Hepatol.* **2015**, *63*, 462–469. [CrossRef]
21. Abdelmalek, M.F.; Suzuki, A.; Guy, C.; Unalp-Arida, A.; Colvin, R.; Johnson, R.J.; Diehl, A.M. Increased fructose consumption is associated with fibrosis severity in patients with nonalcoholic fatty liver disease. *Hepatology* **2010**, *51*, 1961–1971. [CrossRef] [PubMed]

22. Mager, D.R.; Iniguez, I.R.; Gilmour, S.; Yap, J. The effect of a low fructose and low glycemic index/load (FRAGILE) dietary intervention on indices of liver function, cardiometabolic risk factors, and body composition in children and adolescents with nonalcoholic fatty liver disease (NAFLD). *JPEN J. Parenter. Enteral. Nutr.* **2015**, *39*, 73–84. [CrossRef] [PubMed]

23. Cortez-Pinto, H.; Jesus, L.; Barros, H.; Lopes, C.; Moura, M.C.; Camilo, M.E. How different is the dietary pattern in non-alcoholic steatohepatitis patients? *Clin. Nutr.* **2006**, *25*, 816–823. [CrossRef] [PubMed]

24. Le, K.A.; Faeh, D.; Stettler, R.; Ith, M.; Kreis, R.; Vermathen, P.; Boesch, C.; Ravussin, E.; Tappy, L. A 4-wk high-fructose diet alters lipid metabolism without affecting insulin sensitivity or ectopic lipids in healthy humans. *Am. J. Clin. Nutr.* **2006**, *84*, 1374–1379. [CrossRef]

25. Ngo Sock, E.T.; Le, K.A.; Ith, M.; Kreis, R.; Boesch, C.; Tappy, L. Effects of a short-term overfeeding with fructose or glucose in healthy young males. *Br. J. Nutr.* **2010**, *103*, 939–943. [CrossRef]

26. Sobrecases, H.; Le, K.A.; Bortolotti, M.; Schneiter, P.; Ith, M.; Kreis, R.; Boesch, C.; Tappy, L. Effects of short-term overfeeding with fructose, fat and fructose plus fat on plasma and hepatic lipids in healthy men. *Diabetes Metab.* **2010**, *36*, 244–246. [CrossRef]

27. Sevastianova, K.; Santos, A.; Kotronen, A.; Hakkarainen, A.; Makkonen, J.; Silander, K.; Peltonen, M.; Romeo, S.; Lundbom, J.; Lundbom, N.; et al. Effect of short-term carbohydrate overfeeding and long-term weight loss on liver fat in overweight humans. *Am. J. Clin. Nutr.* **2012**, *96*, 727–734. [CrossRef]

28. Browning, J.D.; Baker, J.A.; Rogers, T.; Davis, J.; Satapati, S.; Burgess, S.C. Short-term weight loss and hepatic triglyceride reduction: Evidence of a metabolic advantage with dietary carbohydrate restriction. *Am. J. Clin. Nutr.* **2011**, *93*, 1048–1052. [CrossRef]

29. Haufe, S.; Engeli, S.; Kast, P.; Bohnke, J.; Utz, W.; Haas, V.; Hermsdorf, M.; Mähler, A.; Wiesner, S.; Birkenfeld, A.L.; et al. Randomized comparison of reduced fat and reduced carbohydrate hypocaloric diets on intrahepatic fat in overweight and obese human subjects. *Hepatology* **2011**, *53*, 1504–1514. [CrossRef]

30. Volynets, V.; Machann, J.; Kuper, M.A.; Maier, I.B.; Spruss, A.; Konigsrainer, A.; Bischoff, S.C.; Bergheim, I. A moderate weight reduction through dietary intervention decreases hepatic fat content in patients with non-alcoholic fatty liver disease (NAFLD): A pilot study. *Eur. J. Nutr.* **2013**, *52*, 527–535. [CrossRef]

31. Theytaz, F.; Noguchi, Y.; Egli, L.; Campos, V.; Buehler, T.; Hodson, L.; Patterson, B.W.; Nishikata, N.; Kreis, R.; Mittendorfer, B.; et al. Effects of supplementation with essential amino acids on intrahepatic lipid concentrations during fructose overfeeding in humans. *Am. J. Clin. Nutr.* **2012**, *96*, 1008–1016. [CrossRef] [PubMed]

32. Veldhorst, M.A.; Westerterp-Plantenga, M.S.; Westerterp, K.R. Gluconeogenesis and energy expenditure after a high-protein, carbohydrate-free diet. *Am. J. Clin. Nutr.* **2009**, *90*, 519–526. [CrossRef] [PubMed]

33. Koopman, K.E.; Caan, M.W.; Nederveen, A.J.; Pels, A.; Ackermans, M.T.; Fliers, E.; la Fleur, S.E.; Serlie, M.J. Hypercaloric diets with increased meal frequency, but not meal size, increase intrahepatic triglycerides: A randomized controlled trial. *Hepatology* **2014**, *60*, 545–553. [CrossRef]

34. Madan, S.A.; John, F.; Pyrsopoulos, N.; Pitchumoni, C.S. Nonalcoholic fatty liver disease and carotid artery atherosclerosis in children and adults: A meta-analysis. *Eur. J. Gastroenterol. Hepatol.* **2015**, *27*, 1237–1248. [CrossRef] [PubMed]

35. Malik, V.S.; Popkin, B.M.; Bray, G.A.; Despres, J.P.; Hu, F.B. Sugar-sweetened beverages, obesity, type 2 diabetes mellitus, and cardiovascular disease risk. *Circulation* **2010**, *121*, 1356–1364. [CrossRef]

36. Fung, T.T.; Malik, V.; Rexrode, K.M.; Manson, J.E.; Willett, W.C.; Hu, F.B. Sweetened beverage consumption and risk of coronary heart disease in women. *Am. J. Clin. Nutr.* **2009**, *89*, 1037–1042. [CrossRef]

37. Yang, Q.; Zhang, Z.; Gregg, E.W.; Flanders, W.D.; Merritt, R.; Hu, F.B. Added sugar intake and cardiovascular diseases mortality among US adults. *JAMA Intern. Med.* **2014**, *174*, 516–524. [CrossRef]

38. Bernstein, A.M.; de Koning, L.; Flint, A.J.; Rexrode, K.M.; Willett, W.C. Soda consumption and the risk of stroke in men and women. *Am. J. Clin. Nutr.* **2012**, *95*, 1190–1199. [CrossRef]

39. Eshak, E.S.; Iso, H.; Kokubo, Y.; Saito, I.; Yamagishi, K.; Inoue, M.; Tsugane, S. Soft drink intake in relation to incident ischemic heart disease, stroke, and stroke subtypes in Japanese men and women: The Japan Public Health Centre-based study cohort I. *Am. J. Clin. Nutr.* **2012**, *96*, 1390–1397. [CrossRef]

40. Piepoli, M.F.; Hoes, A.W.; Agewall, S.; Albus, C.; Brotons, C.; Catapano, A.L.; Cooney, M.T.; Corrà, U.; Cosyns, B.; Deaton, C.; et al. 2016 European Guidelines on cardiovascular disease prevention in clinical practice. *Rev. Esp. Cardiol. (Engl. Ed.)* **2016**, *69*, 939. [CrossRef]

41. Rebollo, A.; Roglans, N.; Alegret, M.; Laguna, J.C. Way back for fructose and liver metabolism: Bench side to molecular insights. *World J. Gastroenterol.* **2012**, *18*, 6552–6559. [CrossRef] [PubMed]
42. Jin, R.; Welsh, J.A.; Le, N.A.; Holzberg, J.; Sharma, P.; Martin, D.R.; Vos, M.B. Dietary fructose reduction improves markers of cardiovascular disease risk in Hispanic-American adolescents with NAFLD. *Nutrients* **2014**, *6*, 3187–3201. [CrossRef] [PubMed]
43. Anderson, J.W.; Hanna, T.J.; Peng, X.; Kryscio, R.J. Whole grain foods and heart disease risk. *J. Am. Coll. Nutr.* **2000**, *19*, 291S–299S. [CrossRef] [PubMed]
44. Katcher, H.I.; Legro, R.S.; Kunselman, A.R.; Gillies, P.J.; Demers, L.M.; Bagshaw, D.M.; Kris-Etherton, P.M. The effects of a whole grain-enriched hypocaloric diet on cardiovascular disease risk factors in men and women with metabolic syndrome. *Am. J. Clin. Nutr.* **2008**, *87*, 79–90. [CrossRef] [PubMed]
45. Mellen, P.B.; Walsh, T.F.; Herrington, D.M. Whole grain intake and cardiovascular disease: A meta-analysis. *Nutr. Metab. Cardiovasc. Dis.* **2008**, *18*, 283–290. [CrossRef]
46. White, B. Dietary fatty acids. *Am. Fam. Physician* **2009**, *80*, 345–350.
47. Choque, B.; Catheline, D.; Rioux, V.; Legrand, P. Linoleic acid: Between doubts and certainties. *Biochimie* **2014**, *96*, 14–21. [CrossRef]
48. Cordain, L.; Eaton, S.B.; Sebastian, A.; Mann, N.; Lindeberg, S.; Watkins, B.A.; O'Keefe, J.H.; Brand-Miller, J. Origins and evolution of the Western diet: Health implications for the 21st century. *Am. J. Clin. Nutr.* **2005**, *81*, 341–354. [CrossRef]
49. Donnelly, K.L.; Smith, C.I.; Schwarzenberg, S.J.; Jessurun, J.; Boldt, M.D.; Parks, E.J. Sources of fatty acids stored in liver and secreted via lipoproteins in patients with nonalcoholic fatty liver disease. *J. Clin. Investig.* **2005**, *115*, 1343–1351. [CrossRef]
50. Musso, G.; Gambino, R.; De Michieli, F.; Cassader, M.; Rizzetto, M.; Durazzo, M.; Fagà, E.; Silli, B.; Pagano, G. Dietary habits and their relations to insulin resistance and postprandial lipemia in nonalcoholic steatohepatitis. *Hepatology* **2003**, *37*, 909–916. [CrossRef]
51. Toshimitsu, K.; Matsuura, B.; Ohkubo, I.; Niiya, T.; Furukawa, S.; Hiasa, Y.; Kawamura, M.; Ebihara, K.; Onji, M. Dietary habits and nutrient intake in non-alcoholic steatohepatitis. *Nutrition* **2007**, *23*, 46–52. [CrossRef] [PubMed]
52. Araya, J.; Rodrigo, R.; Videla, L.A.; Thielemann, L.; Orellana, M.; Pettinelli, P.; Poniachik, J. Increase in long-chain polyunsaturated fatty acid n - 6/n - 3 ratio in relation to hepatic steatosis in patients with non-alcoholic fatty liver disease. *Clin. Sci. (Lond.)* **2004**, *106*, 635–643. [CrossRef]
53. Elizondo, A.; Araya, J.; Rodrigo, R.; Poniachik, J.; Csendes, A.; Maluenda, F.; Díaz, J.C.; Signorini, C.; Sgherri, C.; Comporti, M.; et al. Polyunsaturated fatty acid pattern in liver and erythrocyte phospholipids from obese patients. *Obesity (Silver Spring)* **2007**, *15*, 24–31. [CrossRef] [PubMed]
54. Jump, D.B.; Lytle, K.A.; Depner, C.M.; Tripathy, S. Omega-3 polyunsaturated fatty acids as a treatment strategy for nonalcoholic fatty liver disease. *Pharmacol. Ther.* **2018**, *181*, 108–125. [CrossRef] [PubMed]
55. Levy, J.R.; Clore, J.N.; Stevens, W. Dietary n-3 polyunsaturated fatty acids decrease hepatic triglycerides in Fischer 344 rats. *Hepatology* **2004**, *39*, 608–616. [CrossRef]
56. Sekiya, M.; Yahagi, N.; Matsuzaka, T.; Najima, Y.; Nakakuki, M.; Nagai, R.; Ishibashi, S.; Osuga, J.I.; Yamada, N.; Shimano, H. Polyunsaturated fatty acids ameliorate hepatic steatosis in obese mice by SREBP-1 suppression. *Hepatology* **2003**, *38*, 1529–1539. [CrossRef]
57. Depner, C.M.; Traber, M.G.; Bobe, G.; Kensicki, E.; Bohren, K.M.; Milne, G.; Jump, D.B. A metabolomic analysis of omega-3 fatty acid-mediated attenuation of western diet-induced nonalcoholic steatohepatitis in LDLR-/- mice. *PLoS ONE* **2013**, *8*, e83756. [CrossRef]
58. Lytle, K.A.; Wong, C.P.; Jump, D.B. Docosahexaenoic acid blocks progression of western diet-induced nonalcoholic steatohepatitis in obese Ldlr-/- mice. *PLoS ONE* **2017**, *12*, e0173376. [CrossRef]
59. Rosqvist, F.; Iggman, D.; Kullberg, J.; Cedernaes, J.; Johansson, H.E.; Larsson, A.; Johansson, L.; Ahlström, H.; Arner, P.; Dahlman, I.; et al. Overfeeding polyunsaturated and saturated fat causes distinct effects on liver and visceral fat accumulation in humans. *Diabetes* **2014**, *63*, 2356–2368. [CrossRef]
60. Bjermo, H.; Iggman, D.; Kullberg, J.; Dahlman, I.; Johansson, L.; Persson, L.; Berglund, J.; Pulkki, K.; Basu, S.; Uusitupa, M.; et al. Effects of n-6 PUFAs compared with SFAs on liver fat, lipoproteins, and inflammation in abdominal obesity: A randomized controlled trial. *Am. J. Clin. Nutr.* **2012**, *95*, 1003–1012. [CrossRef]

61. Errazuriz, I.; Dube, S.; Slama, M.; Visentin, R.; Nayar, S.; O'Connor, H.; Cobelli, C.; Das, S.K.; Basu, A.; Kremers, W.K.; et al. Randomized Controlled Trial of a MUFA or Fiber-Rich Diet on Hepatic Fat in Prediabetes. *J. Clin. Endocrinol. Metab.* **2017**, *102*, 1765–1774. [CrossRef]
62. Bozzetto, L.; Prinster, A.; Annuzzi, G.; Costagliola, L.; Mangione, A.; Vitelli, A.; Mazzarella, R.; Longobardo, M.; Mancini, M.; Vigorito, C.; et al. Liver fat is reduced by an isoenergetic MUFA diet in a controlled randomized study in type 2 diabetic patients. *Diabetes Care* **2012**, *35*, 1429–1435. [CrossRef] [PubMed]
63. Ryan, M.C.; Itsiopoulos, C.; Thodis, T.; Ward, G.; Trost, N.; Hofferberth, S.; O'Dea, K.; Desmond, P.V.; Johnson, N.A.; Wilson, A.M. The Mediterranean diet improves hepatic steatosis and insulin sensitivity in individuals with non-alcoholic fatty liver disease. *J. Hepatol.* **2013**, *59*, 138–143. [CrossRef] [PubMed]
64. European Association for the Study of the Liver; European Association for the Study of Diabetes; European Association for the Study of Obesity. EASL-EASD-EASO Clinical Practice Guidelines for the management of non-alcoholic fatty liver disease. *Diabetologia* **2016**, *59*, 1121–1140. [CrossRef] [PubMed]
65. Sui, Y.H.; Luo, W.J.; Xu, Q.Y.; Hua, J. Dietary saturated fatty acid and polyunsaturated fatty acid oppositely affect hepatic NOD-like receptor protein 3 inflammasome through regulating nuclear factor-kappa B activation. *World J. Gastroenterol.* **2016**, *22*, 2533–2544. [CrossRef]
66. Jasirwan, C.O.M.; Lesmana, C.R.A.; Hasan, I.; Sulaiman, A.S.; Gani, R.A. The role of gut microbiota in non-alcoholic fatty liver disease: Pathways of mechanisms. *Biosci. Microbiota Food Health* **2019**, *38*, 81–88. [CrossRef]
67. Meex, R.C.R.; Blaak, E.E. Mitochondrial Dysfunction is a Key Pathway that Links Saturated Fat Intake to the Development and Progression of NAFLD. *Mol. Nutr. Food. Res.* **2020**, e1900942. [CrossRef]
68. Lottenberg, A.M.; Afonso Mda, S.; Lavrador, M.S.; Machado, R.M.; Nakandakare, E.R. The role of dietary fatty acids in the pathology of metabolic syndrome. *J. Nutr. Biochem.* **2012**, *23*, 1027–1040. [CrossRef]
69. Lytle, K.A.; Depner, C.M.; Wong, C.P.; Jump, D.B. Docosahexaenoic acid attenuates Western diet-induced hepatic fibrosis in Ldlr-/- mice by targeting the TGFbeta-Smad3 pathway. *J. Lipid. Res.* **2015**, *56*, 1936–1946. [CrossRef]
70. Collaborators, G.B.D.R.F.; Forouzanfar, M.H.; Alexander, L.; Anderson, H.R.; Bachman, V.F.; Biryukov, S.; Brauer, M.; Burnett, R.; Casey, D.; Coates, M.M.; et al. Global, regional, and national comparative risk assessment of 79 behavioural, environmental and occupational, and metabolic risks or clusters of risks in 188 countries, 1990–2013: A systematic analysis for the Global Burden of Disease Study 2013. *Lancet* **2015**, *386*, 2287–2323. [CrossRef]
71. Linseisen, J.; Welch, A.A.; Ocke, M.; Amiano, P.; Agnoli, C.; Ferrari, P.; Sonestedt, E.; Chajès, V.; Bueno-de-Mesquita, H.B.; Kaaks, R.; et al. Dietary fat intake in the European Prospective Investigation into Cancer and Nutrition: Results from the 24-h dietary recalls. *Eur. J. Clin. Nutr.* **2009**, *63*, S61–S80. [CrossRef] [PubMed]
72. Molendi-Coste, O.; Legry, V.; Leclercq, I.A. Why and How Meet n-3 PUFA Dietary Recommendations? *Gastroenterol. Res. Pract.* **2011**, *2011*, 364040. [CrossRef] [PubMed]
73. Simopoulos, A.P. The importance of the ratio of omega-6/omega-3 essential fatty acids. *Biomed. Pharmacother.* **2002**, *56*, 365–379. [CrossRef]
74. Das, U.N. Essential fatty acids and their metabolites could function as endogenous HMG-CoA reductase and ACE enzyme inhibitors, anti-arrhythmic, anti-hypertensive, anti-atherosclerotic, anti-inflammatory, cytoprotective, and cardioprotective molecules. *Lipids Health Dis.* **2008**, *37*. [CrossRef] [PubMed]
75. Berryman, C.E.; Preston, A.G.; Karmally, W.; Deckelbaum, R.J.; Kris-Etherton, P.M. Effects of almond consumption on the reduction of LDL-cholesterol: A discussion of potential mechanisms and future research directions. *Nutr. Rev.* **2011**, *69*, 171–185. [CrossRef]
76. Martin de Santa Olalla, L.; Sanchez Muniz, F.J.; Vaquero, M.P. N-3 fatty acids in glucose metabolism and insulin sensitivity. *Nutr. Hosp.* **2009**, *24*, 113–127.
77. Harris, W.S.; Mozaffarian, D.; Lefevre, M.; Toner, C.D.; Colombo, J.; Cunnane, S.C.; Holden, J.M.; Klurfeld, D.M.; Morris, M.C.; Whelan, J. Towards establishing dietary reference intakes for eicosapentaenoic and docosahexaenoic acids. *J. Nutr.* **2009**, *139*, 804S–819S. [CrossRef]
78. Campos, H.; Baylin, A.; Willett, W.C. Alpha-linolenic acid and risk of nonfatal acute myocardial infarction. *Circulation* **2008**, *118*, 339–345. [CrossRef]
79. Yashodhara, B.M.; Umakanth, S.; Pappachan, J.M.; Bhat, S.K.; Kamath, R.; Choo, B.H. Omega-3 fatty acids: A comprehensive review of their role in health and disease. *Postgrad. Med. J.* **2009**, *85*, 84–90. [CrossRef]
80. Eaton, S.B.; Konner, M.J.; Cordain, L. Diet-dependent acid load, Paleolithic [corrected] nutrition, and evolutionary health promotion. *Am. J. Clin. Nutr.* **2010**, *91*, 295–297. [CrossRef]

81. Nagata, C.; Takatsuka, N.; Shimizu, H. Soy and fish oil intake and mortality in a Japanese community. *Am. J. Epidemiol.* **2002**, *156*, 824–831. [CrossRef] [PubMed]
82. De Lorgeril, M.; Salen, P.; Martin, J.L.; Monjaud, I.; Delaye, J.; Mamelle, N. Mediterranean diet, traditional risk factors, and the rate of cardiovascular complications after myocardial infarction: Final report of the Lyon Diet Heart Study. *Circulation* **1999**, *99*, 779–885. [CrossRef] [PubMed]
83. Masterton, G.S.; Plevris, J.N.; Hayes, P.C. Review article: Omega-3 fatty acids—A promising novel therapy for non-alcoholic fatty liver disease. *Aliment. Pharmacol. Ther.* **2010**, *31*, 679–692. [CrossRef] [PubMed]
84. Perrone, M.A.; Gualtieri, P.; Gratteri, S.; Ali, W.; Sergi, D.; Muscoli, S.; Cammarano, A.; Bernardini, S.; Renzo, L.D.; Romeo, F. Effects of postprandial hydroxytyrosol and derivates on oxidation of LDL, cardiometabolic state and gene expression: A nutrigenomic approach for cardiovascular prevention. *J. Cardiovasc. Med. (Hagerstown)* **2019**, *20*, 419–426. [CrossRef] [PubMed]
85. Gentilcore, D.; Chaikomin, R.; Jones, K.L.; Russo, A.; Feinle-Bisset, C.; Wishart, J.M.; Rayner, C.K.; Horowitz, M. Effects of fat on gastric emptying of and the glycemic, insulin, and incretin responses to a carbohydrate meal in type 2 diabetes. *J. Clin. Endocrinol. Metab.* **2006**, *91*, 2062–2067. [CrossRef] [PubMed]
86. Eckel, R.H.; Jakicic, J.M.; Ard, J.D.; de Jesus, J.M.; Houston Miller, N.; Hubbard, V.S.; Lee, I.M.; Lichtenstein, A.H.; Loria, C.M.; Millen, B.E.; et al. 2013 AHA/ACC guideline on lifestyle management to reduce cardiovascular risk: A report of the American College of Cardiology/American Heart Association Task Force on Practice Guidelines. *J. Am. Coll. Cardiol.* **2014**, *63*, 2960–2984. [CrossRef]
87. Chalvon-Demersay, T.; Even, P.C.; Tome, D.; Chaumontet, C.; Piedcoq, J.; Gaudichon, C.; Azzout-Marniche, D. Low-protein diet induces, whereas high-protein diet reduces hepatic FGF21 production in mice, but glucose and not amino acids up-regulate FGF21 in cultured hepatocytes. *J. Nutr. Biochem.* **2016**, *36*, 60–67. [CrossRef]
88. Pichon, L.; Huneau, J.F.; Fromentin, G.; Tome, D. A high-protein, high-fat, carbohydrate-free diet reduces energy intake, hepatic lipogenesis, and adiposity in rats. *J. Nutr.* **2006**, *136*, 1256–1260. [CrossRef]
89. Zelber-Sagi, S.; Nitzan-Kaluski, D.; Goldsmith, R.; Webb, M.; Blendis, L.; Halpern, Z.; Oren, R. Long term nutritional intake and the risk for non-alcoholic fatty liver disease (NAFLD): A population based study. *J. Hepatol.* **2007**, *47*, 711–717. [CrossRef]
90. Cruz-Jentoft, A.J.; Bahat, G.; Bauer, J.; Boirie, Y.; Bruyere, O.; Cederholm, T.; Cooper, C.; Landi, F.; Rolland, Y.; Sayer, A.A.; et al. Sarcopenia: Revised European consensus on definition and diagnosis. *Age Ageing* **2019**, *48*, 601. [CrossRef]
91. Lee, Y.H.; Jung, K.S.; Kim, S.U.; Yoon, H.J.; Yun, Y.J.; Lee, B.W.; Kang, E.S.; Han, K.H.; Lee, H.C.; Cha, B.S. Sarcopaenia is associated with NAFLD independently of obesity and insulin resistance: Nationwide surveys (KNHANES 2008–2011). *J. Hepatol.* **2015**, *63*, 486–493. [CrossRef] [PubMed]
92. Tamura, Y.; Omura, T.; Toyoshima, K.; Araki, A. Nutrition Management in Older Adults with Diabetes: A Review on the Importance of Shifting Prevention Strategies from Metabolic Syndrome to Frailty. *Nutrients* **2020**, *12*, 3367. [CrossRef] [PubMed]
93. Liu, X.; Hu, Z.; Xu, X.; Li, Z.; Chen, Y.; Dong, J. The associations of plant-based protein intake with all-cause and cardiovascular mortality in patients on peritoneal dialysis. *Nutr. Metab. Cardiovasc. Dis.* **2020**, *30*, 967–976. [CrossRef] [PubMed]
94. Zhubi-Bakija, F.; Bajraktari, G.; Bytyci, I.; Mikhailidis, D.P.; Henein, M.Y.; Latkovskis, G.; Rexhaj, Z.; Zhubi, E.; Banach, M.; International Lipid Expert Panel (ILEP). The impact of type of dietary protein, animal versus vegetable, in modifying cardiometabolic risk factors: A position paper from the International Lipid Expert Panel (ILEP). *Clin. Nutr.* **2020**. [CrossRef] [PubMed]
95. Fang, X.; An, P.; Wang, H.; Wang, X.; Shen, X.; Li, X.; Min, J.; Liu, S.; Wang, F. Dietary intake of heme iron and risk of cardiovascular disease: A dose-response meta-analysis of prospective cohort studies. *Nutr. Metab. Cardiovasc. Dis.* **2015**, *25*, 24–35. [CrossRef] [PubMed]
96. Pisano, G.; Lombardi, R.; Fracanzani, A.L. Vascular Damage in Patients with Nonalcoholic Fatty Liver Disease: Possible Role of Iron and Ferritin. *Int. J. Mol. Sci.* **2016**, *17*, 675. [CrossRef] [PubMed]
97. Kim, Y.; Hwang, S.W.; Kim, S.; Lee, Y.S.; Kim, T.Y.; Lee, S.H.; Kim, S.J.; Yoo, H.J.; Kim, E.N.; Kweon, M.N. Dietary cellulose prevents gut inflammation by modulating lipid metabolism and gut microbiota. *Gut Microbes* **2020**, *11*, 944–961. [CrossRef]
98. Di Caro, V.; Cummings, J.L.; Alcamo, A.M.; Piganelli, J.D.; Clark, R.S.B.; Morowitz, M.J.; Aneja, R.K. Dietary Cellulose Supplementation Modulates the Immune Response in a Murine Endotoxemia Model. *Shock* **2019**, *51*, 526–534. [CrossRef]

99. Chambers, E.S.; Byrne, C.S.; Morrison, D.J.; Murphy, K.G.; Preston, T.; Tedford, C.; Garcia-Perez, I.; Fountana, S.; Serrano-Contreras, J.I.; Holmes, E.; et al. Dietary supplementation with inulin-propionate ester or inulin improves insulin sensitivity in adults with overweight and obesity with distinct effects on the gut microbiota, plasma metabolome and systemic inflammatory responses: A randomised cross-over trial. *Gut* **2019**, *68*, 1430–1438. [CrossRef]
100. Jayachandran, M.; Chen, J.; Chung, S.S.M.; Xu, B. A critical review on the impacts of beta-glucans on gut microbiota and human health. *J. Nutr. Biochem.* **2018**, *61*, 101–110. [CrossRef]
101. Miedema, M.D.; Petrone, A.; Shikany, J.M.; Greenland, P.; Lewis, C.E.; Pletcher, M.J.; Gaziano, J.M.; Djousse, L. Association of Fruit and Vegetable Consumption During Early Adulthood With the Prevalence of Coronary Artery Calcium After 20 Years of Follow-Up: The Coronary Artery Risk Development in Young Adults (CARDIA) Study. *Circulation* **2015**, *132*, 1990–1998. [CrossRef] [PubMed]
102. Dauchet, L.; Amouyel, P.; Hercberg, S.; Dallongeville, J. Fruit and vegetable consumption and risk of coronary heart disease: A meta-analysis of cohort studies. *J. Nutr.* **2006**, *136*, 2588–2593. [CrossRef] [PubMed]
103. Barrera, F.; George, J. The role of diet and nutritional intervention for the management of patients with NAFLD. *Clin. Liver Dis.* **2014**, *18*, 91–112. [CrossRef] [PubMed]
104. Loffredo, L.; Perri, L.; Di Castelnuovo, A.; Iacoviello, L.; De Gaetano, G.; Violi, F. Supplementation with vitamin E alone is associated with reduced myocardial infarction: A meta-analysis. *Nutr. Metab. Cardiovasc. Dis.* **2015**, *25*, 354–363. [CrossRef] [PubMed]
105. Joris, P.J.; Mensink, R.P. Effects of supplementation with the fat-soluble vitamins E and D on fasting flow-mediated vasodilation in adults: A meta-analysis of randomized controlled trials. *Nutrients* **2015**, *7*, 1728–1743. [CrossRef] [PubMed]
106. Cicero, A.F.G.; Colletti, A.; Bellentani, S. Nutraceutical Approach to Non-Alcoholic Fatty Liver Disease (NAFLD): The Available Clinical Evidence. *Nutrients* **2018**, *10*, 1153. [CrossRef] [PubMed]
107. Harrison, S.A.; Torgerson, S.; Hayashi, P.; Ward, J.; Schenker, S. Vitamin E and vitamin C treatment improves fibrosis in patients with nonalcoholic steatohepatitis. *Am. J. Ogastroenterol.* **2003**, *98*, 2485–2490. [CrossRef]
108. Foster, T.; Budoff, M.J.; Saab, S.; Ahmadi, N.; Gordon, C.; Guerci, A.D. Atorvastatin and antioxidants for the treatment of nonalcoholic fatty liver disease: The St Francis Heart Study randomized clinical trial. *Am. J. Ogastroenterol.* **2011**, *106*, 71–77. [CrossRef]
109. Benetti, E.; Mastrocola, R.; Chiazza, F.; Nigro, D.; D'Antona, G.; Bordano, V.; Fantozzi, R.; Aragno, M.; Collino, M.; Minetto, M.A. Effects of vitamin D on insulin resistance and myosteatosis in diet-induced obese mice. *PLoS ONE* **2018**, *13*, e0189707. [CrossRef]
110. Keane, J.T.; Elangovan, H.; Stokes, R.A.; Gunton, J.E. Vitamin D and the Liver-Correlation or Cause? *Nutrients* **2018**, *10*, 496. [CrossRef]
111. Barchetta, I.; Del Ben, M.; Angelico, F.; Di Martino, M.; Fraioli, A.; La Torre, G.; Saulle, R.; Perri, L.; Morini, S.; Tiberti, C.; et al. No effects of oral vitamin D supplementation on non-alcoholic fatty liver disease in patients with type 2 diabetes: A randomized, double-blind, placebo-controlled trial. *BMC Med.* **2016**, *14*, 92. [CrossRef] [PubMed]
112. Fodor, D.; Albu, A.; Poanta, L.; Porojan, M. Vitamin K and vascular calcifications. *Acta. Physiol. Hung.* **2010**, *97*, 256–266. [CrossRef] [PubMed]
113. Shea, M.K.; Booth, S.L.; Miller, M.E.; Burke, G.L.; Chen, H.; Cushman, M.; Tracy, R.P.; Kritchevsky, S.B. Association between circulating vitamin K1 and coronary calcium progression in community-dwelling adults: The Multi-Ethnic Study of Atherosclerosis. *Am. J. Clin. Nutr.* **2013**, *98*, 197–208. [CrossRef] [PubMed]
114. Panahi, Y.; Kianpour, P.; Mohtashami, R.; Jafari, R.; Simental-Mendia, L.E.; Sahebkar, A. Curcumin Lowers Serum Lipids and Uric Acid in Subjects With Nonalcoholic Fatty Liver Disease: A Randomized Controlled Trial. *J. Cardiovasc. Pharmacol.* **2016**, *68*, 223–229. [CrossRef] [PubMed]
115. Selmanovic, S.; Beganlic, A.; Salihefendic, N.; Ljuca, F.; Softic, A.; Smajic, E. Therapeutic Effects of Curcumin on Ultrasonic Morphological Characteristics of Liver in Patients with Metabolic Syndrome. *Acta Inform. Med.* **2017**, *25*, 169–174. [CrossRef]
116. Xiao, J.; Sheng, X.; Zhang, X.; Guo, M.; Ji, X. Curcumin protects against myocardial infarction-induced cardiac fibrosis via SIRT1 activation in vivo and in vitro. *Drug Des. Dev Ther.* **2016**, *10*, 1267–1277. [CrossRef]
117. Wongcharoen, W.; Jai-Aue, S.; Phrommintikul, A.; Nawarawong, W.; Woragidpoonpol, S.; Tepsuwan, T.; Sukonthasarn, A.; Apaijai, N.; Chattipakorn, N. Effects of curcuminoids on frequency of acute myocardial infarction after coronary artery bypass grafting. *Am. J. Cardiol.* **2012**, *110*, 40–44. [CrossRef]

118. Wu, X.; Huang, L.; Zhou, X.; Liu, J. Curcumin protects cardiomyopathy damage through inhibiting the production of reactive oxygen species in type 2 diabetic mice. *Biochem. Biophys. Res. Commun.* **2020**, *530*, 15–21. [CrossRef]
119. Banez, M.J.; Geluz, M.I.; Chandra, A.; Hamdan, T.; Biswas, O.S.; Bryan, N.S.; Von Schwarz, E.R. A systemic review on the antioxidant and anti-inflammatory effects of resveratrol, curcumin, and dietary nitric oxide supplementation on human cardiovascular health. *Nutr. Res.* **2020**, *78*, 11–26. [CrossRef]
120. Perez-Jimenez, J.; Fezeu, L.; Touvier, M.; Arnault, N.; Manach, C.; Hercberg, S.; Galan, P.; Scalbert, A. Dietary intake of 337 polyphenols in French adults. *Am. J. Clin. Nutr.* **2011**, *93*, 1220–1228. [CrossRef]
121. Annuzzi, G.; Bozzetto, L.; Costabile, G.; Giacco, R.; Mangione, A.; Anniballi, G.; Vitale, M.; Vetrani, C.; Cipriano, P.; Corte, G.D.; et al. Diets naturally rich in polyphenols improve fasting and postprandial dyslipidemia and reduce oxidative stress: A randomized controlled trial. *Am. J. Clin. Nutr.* **2014**, *99*, 463–471. [CrossRef] [PubMed]
122. Sakata, R.; Nakamura, T.; Torimura, T.; Ueno, T.; Sata, M. Green tea with high-density catechins improves liver function and fat infiltration in non-alcoholic fatty liver disease (NAFLD) patients: A double-blind placebo-controlled study. *Int. J. Mol. Med.* **2013**, *32*, 989–994. [CrossRef] [PubMed]
123. Poulsen, M.M.; Vestergaard, P.F.; Clasen, B.F.; Radko, Y.; Christensen, L.P.; Stodkilde-Jorgensen, H.; Møller, N.; Jessen, N.; Pedersen, S.B.; Jørgensen, J.O.L. High-dose resveratrol supplementation in obese men: An investigator-initiated, randomized, placebo-controlled clinical trial of substrate metabolism, insulin sensitivity, and body composition. *Diabetes* **2013**, *62*, 1186–1195. [CrossRef] [PubMed]
124. Della Pepa, G.; Vetrani, C.; Lombardi, G.; Bozzetto, L.; Annuzzi, G.; Rivellese, A.A. Isocaloric Dietary Changes and Non-Alcoholic Fatty Liver Disease in High Cardiometabolic Risk Individuals. *Nutrients* **2017**, *9*, 1065. [CrossRef]
125. Wijarnpreecha, K.; Thongprayoon, C.; Ungprasert, P. Coffee consumption and risk of nonalcoholic fatty liver disease: A systematic review and meta-analysis. *Eur. J. Gastroenterol. Hepatol.* **2017**, *29*, e8–e12. [CrossRef]
126. Schwimmer, J.B.; Celedon, M.A.; Lavine, J.E.; Salem, R.; Campbell, N.; Schork, N.J.; Shiehmorteza, M.; Yokoo, T.; Chavez, A.; Middleton, M.S.; et al. Heritability of nonalcoholic fatty liver disease. *Gastroenterology* **2009**, *136*, 1585–1592. [CrossRef]
127. Dongiovanni, P.; Donati, B.; Fares, R.; Lombardi, R.; Mancina, R.M.; Romeo, S.; Valenti, L. PNPLA3 I148M polymorphism and progressive liver disease. *World J. Gastroenterol.* **2013**, *19*, 6969–6978. [CrossRef]
128. Romeo, S.; Kozlitina, J.; Xing, C.; Pertsemlidis, A.; Cox, D.; Pennacchio, L.A.; Boerwinkle, E.; Cohen, J.C.; Hobbs, H.H. Genetic variation in PNPLA3 confers susceptibility to nonalcoholic fatty liver disease. *Nat. Genet.* **2008**, *40*, 1461–1465. [CrossRef]
129. Kozlitina, J.; Smagris, E.; Stender, S.; Nordestgaard, B.G.; Zhou, H.H.; Tybjaerg-Hansen, A.; Vogt, T.F.; Hobbs, H.H.; Cohen, J.C. Exome-wide association study identifies a TM6SF2 variant that confers susceptibility to nonalcoholic fatty liver disease. *Nat. Genet.* **2014**, *46*, 352–356. [CrossRef]
130. Mancina, R.M.; Dongiovanni, P.; Petta, S.; Pingitore, P.; Meroni, M.; Rametta, R.; Borén, J.; Montalcini, T.; Pujia, A.; Wiklund, O.; et al. The MBOAT7-TMC4 Variant rs641738 Increases Risk of Nonalcoholic Fatty Liver Disease in Individuals of European Descent. *Gastroenterology* **2016**, *150*, 1219–1230. [CrossRef]
131. Beer, N.L.; Tribble, N.D.; McCulloch, L.J.; Roos, C.; Johnson, P.R.; Orho-Melander, M.; Gloyn, A.L. The P446L variant in GCKR associated with fasting plasma glucose and triglyceride levels exerts its effect through increased glucokinase activity in liver. *Hum. Mol. Genet.* **2009**, *18*, 4081–4088. [CrossRef] [PubMed]
132. Chen, Y.Y.; Wang, B.N.; Yu, X.P. Correlation between the 677C>T polymorphism in the methylene tetrahydrofolate reductase gene and serum homocysteine levels in coronary heart disease. *Genet. Mol. Res.* **2016**, *15*. [CrossRef] [PubMed]
133. Raina, J.K.; Sharma, M.; Panjaliya, R.K.; Bhagat, M.; Sharma, R.; Bakaya, A.; Kumar, P. Methylenetetrahydrofolate reductase C677T and methionine synthase A2756G gene polymorphisms and associated risk of cardiovascular diseases: A study from Jammu region. *Indian Heart J.* **2016**, *68*, 421–430. [CrossRef]
134. Do, R.; Stitziel, N.O.; Won, H.H.; Jorgensen, A.B.; Duga, S.; Angelica Merlini, P.; Kiezun, A.; Farrall, M.; Goel, A.; Zuk, O.; et al. Exome sequencing identifies rare LDLR and APOA5 alleles conferring risk for myocardial infarction. *Nature* **2015**, *518*, 102–106. [CrossRef]
135. Knoblauch, H.; Bauerfeind, A.; Toliat, M.R.; Becker, C.; Luganskaja, T.; Gunther, U.P.; Rohde, K.; Schuster, H.; Junghans, C.; Luft, F.C.; et al. Haplotypes and SNPs in 13 lipid-relevant genes explain most of the genetic variance in high-density lipoprotein and low-density lipoprotein cholesterol. *Hum. Mol. Genet.* **2004**, *13*, 993–1004. [CrossRef] [PubMed]

136. Zhang, Y.; Tang, H.Q.; Peng, W.J.; Zhang, B.B.; Liu, M. Meta-analysis for the Association of Apolipoprotein E epsilon2/epsilon3/epsilon4 Polymorphism with Coronary Heart Disease. *Chin. Med. J. (Engl.)* **2015**, *128*, 1391–1398. [CrossRef]
137. Hesketh, J. Personalised nutrition: How far has nutrigenomics progressed? *Eur. J. Clin. Nutr.* **2013**, *67*, 430–435. [CrossRef]
138. Stender, S.; Kozlitina, J.; Nordestgaard, B.G.; Tybjaerg-Hansen, A.; Hobbs, H.H.; Cohen, J.C. Adiposity amplifies the genetic risk of fatty liver disease conferred by multiple loci. *Nat. Genet.* **2017**, *49*, 842–847. [CrossRef]
139. Tian, C.; Stokowski, R.P.; Kershenobich, D.; Ballinger, D.G.; Hinds, D.A. Variant in PNPLA3 is associated with alcoholic liver disease. *Nat. Genet.* **2010**, *42*, 21–23. [CrossRef]
140. Davis, J.N.; Le, K.A.; Walker, R.W.; Vikman, S.; Spruijt-Metz, D.; Weigensberg, M.J.; Allayee, H.; Goran, M.I. Increased hepatic fat in overweight Hispanic youth influenced by interaction between genetic variation in PNPLA3 and high dietary carbohydrate and sugar consumption. *Am. J. Clin. Nutr.* **2010**, *92*, 1522–1527. [CrossRef]
141. Nobili, V.; Liccardo, D.; Bedogni, G.; Salvatori, G.; Gnani, D.; Bersani, I.; Alisi, A.; Valenti, L.; Raponi, M. Influence of dietary pattern, physical activity, and I148M PNPLA3 on steatosis severity in at-risk adolescents. *Genes Nutr.* **2014**, *9*, 392. [CrossRef] [PubMed]
142. Santoro, N.; Savoye, M.; Kim, G.; Marotto, K.; Shaw, M.M.; Pierpont, B.; Caprio, S. Hepatic fat accumulation is modulated by the interaction between the rs738409 variant in the PNPLA3 gene and the dietary omega6/omega3 PUFA intake. *PLoS ONE* **2012**, *7*, e37827. [CrossRef] [PubMed]
143. Scorletti, E.; West, A.L.; Bhatia, L.; Hoile, S.P.; McCormick, K.G.; Burdge, G.C.; Lillycrop, K.A.; Clough, G.F.; Calder, P.C.; Byrne, C.D. Treating liver fat and serum triglyceride levels in NAFLD, effects of PNPLA3 and TM6SF2 genotypes: Results from the WELCOME trial. *J. Hepatol.* **2015**, *63*, 1476–1483. [CrossRef] [PubMed]
144. Musso, G.; Cipolla, U.; Cassader, M.; Pinach, S.; Saba, F.; De Michieli, F.; Paschetta, E.; Bongiovanni, D.; Framarin, L.; Leone, N.; et al. TM6SF2 rs58542926 variant affects postprandial lipoprotein metabolism and glucose homeostasis in NAFLD. *J. Lipid Res.* **2017**, *58*, 1221–1229. [CrossRef]
145. O'Hare, E.A.; Yang, R.; Yerges-Armstrong, L.M.; Sreenivasan, U.; McFarland, R.; Leitch, C.C.; Wilson, M.H.; Narina, S.; Gorden, A.; Ryan, K.A.; et al. TM6SF2 rs58542926 impacts lipid processing in liver and small intestine. *Hepatology* **2017**, *65*, 1526–1542. [CrossRef]
146. Meroni, M.; Dongiovanni, P.; Longo, M.; Carli, F.; Baselli, G.; Rametta, R.; Pelusi, S.; Badiali, S.; Maggioni, M.; Gaggini, M.; et al. Mboat7 down-regulation by hyper-insulinemia induces fat accumulation in hepatocytes. *EBioMedicine* **2020**, *52*, 102658. [CrossRef]
147. Nettleton, J.A.; McKeown, N.M.; Kanoni, S.; Lemaitre, R.N.; Hivert, M.F.; Ngwa, J.; van Rooij, F.J.A.; Sonestedt, E.; Wojczynski, M.K.; Ye, A.; et al. Interactions of dietary whole-grain intake with fasting glucose- and insulin-related genetic loci in individuals of European descent: A meta-analysis of 14 cohort studies. *Diabetes Care* **2010**, *33*, 2684–2691. [CrossRef]
148. Corella, D.; Carrasco, P.; Sorli, J.V.; Estruch, R.; Rico-Sanz, J.; Martinez-Gonzalez, M.A.; Salas-Salvadó, J.; Covas, M.I.; Coltell, O.; Arós, F.; et al. Mediterranean diet reduces the adverse effect of the TCF7L2-rs7903146 polymorphism on cardiovascular risk factors and stroke incidence: A randomized controlled trial in a high-cardiovascular-risk population. *Diabetes Care* **2013**, *36*, 3803–3811. [CrossRef]
149. Tortosa-Caparros, E.; Navas-Carrillo, D.; Marin, F.; Orenes-Pinero, E. Anti-inflammatory effects of omega 3 and omega 6 polyunsaturated fatty acids in cardiovascular disease and metabolic syndrome. *Crit. Rev. Food Sci. Nutr.* **2017**, *57*, 3421–3429. [CrossRef]
150. Ordovas, J.M.; Corella, D.; Cupples, L.A.; Demissie, S.; Kelleher, A.; Coltell, O.; Wilson, P.W.F.; Schaefer, E.J.; Tucker, K. Polyunsaturated fatty acids modulate the effects of the APOA1 G-A polymorphism on HDL-cholesterol concentrations in a sex-specific manner: The Framingham Study. *Am. J. Clin. Nutr.* **2002**, *75*, 38–46. [CrossRef]
151. Egert, S.; Boesch-Saadatmandi, C.; Wolffram, S.; Rimbach, G.; Muller, M.J. Serum lipid and blood pressure responses to quercetin vary in overweight patients by apolipoprotein E genotype. *J. Nutr.* **2010**, *140*, 278–284. [CrossRef] [PubMed]
152. Yang, Y.; Ruiz-Narvaez, E.; Kraft, P.; Campos, H. Effect of apolipoprotein E genotype and saturated fat intake on plasma lipids and myocardial infarction in the Central Valley of Costa Rica. *Hum. Biol.* **2007**, *79*, 637–647. [CrossRef] [PubMed]

153. Arigony, A.L.; de Oliveira, I.M.; Machado, M.; Bordin, D.L.; Bergter, L.; Pra, D.; Henriques, J.A.P. The influence of micronutrients in cell culture: A reflection on viability and genomic stability. *Biomed. Res. Int.* **2013**, *2013*, 597282. [CrossRef] [PubMed]
154. Santos, J.D.B.; Mendonca, A.A.S.; Sousa, R.C.; Silva, T.G.S.; Bigonha, S.M.; Santos, E.C.; Gonçalves, R.V.; Novaes, R.D. Food-drug interaction: Anabolic steroids aggravate hepatic lipotoxicity and nonalcoholic fatty liver disease induced by trans fatty acids. *Food Chem. Toxicol.* **2018**, *116*, 360–368. [CrossRef]
155. Nakajima, T.; Moriguchi, M.; Katagishi, T.; Sekoguchi, S.; Nishikawa, T.; Takashima, H.; Kimura, H.; Minami, M.; Itoh, Y.; Kagawa, K.; et al. Premature telomere shortening and impaired regenerative response in hepatocytes of individuals with NAFLD. *Liver Int.* **2006**, *26*, 23–31. [CrossRef]
156. Garcia-Calzon, S.; Martinez-Gonzalez, M.A.; Razquin, C.; Corella, D.; Salas-Salvado, J.; Martinez, J.A.; Zalba, J.; Marti, A. Pro12Ala polymorphism of the PPARgamma2 gene interacts with a mediterranean diet to prevent telomere shortening in the PREDIMED-NAVARRA randomized trial. *Circ. Cardiovasc. Genet.* **2015**, *8*, 91–99. [CrossRef]
157. Ferguson, L.R.; De Caterina, R.; Gorman, U.; Allayee, H.; Kohlmeier, M.; Prasad, C.; Choi, M.S.; Curi, R.; De Luis, D.A.; Gil, A.; et al. Guide and Position of the International Society of Nutrigenetics/Nutrigenomics on Personalised Nutrition: Part 1-Fields of Precision Nutrition. *J. Nutrigenet. Nutr.* **2016**, *9*, 12–27. [CrossRef]
158. Navarro-Ibarra, M.J.; Hernandez, J.; Caire-Juvera, G. Diet, physical activity and telomere length in adults. *Nutr. Hosp.* **2019**, *36*, 1403–1417. [CrossRef]
159. Muller, M.; Kersten, S. Nutrigenomics: Goals and strategies. *Nat. Rev. Genet.* **2003**, *4*, 315–322. [CrossRef]
160. Alsaleh, A.; O'Dell, S.D.; Frost, G.S.; Griffin, B.A.; Lovegrove, J.A.; Jebb, S.A.; Sanders, T.A.B.; RISCK Study investigators. Interaction of PPARG Pro12Ala with dietary fat influences plasma lipids in subjects at cardiometabolic risk. *J. Lipid Res.* **2011**, *52*, 2298–2303. [CrossRef]
161. Volcik, K.A.; Nettleton, J.A.; Ballantyne, C.M.; Boerwinkle, E. Peroxisome proliferator-activated receptor [alpha] genetic variation interacts with n-6 and long-chain n-3 fatty acid intake to affect total cholesterol and LDL-cholesterol concentrations in the Atherosclerosis Risk in Communities Study. *Am. J. Clin. Nutr.* **2008**, *87*, 1926–1931. [CrossRef] [PubMed]
162. Razquin, C.; Alfredo Martinez, J.; Martinez-Gonzalez, M.A.; Corella, D.; Santos, J.M.; Marti, A. The Mediterranean diet protects against waist circumference enlargement in 12Ala carriers for the PPARgamma gene: 2 years' follow-up of 774 subjects at high cardiovascular risk. *Br. J. Nutr.* **2009**, *102*, 672–679. [CrossRef] [PubMed]
163. Meroni, M.; Longo, M.; Erconi, V.; Valenti, L.; Gatti, S.; Fracanzani, A.L.; Dongiovanni, P. mir-101-3p Downregulation Promotes Fibrogenesis by Facilitating Hepatic Stellate Cell Transdifferentiation During Insulin Resistance. *Nutrients* **2019**, *11*, 2597. [CrossRef] [PubMed]
164. Pirola, C.J.; Gianotti, T.F.; Burgueno, A.L.; Rey-Funes, M.; Loidl, C.F.; Mallardi, P.; Martino, J.S.; Castaño, G.O.; Sookoian, S. Epigenetic modification of liver mitochondrial DNA is associated with histological severity of nonalcoholic fatty liver disease. *Gut* **2013**, *62*, 1356–1363. [CrossRef] [PubMed]
165. Podrini, C.; Borghesan, M.; Greco, A.; Pazienza, V.; Mazzoccoli, G.; Vinciguerra, M. Redox homeostasis and epigenetics in non-alcoholic fatty liver disease (NAFLD). *Curr. Pharm. Des.* **2013**, *19*, 2737–2746. [CrossRef]
166. Wang, L.J.; Zhang, H.W.; Zhou, J.Y.; Liu, Y.; Yang, Y.; Chen, X.L.; Zhu, C.H.; Zheng, R.D.; Ling, W.H.; Zhu, H.L. Betaine attenuates hepatic steatosis by reducing methylation of the MTTP promoter and elevating genomic methylation in mice fed a high-fat diet. *J. Nutr. Biochem.* **2014**, *25*, 329–336. [CrossRef]
167. Pooya, S.; Blaise, S.; Moreno Garcia, M.; Giudicelli, J.; Alberto, J.M.; Gueant-Rodriguez, R.M.; Jeannesson, E.; Gueguen, N.; Bressenot, A.; Nicolas, B.; et al. Methyl donor deficiency impairs fatty acid oxidation through PGC-1alpha hypomethylation and decreased ER-alpha, ERR-alpha, and HNF-4alpha in the rat liver. *J. Hepatol.* **2012**, *57*, 344–351. [CrossRef]
168. Cordero, P.; Milagro, F.I.; Campion, J.; Martinez, J.A. Maternal methyl donors supplementation during lactation prevents the hyperhomocysteinemia induced by a high-fat-sucrose intake by dams. *Int. J. Mol. Sci.* **2013**, *14*, 24422–24437. [CrossRef]
169. Whayne, T.F. Epigenetics in the development, modification, and prevention of cardiovascular disease. *Mol. Biol. Rep.* **2015**, *42*, 765–776. [CrossRef]
170. Chang, H.C.; Guarente, L. SIRT1 and other sirtuins in metabolism. *Trends Endocrinol. Metab.* **2014**, *25*, 138–145. [CrossRef]

171. Lee, J.H.; Friso, S.; Choi, S.W. Epigenetic mechanisms underlying the link between non-alcoholic fatty liver diseases and nutrition. *Nutrients* **2014**, *6*, 3303–3325. [CrossRef] [PubMed]
172. Tan, J.; McKenzie, C.; Potamitis, M.; Thorburn, A.N.; Mackay, C.R.; Macia, L. The role of short-chain fatty acids in health and disease. *Adv. Immunol.* **2014**, *121*, 91–119. [CrossRef] [PubMed]
173. Long, J.K.; Dai, W.; Zheng, Y.W.; Zhao, S.P. miR-122 promotes hepatic lipogenesis via inhibiting the LKB1/AMPK pathway by targeting Sirt1 in non-alcoholic fatty liver disease. *Mol. Med.* **2019**, *25*, 26. [CrossRef] [PubMed]
174. Zhang, L.; Hou, D.; Chen, X.; Li, D.; Zhu, L.; Zhang, Y.; Li, J.; Bian, Z.; Liang, X.Y.; Cai, X.; et al. Exogenous plant MIR168a specifically targets mammalian LDLRAP1: Evidence of cross-kingdom regulation by microRNA. *Cell Res.* **2012**, *22*, 107–126. [CrossRef] [PubMed]
175. Palmer, J.D.; Soule, B.P.; Simone, B.A.; Zaorsky, N.G.; Jin, L.; Simone, N.L. MicroRNA expression altered by diet: Can food be medicinal? *Ageing Res. Rev.* **2014**, *17*, 16–24. [CrossRef] [PubMed]
176. Wankhade, U.D.; Zhong, Y.; Kang, P.; Alfaro, M.; Chintapalli, S.V.; Thakali, K.M.; Shankar, K. Enhanced offspring predisposition to steatohepatitis with maternal high-fat diet is associated with epigenetic and microbiome alterations. *PLoS ONE* **2017**, *12*, e0175675. [CrossRef] [PubMed]

2

Coconuts and Health: Different Chain Lengths of Saturated Fats Require Different Consideration

Susan Hewlings [1,2]

[1] Department of Nutrition and Dietetics, Central Michigan University, Mount Pleasant, MI 48859, USA; hewli1sj@cmich.edu

[2] GRAS Associates/Nutrasource, Guelph, ON N1G 0B, Canada

Abstract: The diet heart hypothesis has driven nutrition recommendations and policy for decades. Recent studies have questioned the hypothesis and sparked great controversy over the assumed connection between saturated fat intake and heart disease. Recent evidence suggests that dietary patterns should be the focus of dietary recommendations, not any one food or nutrient. Furthermore, to classify foods as simply saturated fat, polyunsaturated or monounsaturated fats is to ignore the many other potential nutrients and health benefits. Coconut is classified as a saturated fat and therefore listed as a food to limit to reduce heart disease risk. However, different saturated fats, medium-chain or long-chain, act differently metabolically and thus have different health effects. The medium-chain fatty acids predominate in coconut are absorbed differently and have been associated with several health benefits, including improvements in cognitive function and a more favorable lipid profile compared to longer chain fatty acids. Coconuts provide a healthful source of saturated fats and should not be considered the same as foods with longer chain saturated fats. Future recommendations should take this research into consideration. It is the purpose of this review to discuss the research regarding the connection between saturated fat intake, specifically coconut consumption, and health, while focusing on dietary patterns and lifestyle behaviors.

Keywords: saturated fats; coconut; medium-chain fatty acids; lauric acid; cardiovascular disease

---

1. Introduction

There is a long-standing dogma in public health nutrition that elevated serum total cholesterol, particularly of low-density lipoproteins (LDL-C), increases risk of cardiovascular disease (CVD)/coronary heart disease (CHD). It is also believed that higher high-density lipoprotein cholesterol (HDL-C) decreases risk. Lowering LDL-C has, thus, been at the center of recommendations for reducing cardiovascular disease risk. Connected to this is a long-standing deduction that increased intake of saturated fat increases risk of CVD, and therefore, recommendations to decrease saturated fat intake have also been a part of recommendations for decreasing CVD risk [1,2]. Much of the research linking saturated fat intake to higher LDL-C levels to cardiovascular disease risk has assumed this relationship as part of what is referred to as the diet heart hypothesis [3]. However, the effect of different fats on LDL cholesterol needs to be interpreted cautiously. Without considering CVD risk outcome within the context of the dietary pattern, it is difficult to draw conclusions exclusively from effects on blood lipid levels, especially following short term dietary interventions. Furthermore, it has been shown that in most individuals, reducing saturated fat in the diet reduces large LDL particles subspecies rather than the smaller LDL particles [4]. The smaller particles demonstrate a higher association with CVD risk than do the larger LDL particles [5].

Nonetheless, because of this suggested association, the American Heart Association (AHA) and other major organizations have recommended that individuals decrease their saturated fat intake to reduce their risk of CVD [6–8]. However, the saturated fat intake and CVD connection is one of the most debated modern day nutrition beliefs [9–13]. Some studies have shown that this assumption of a direct causal relationship is not completely correct. Lowering saturated fat intake does not always lead to an improved lipid profile, especially if the saturated fat is replaced with carbohydrates [11,12,14]. This points to the importance of considering the replacement fat, as well as the comparator fat or fat source, when interpreting studies related to fatty acids and disease outcomes [15]. Amid this controversy, the AHA and other organizations maintain their overall recommendations to lower saturated fat intake while further clarifying that what the saturated fats are replaced with is important, and that replacement should be with vegetable based polyunsaturated and monounsaturated fatty acids. The AHA has gone on to clarify that different types of polyunsaturated fats, omega 6 and omega 3, as well as different types of saturated fats may have different effects on cholesterol [6]. Within this discussion the consumption of coconut oil is addressed and the AHA's recommends that individuals avoid consumption of coconut oil. However, the discussion omits research related to the potential benefits of the other nutrients provided by coconut, as well as discussion of the unique properties of lauric acid, the type of saturated fat provided by coconut compared to other saturated fatty acids (SFAs) [16]. Evidence from large observational studies suggests that different SFAs with different physical, chemical, and metabolic structures have different metabolic and health effects, particularly related to blood lipids, glucose-insulin homeostasis, insulin resistance, and diabetes [17,18].

The controversy has evolved from the considerable debate over the last few decades surrounding total fat, particularly saturated fat, and its role in weight management and disease recommendations. Much of the debate has focused on how much saturated fat should be part of a healthy diet [19]. A separate but related controversy is the recent evidence challenging the connection of HDL-C and CVD. While beyond the scope of this review to discuss in detail, the debate centers on whether HDL-C should be a target for intervention and whether recommendations should be centered on a specific target of HDL-C. However, it is agreed that the concentration of HDL-C is an independent, inverse predictor of the risk of having a cardiovascular event; therefore, research should focus on more robust biomarkers and genetic differences [20]. Despite this ongoing debate, it is important to recognize that dietary fats are essential nutrients that play an important role in critical physiological functions including storing energy, supplying essential fatty acids, absorbing and transporting fat-soluble vitamins, protecting and insulating vital organs, providing flavor and satiety in food, providing for cell membrane structure, and serving as a precursor to steroid hormones. However, an abundance of fat in the diet is associated with increased body weight for many reasons, including its caloric density, providing approximately 9 kcal/g compared to approximately 4 kcal/g provided by carbohydrates and proteins [21]. Furthermore, many studies link diets high in fats, especially saturated fats, to many lifestyle diseases such as obesity, heart disease, and cancer [1,22,23]. What has not been clearly identified in the literature and in the recommendations is the food source of the saturated fat and that not all foods classified as saturated fats contain the same fatty acid profiles.

The coconut palm (*Cocos nucifera*) is common across the tropics and subtropics, and while it has become a symbol for warm, sunny vacation locations, it is an important crop for many communities globally, particularly the many islands of the Pacific. It is not just a food source; it provides fiber, timber, fuel, and medicine. It was first used worldwide as an oil when Europeans arrived in the Pacific Islands in the 19th century when it became the first vegetable oil used in world trade [24]. The pharmacological effects of the coconut vary depending on which part of the plant or fruit is being studied or which form consumed (oil, milk, flesh). Production methods (detailed by

Krishna et al., 2010 [25]) for extracting coconut oil can vary as well. However, the wet processing method used to extract virgin coconut oil (VCO) is thought to be superior and VCO is thought to have superior health benefits because of its greater phenolic compounds and associated antioxidant properties, while fatty acid profiles seem unaffected by processing [25–27]. A recent systematic review reported that antioxidant activity has been identified in the endocarp and coconut water, while the fiber was shown to have antibacterial, antiparasitic, and anti-inflammatory effects [28]. Because of these many bioactive compounds and reported benefits, coconut's use in a variety of products has gained popularity. It is used in skin care products, cooking oils, sweeteners, beverages, and more. The coconut crop is said to provide sustainable agriculture supporting the three pillars of society, economy, and environment [29]. Despite the many benefits associated with coconut, recommendations for an increase in consumption remain controversial. This controversial recommendation is tied to the debate surrounding saturated fat recommendations and the high saturated fat content of coconut oil, which is about 92%, of which 62–70% is medium-chain triglyceride (MCT) [25,30,31].

The challenge in addressing the issue of whether consumption of coconut, or any other single food, unfavorably effects lipid profiles or cardiovascular disease risk is that food sources typically contain more than one nutrient and diets contain many foods. Therefore, discovering a relationship between any one food and disease must take into consideration the complex nature of dietary and lifestyle patterns that ultimately influence disease outcomes [32].

It is the purpose of this review to discuss the research regarding the connection between saturated fat intake, specifically coconut consumption, and health while understanding that the connection undoubtedly involves more than one food and is more likely reflective of dietary patterns and lifestyle behaviors. However, this is not to say there is no value in exploring the health effects of any given food in the context of a dietary pattern. PubMed and Google Scholar were searched for the following terms: "coconut", "coconut and health", "*Cocos nucifera* and health", "coconut and cardiovascular disease", "coconut and Alzheimer's disease", "coconut antimicrobial", "coconut and antiviral", and "lauric acid and health".

2. Coconut Oil

In assessing the relationship between a single food or dietary pattern, it is important to consider the complete nutrient composition of the food(s) being analyzed, even when considering the different forms of the same food [33]. Coconut oil is consumed in three main forms: refined coconut oil, copra oil, and VCO. While the fatty acid profile is the same among the different types, VCO contains a higher amount of monoglycerides and antioxidants and other phytonutrients because of differences in processing [26,34].

Saturated fatty acids are not a single family of fats but comprise three sub-groups: short- (C2–C6), medium- (C6–C12), and long-chain (C14–C24) fatty acids. Although all three sub-groups are currently considered saturated fatty acids and are, thus, grouped together in interpreting diet and disease relationships and in making diet recommendations for health, they are distinctly different. Coconut oil is made up of about 92% saturated fats and 9% unsaturated fats. However, these saturated fats differ from the saturated fats in animal fats. The fats in coconut oil are 65% medium-chain and predominantly (~48%) lauric acid (C12) (see Figure 1) [33].

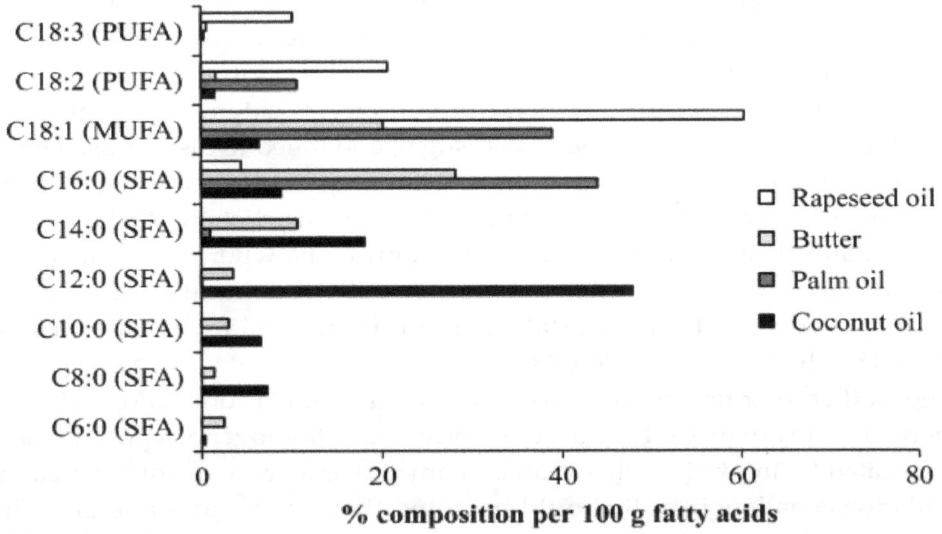

Figure 1. Fatty acid composition of virgin coconut oil compared to other food sources [35]. (With permission from John Wiley and Sons INC., Nutrition Bulletin.)

As Figure 1 demonstrates, though butter and coconut oil are both classified as saturated fat, they have very different fatty acid profiles. Coconut oil is the highest natural source of lauric acid. Lauric acid and its derivative monolaurin constitute around 50% of coconut fat-derived lipids [36]. The shorter chain length influences absorption such that medium-chain fatty acids are mostly absorbed intact and transferred via the portal vein directly to the liver on a mixed diet. Medium-chain fatty acids (MCFA) are partly metabolized in the mitochondria of the liver to produce ketone bodies, including 3-β-hydroxybutyrate, acetoacetic acid, and acetone, which are then transported to the organs of the body such as the brain, which can use ketones for energy production [30]. Due to the high concentration of lauric, capric, and caprylic acids, it has been suggested that coconut oil has unique properties different from other foods high in SFAs [37]. It should be noted that the majority of research on MCFAs has been focused on C8:0 and C10:0 fatty acids, although C6:0 to C12:0 are also considered MCFAs, based on their similar properties [33,38]. Because of their absorption characteristics, MCTs have been used since the 1960s in clinical formulas for adult and infant patients who have issues with the absorption of longer chain fats. Because C12:0 diffuses into the mitochondrial membrane without requiring the carrier carnitine, unlike longer chain fatty acids, it has historically been used for sports nutrition products when quicker absorption and utilization are desirable [39]. Lauric acid can be classified as either a long-chain or MCFA, depending on digestion and absorption and what else is being consumed in the diet. For example, it has been reported that when subjects consume a diet containing different fats, MCFAs tend to be channeled towards the portal vein. However, when the diet is mainly MCFA, some of these may also be incorporated into chylomicrons, suggesting the body adjusts based on the fat content of the diet [40]. This may explain some of the conflicting results that are reported in the literature [33]. Because of these differences in properties and its health benefits, lauric acid should not be considered the same as other longer-chain saturated fatty acids, such as palmitic acid (C16:0) and stearic acid (C18:0), which are much more prominent in butter and animal fats. For example, it has been reported that coconut oil consumption leads to a more favorable lipid profile compared to consumption of butter [38].

3. Cardiovascular Risk Factors

3.1. Saturated Fat and CVD/CHD

There is debate surrounding the role of SFA in the development of CVD, and since coconut oil is largely saturated fat (92%), its consumption has also been discouraged due to "guilt by association".

Several studies suggest no relationship between saturated fat consumption and CVD. For example, a meta-analysis of prospective cohort studies found no significant evidence that dietary saturated fat is associated with an increased risk of cardiovascular disease [11]. However, the study had limitations in that it compared diets high in saturated fat to commonly eaten diets high in carbohydrates, specifically high in refined carbohydrate and added sugar, and failed to distinguish between the type of carbohydrate being substituted. Consistent with these findings, a prospective cohort study (the PURE study) conducted over 10 years of 135,335 individuals assessing dietary intake with validated food frequency questionnaires from 18 countries, on five continents, where overnutrition is common in some and undernutrition in others, found that high carbohydrate intake (>60% total calories) was associated with increased risk of total mortality. In addition, total fat as well as saturated fat and unsaturated fat intake, which were considered separately, were associated with lower mortality rate [41]. The authors suggest that their findings contradict those reporting a connection between saturated fat and CVD [22] because many of these studies were conducted in homogenous populations where CVD is prevalent and saturated fat intake is higher than in many lower income countries, making applicability to diverse populations challenging. It should be noted that many participants in the PURE study consumed as high as 77% of their daily calories from carbohydrates, which could explain some of the findings related to carbohydrate intake and mortality. They did not differentiate types of carbohydrates either, which limits interpretation [41]. Similarly, a meta-analysis of observational cohort studies (3–12 depending on the association) reported no association between higher intake of SFA and all-cause mortality, CHD, CHD mortality, ischemic stroke, or type 2 diabetes among healthy adults [14]. A meta-analysis of 21 prospective epidemiological studies ranging from 6–21 years in length using various dietary assessment tools reported no association between SFA intake and CVD or stroke, even when controlling for energy intake [11]. In contrast, were the findings of a prospective cohort study followed 84,628 women (Nurses' Health Study, 1980 to 2010), and 42,908 men (Health Professionals Follow-up Study, 1986 to 2010) who were free of diabetes, cardiovascular disease, and cancer at baseline. Diet was assessed by semiquantitative food frequency questionnaire every 4 years, and saturated fat intake, unsaturated fat intake, and sources of carbohydrates were compared in relation to risk of CVD. They documented 7667 incident cases of CHD and found that replacing SFA with monounsaturated fatty acids (MUFAs), polyunsaturated fatty acids (PUFAs), or carbohydrate from whole grain is associated with lower CVD risk [23]. Furthermore, when reviewing studies using a multivariable regression analysis that isolates the effects of specific nutrient exchanges, replacing 5% energy intake from SFAs with equivalent energy intake from MUFAs, PUFAs, or whole grain sources of carbohydrate was associated with a significantly lower risk of CHD [16]. The results of these studies strongly support careful examination of the balance of nutrients such that with what one replaces the decreased nutrient is an important aspect of assessing study outcomes, in this case with what one replaces saturated fat appears to influence disease risk. This is supported by results from two large prospective cohort studies (the Health Professionals Follow up and the Nurses' Health Study), as neither found significant associations between saturated fatty acid intake and risk of cardiovascular disease when they controlled for the replacement nutrients [22,23,42]. In addition, the source of the SFA should be considered. A report from the Rotterdam prospective cohort study of 4722 Dutch men and women over 55 years of age found that higher intake of palmitic acid was associated with a higher risk of CHD, while SFAs with other carbon chain lengths were not. Substitution of total SFA with animal protein was also associated with CHD, while no association was found between total SFA intake and CHD risk regardless of food source [43]. Similarly, results from the Atherosclerosis Risk in Communities (ARIC) study suggest that consumption of plant-based protein and fats were associated with lower mortality, while proteins and fats from animal sources were associated with increased mortality, suggesting that the sources of food and thus SFA chain length may impact disease risk [44]. In a 10.6 years prospective cohort study of 195,658 participants from the UK Biobank, there was no evidence that saturated fat intake was associated with incident CVD, while substitution of polyunsaturated for saturated fat was associated with higher CVD risk. They also reported a positive correlation between saturated fat intake and all-cause mortality at intakes above average consumption. Interestingly, results from this study suggest that the dietary intake with the lowest hazard ratio for all-cause mortality consisted of a high intake of fiber (10 to 30 g/day), protein (14% to 30%), and monounsaturated fat (10% to 25%) and moderate intake of polyunsaturated fat (5% to <7%) and starch (20% to <30%) [45].

3.2. *Type of Fat*

The information from the Rotterdam and ARIC studies suggests that in addition to considering what the SFA is replaced, it is important to consider the type of saturated fats as well. It has been suggested that lauric acid and coconut oil do have an impact on lipoproteins. A systematic review and regression analysis published by the World Health Organization of SFAs on lipid profile and lipoproteins found that reducing SFA intake with cis-PUFA (of mostly linoleic acid or α-linolenic acid) or cis-MUFA (predominantly oleic acid) were more favorable than replacing SFA with a mixture of carbohydrates. Cis-PUFA replacement had more favorable effects on total and LDL cholesterol and triglycerides. The effects were seen even at low saturated fat intake. Increased intake of lauric, myristic, or palmitic acid raised serum total, LDL, and HDL cholesterol levels, and lowered triglyceride levels more than complex carbohydrate replacement, while increased intake of stearic acid did not have a significant effect. Lauric acid decreased the total cholesterol to HDL cholesterol and LDL cholesterol to HDL cholesterol ratios compared to a mixture of carbohydrates. The studies included in this analysis utilized tightly controlled diet interventions were short term (3–5-weeks), and included a range of SFA intakes, from 1.6–24.4%. While this allows for precise detection of effects, it may not reflect real world changes in diet, which typically involve more than one nutrient. Furthermore, long-term effects are not reflected in the short-term studies. The authors point out that intakes of lauric and myristic acid in the included studies was low (i.e., mean of 1.2% of total energy intake). They suggest that "in order to obtain more insight into the effects of these two SFA on the serum lipoprotein profile at higher intakes, more well-controlled intervention studies at higher intakes are needed" [46]. In a systematic review and meta-analysis, coconut oil was found to significantly increase HDL-C when compared with plant oils and animal oils and it significantly increased LDL-C compared with plants oils and lowered LDL-C compared with animal oils [37]. Similarly, two studies which used VCO as the coconut source reported significantly elevated HDL-C and no significant changes in LDL-C when comparing subjects consuming VCO to those consuming a virgin olive oil/butter/standard diet [47,48]. In another study, coconut oil was found to be positively associated with HDL-C levels in menopausal women in the Philippines [49].

In a randomized trial, participants were randomized to 1 of 3 groups, extra VCO, virgin olive oil, or butter and asked to add 50 g of one of these fats per day for four weeks into their normal diet or consume it as a supplement. This study found that LDL-C concentrations were significantly increased in the butter group compared with the extra VCO or olive oil group. No differences in LDL-C were observed in coconut oil compared with olive oil. Coconut oil also significantly increased HDL-C compared with butter or olive oil [47]. Similarly, in a study comparing coconut oil, butter, and safflower oil on lipids and lipoproteins in free-living subjects with moderately elevated cholesterol levels, it was found that the coconut oil and butter diets significantly increased total cholesterol and LDL-C relative to safflower oil; however, total cholesterol and LDL-C were significantly higher on the diet containing butter than on the diet containing coconut oil. The authors concluded that "coconut oil rich in lauric acid has a lesser effect than butter, which is high in palmitic acid, on total and LDL cholesterol in hypercholesterolemic men and women" [50].

A recent systematic review and meta-analysis assessing the effect of coconut oil consumption on blood lipids and other cardiovascular risk factors compared with other cooking oils included 16 articles published through June 2019. Coconut oil consumption significantly increased LDL-C by 10.47 mg/dL and HDL-C by 4.00 mg/dL as compared with non-tropical vegetable oils [51]. It should be noted that the authors did not compare coconut consumption to animal sources of saturated fat and they included shorter term studies with no evidence of cardiovascular outcomes.

A previous review conducted a network meta-analysis, which may be more appropriate for comparing multiple treatments, in order to compare the effects of 13 different oils (safflower, sunflower, rapeseed, hempseed, flaxseed, corn, olive, soybean, palm, coconut oil, beef fat, lard, and butter) across randomized trials on established blood lipid factors. Fifty-four trials with 2065 participants published between 1984 and 2018 were included in the analysis. Coconut oil was ranked best to improve HDL-C. The analysis showed that all vegetable oils including coconut oil were more effective in reducing total cholesterol (−0.49 to −0.18 mmol/L) and LDL-C (−0.42 to −0.23 mmol/L) compared with butter [52].

A systematic review was conducted to assess the effect of coconut consumption on cardiovascular risk factors and outcomes in humans. The review included 8 clinical trials and 13 observational studies examining the effects of coconut oil or coconut products on serum lipids. The authors reported that in most studies, coconut oil raised total and LDL-C to a greater extent than cis unsaturated plant oils, but to a lesser extent than butter, suggesting that while coconut oil consumption may offer some benefits compared to other saturated fats, they most likely do not offer a benefit compared to other vegetable fats. However, this is not to say that consumption of coconut unfavorably raises serum lipids. For example, the observational studies included in the review suggested that consumption of coconut flesh or squeezed coconut in the context of traditional dietary patterns does not lead to adverse cardiovascular outcomes. This is an important observation, as it addresses the modern view of the effects of dietary intake on disease outcomes from the perspective of dietary patterns as opposed to one particular food or nutrient. Thus, considering all nutrients, phytochemicals, and other bioactive substances provided by foods that make up dietary patterns [38]. This is an important step forward to providing more appropriate guidelines and recommendations

To summarize, evidence suggests that the saturated fat lipid CVD risk connection is being appropriately challenged, please see a summary of included studies in Table 1. As discussed above, it appears that the connection is not as linear, nor as simple as previously suggested in several ways. It is not as simple as just decrease saturated fat and then disease risk decreases, it appears that with what one replaces the saturated fat is of great importance, in that replacing saturated fat with carbohydrates does not seem to be as advantageous as replacing it with vegetable sources of mono and poly unsaturated fats. Additionally, recent research has shown that not all saturated fats are the same, and therefore, do not have the same effect on CVD risk. Shorter chain saturated fats from vegetable sources appear to have a more beneficial effect on blood lipid profiles and potentially any associated CVD/CHD risk than do longer chains. Coconuts are classified as a saturated fat, although the majority of fats contained in the coconut are medium-chain, and therefore, appear to have a more favorable impact on blood lipids and CVD/CHD risk than animal based saturated fats that are of a longer chain such as beef fat and butter. Oils contain more than just the fatty acids that comprise them, and other nutrients, such as polyphenols and vitamins, may also have an impact on aspects of health in addition to their impact on CVD risk. More research is needed in order to accurately differentiate the types of saturated fats and their impact on health outcomes. Within such research, it would be important to consider all bioactive ingredients within the various sources such that all beneficial compounds are considered in addition to the fatty acid content. It is critical that future revisions of public health policy and dietary recommendations consider such evidence.

Table 1. Summary of studies related to fats and CVD.

Author	Type of Study	Purpose	Included	Conclusion
[11]	Meta-Analysis of prospective epidemiological studies	21 studies related to the association of dietary saturated fat with CHD, stroke, CVD; CHD inclusive of stroke.	5–23 years of follow-up of 347,747 subjects	No significant evidence that saturated fat is associated with increased risk of CHD or CVD
[41]	Epidemiological Cohort	Associations between consumption of carbohydrate, total fat, and each type of fat with cardiovascular disease and total mortality.	Dietary intake of 135,335 individuals aged 35–70 years, in 18 countries; median follow-up 74 years,	↑ Carbohydrate intake associated with ↑ risk of total mortality; total fat and types of fat related to ↓ total mortality. Total fat and types of fat not associated with CVD, myocardial infarction, or cardiovascular disease mortality, saturated fat had an inverse association with stroke.
[22]	Prospective Cohort	Associations between intakes of individual SFAs and their food sources in relation to the risk of CHD.	80,082 women aged 34–59 Nurse's Health Study; 14-year follow up	Short- to medium-chain fats not associated with CHD risk; intake of longer chain = ↑ risk; ratio of PUFA to SFA inversely associated with CHD risk.
[14]	Meta-Analysis of observational studies	Associations between intake of saturated fat and trans unsaturated fat and all cause mortality, CVD and associated mortality, CHD and associated mortality, ischemic stroke, and type 2 diabetes.	41 studies on saturated fats and health outcomes in prospective cohort studies published between 1981 and 2014; 67 data points; 20 studies with 28 data points for trans fats	Saturated fats are not associated with all cause mortality, CVD, CHD, ischemic stroke, or type 2 diabetes, but the evidence is heterogeneous with methodological limitations. Trans fats are associated with all cause mortality, total CHD, and CHD mortality.
[23]	Prospective Cohort	Associations of SFAs compared to PUFAs and carbohydrates to CHD risk.	84,628 women 42,908 men 24–30 year follow up	↑ Intake of PUFAs and whole grains = ↓ risk of CHD; replacing 5% of energy intake from SFAs with PUFAs, MUFAs, or carbohydrates from whole grains was associated with a 25%, 15%, and 9% ↓ risk of CHD.
[42]	Prospective Cohort	Association between fat intake and CHD.	43,757 men aged 40 to 75 years; 6 year follow up	SFA intake not associated with CHD once corrected for fiber intake; ↑ linolenic acid = ↓ risk CHD.
[43]	Prospective Cohort	Association between dietary SFA and CHD depends on the food source, the carbon chain length of SFA, and the substituting macronutrient.	4722 Dutch men and women > 55 years; 16.3 year follow up	↑ Intake of palmitic acid ↑ risk; other SFAs are not associated with CHD; no effect of food source of SFA; replacement of SFA with animal protein ↑ risk; replacement with other macronutrients not associated with risk.

Table 1. *Cont.*

Author	Type of Study	Purpose	Included	Conclusion
[44]	Prospective Cohort and Meta-Analysis	Association between carbohydrate intake and mortality.	15,428 aged 55–64 years ARIC study; 25 year follow up	U-shaped relationship between carbohydrate intake and mortality; low carbohydrate intake with animal protein increased risk, while with high plant protein decreased risk.
[45]	Prospective population study	Association of macronutrient intake with all cause mortality and CVD, and the implications for dietary advice.	195,658 adults 10.6 year follow up	Carbohydrate intake > 50% ↑ association with mortality; ↑ intake of MUFA, ↓ intake of PUFA, ↓ intake of SFA = ↓ risk of mortality.
[46]	Systematic Review and Meta-Analysis of RCTs	Assess the impact of phytosterol (PS) supplementation on serum Lp(a) and FFA concentration.	12 effect sizes from 7 different studies	PS supplementation = ↓ in Lp(a) and FFA.
[37]	Systematic Review and Meta-Analysis	Examine the evidence surrounding coconut oil consumption and its impact on cardiovascular health.	12 studies	Compared with plant oils and animal oils, coconut oil ↑ HDL-C by 0.57 mg/dL and 0.33 mg/dL. Coconut oil significantly ↑ LDL-C by 0.26 mg/dL compared with plant oils and ↓ LDL-C (48.1%) compared with animal oils. No effects on triglyceride. Better lipid profiles were demonstrated with the virgin form of coconut oil.
[49]	Prospective Cohort	Association between coconut oil intake and plasma lipid profiles.	1896 Filipino women aged 35–69 years	In pre-menopausal women, dietary coconut oil use was associated with TC and HDL-C, not in post-menopausal women; coconut oil did not elevate TC, triglyceride levels, and TC/HDL.
[47]	RCT	Compare changes in blood lipid profile, weight, fat distribution, and metabolic markers after four weeks of consumption of 50 g daily of extra virgin coconut oil, butter, or extra virgin olive oil.	91 men and women	LDL-C significantly increased on butter compared with coconut oil and with olive oil, no differences in change of LDL-C in coconut oil compared with olive oil. Coconut oil significantly increased HDL-C compared with butter or olive oil. Butter significantly increased TC/HDL-C ratio and non-HDL-C compared with coconut oil, while coconut oil did not significantly differ from olive oil for TC/HDL-C and non-HDL-C. No significant differences in changes in weight, BMI, central adiposity, fasting blood glucose, and systolic or diastolic blood pressure in any group.

Table 1. *Cont.*

Author	Type of Study	Purpose	Included	Conclusion
[50]	RCT cross over	Compare the effects of coconut oil, butter, and safflower oil on lipids and lipoproteins of moderately hypercholesterolemic subjects.	13 men and 15 women with a plasma total cholesterol between 5.5 and 7.9 mmol/L and plasma triacylglycerols (TAG) less than 3 mmol/L consumed 50% of fat from butter, coconut oil, or safflower oil	Coconut oil and butter diets increased TC and LDL-C compared to safflower oil; the levels of both were significantly lower in the coconut oil than on the butter diet.
[51]	Systematic Review and Meta-Analysis	A systematic review of the effect of coconut oil consumption on blood lipids and other cardiovascular risk factors compared with other cooking oils using data from clinical trials.	16 articles included in the meta-analysis	Coconut oil increased LDL-cholesterol by 10.47 mg/dL and HDL-cholesterol by 4.00 mg/dL compared with nontropical vegetable oils. Coconut oil consumption did not significantly affect markers of glycemia, inflammation, and adiposity as compared with nontropical vegetable oils.
[52]	Systematic Review and Network meta-Analysis	Compare the effects of different oils/solid fats on blood lipids.	54 RCTs 2065 subjects included	Safflower oil ↓ in TC and LDL-C the most, followed by rapeseed oil and sunflower oil; soybean oil was the most effective oil to ↓ TG, followed by corn oil and palm oil; butter and lard were ranked worst for TC and LDL-C reduction; coconut oil was ranked best to ↑ HDL-C, followed by palm oil and beef fat. The NMA showed that all vegetable oils were more effective in reducing TC and LDL-C compared with butter.

4. Alzheimer's Disease

While the majority of research and discussion surrounding the effects of coconut consumption on health have focused on cardiovascular health, there is evidence that coconut consumption may positively impact other diseases. Alzheimer's disease (AD) is a progressive neurogenerative disease and is the most common type of dementia [53]. While an exact cause is not known, lifestyle factors similar to those associated with CVD have been suggested to be associated with an increased risk of AD. Chronic inflammation and increased oxidative stress are thought to be at the center of lifestyle factors that increase AD risk [54]. Therefore, dietary patterns as well as individual foods and nutrients have been investigated for their potential role in the prevention of AD [55]. One such food is coconut. There are a multitude of claims, case studies [56], small clinical trials [57], and anecdotal evidence in the lay literature, but well-controlled clinical trials in humans to support any efficacious claims are lacking [58]. However, a reasonable mechanism of action does seem to support further investigation into the role coconut oil, and the MCTs it contains, may play in improving cognition in those suffering from early stage cognitive dysfunction [30]. In addition to its neuroprotective antioxidant properties, coconut contains high levels of MCFA, which lead to ketone body formation. The ketones are then thought to offset an early sign of AD, brain glucose hypometabolism, by providing an alternative energy source [59,60]. A pilot study was conducted to assess cognitive changes in 44 subjects with AD. Patients ($n = 22$) received a coconut-enriched Mediterranean diet for 21 days and the control ($n = 22$) received an isocaloric Mediterranean diet with no coconut. Those consuming the coconut enriched diet experienced significant improvements in episodic, temporal orientation and semantic memory. The improvements were greater in women with mild-moderate state AD [57]. While there are no large clinical trials or cohort studies to make recommendations for consuming coconut oil to improve cognitive function, information from mechanism of action and small studies supports further research in this area [30,55].

5. Antimicrobial/Antiviral

Coconut has a long history of use as both a food and medicine throughout the world. Its use in Ayurvedic medicine was documented 4000 years ago [61]. The MCFAs are said to be beneficial in destroying a wide assortment of lipid-coated bacteria by disintegrating their lipid membrane [62]. Coconut oil has been shown to demonstrate antifungal and antimicrobial properties, specifically against *P. aeruginosa*, *E. coli*, *Proteus vulgaris*, and *Bacillus subtilis* [63,64] and on Vibrio bacteria [65]. Lauric acid, capric acid, and caprylic acid have been shown to inhibit bacterial growth [66–68]. It has also been shown to have a significant effect on polymicrobial dental biofilm activity [69]. In viruses they are thought to interfere with signal transduction and interfere with the virus assembly and maturation [62,70]. In summary, the use of VCO for its antimicrobial and antiviral benefits have a long history of use and several studies have supported its use, warranting further studies in humans to further define its antimicrobial and antiviral benefits.

6. Conclusions

The coconut palm is an important crop for communities globally both as a food source as well as for fiber, timber, and medicine. It contains several bioactive compounds, particularly extra virgin coconut oil. Many of its health benefits have been overlooked due to its fatty acid composition. It contains primarily saturated fatty acids. The consumption of a diet high in saturated fatty acids has been connected to an increased risk of CVD and other major lifestyle disease. Therefore, historically, public health recommendations have focused on messages encouraging the public to decrease consumption of saturated fats, including coconuts. However, the connection between saturated fat consumption and CVD has been questioned recently. When determining if decreasing saturated fat intake improves lipid profiles and potentially CVD risk it is clear that what the saturated fat is replaced with is critical to interpreting the results. Replacing the fat with vegetable fats appears to be more beneficial than replacing them with simple carbohydrates. This is not surprising considering the negative health implications of consuming excess simple carbohydrates. While diet–disease relationships cannot be definitively identified based on one food or food group, it is clearly important to identify food sources of nutrients when assessing such relationships. For example, there is significant data to support differentiating different food sources of saturated fats to clarify the unique nutrients of each source and the associated health impact. This would be similar to the approach taken with different types of polyunsaturated fats, whereby omega 3 and omega 6 polyunsaturated fats are recognized for their unique properties and health impact. Taking the same approach with different types and sources of saturated fatty acids is warranted when one considers the unique nutrient composition of the coconut compared to other saturated fat sources, such as beef. Beef contains mainly the longer chain saturated fatty acids while coconut contains medium-chain. The medium-chain fatty acids are absorbed differently and have been associated with several health benefits including improvements in cognitive function and a more favorable lipid profile compared to longer chain fatty acids. In the context of a dietary pattern that has been associated with health benefits such as the Mediterranean diet, coconuts may, therefore, provide a healthful source of saturated fats while also providing phenols and antioxidants. While the evidence related to the connection between saturated fat intake and heart disease may be inconclusive and thus not be in full support of reversing suggestion to avoid saturated fats, certainly a revision is justified. A more in-depth investigation of the connection between different types of saturated fat and disease is warranted. Future recommendations and guidelines should take all aspects of the research into consideration when compiling revisions and associated policy.

References

1. Keys, A.; Anderson, J.T.; Grande, F. Prediction of serum-cholesterol responses of man to changes in fats in the diet. *Lancet* **1957**, *273*, 959–966. [CrossRef]
2. Hooper, L.; Martin, N.; Jimoh, O.F.; Kirk, C.; Foster, E.; Abdelhamid, A.S. Reduction in saturated fat intake for cardiovascular disease. *Cochrane Database Syst. Rev.* **2020**, *5*, Cd011737. [CrossRef] [PubMed]
3. Forouhi, N.G.; Krauss, R.M.; Taubes, G.; Willett, W. Dietary fat and cardiometabolic health: Evidence, controversies, and consensus for guidance. *BMJ* **2018**, *361*, k2139. [CrossRef] [PubMed]
4. Bergeron, N.; Chiu, S.; Williams, P.T.; M King, S.; Krauss, R.M. Effects of red meat, white meat, and nonmeat protein sources on atherogenic lipoprotein measures in the context of low compared with high saturated fat intake: A randomized controlled trial. *Am. J. Clin. Nutr.* **2019**, *110*, 24–33. [CrossRef] [PubMed]
5. Krauss, R.M. All low-density lipoprotein particles are not created equal. *Am. Heart Assoc.* **2014**, *34*, 959–961. [CrossRef] [PubMed]
6. Arnett, D.K.; Blumenthal, R.S.; Albert, M.A.; Buroker, A.B.; Goldberger, Z.D.; Hahn, E.J.; Himmelfarb, C.D.; Khera, A.; Lloyd-Jones, D.; McEvoy, J.W.; et al. 2019 ACC/AHA Guideline on the Primary Prevention of Cardiovascular Disease: Executive Summary: A Report of the American College of Cardiology/American Heart Association Task Force on Clinical Practice Guidelines. *Circulation* **2019**, *140*, 563–595. [CrossRef]
7. Central Committee for Medical and Community Program of the American Heart Association. Dietary fat and its relation to heart attacks and strokes. Report by the Central Committee for Medical and Community Program of the American Heart Association. *JAMA* **1961**, *175*, 389–391. [CrossRef]
8. Eckel, R.H.; Jakicic, J.M.; Ard, J.D.; de Jesus, J.M.; Houston Miller, N.; Hubbard, V.S.; Lee, I.M.; Lichtenstein, A.H.; Loria, C.M.; Millen, B.E.; et al. 2013 AHA/ACC guideline on lifestyle management to reduce cardiovascular risk: A report of the American College of Cardiology/American Heart Association Task Force on Practice Guidelines. *Circulation* **2014**, *129*, 76–99. [CrossRef]
9. Mozaffarian, D.; Micha, R.; Wallace, S. Effects on coronary heart disease of increasing polyunsaturated fat in place of saturated fat: A systematic review and meta-analysis of randomized controlled trials. *PLoS Med.* **2010**, *7*, e1000252. [CrossRef]

10. Farvid, M.S.; Ding, M.; Pan, A.; Sun, Q.; Chiuve, S.E.; Steffen, L.M.; Willett, W.C.; Hu, F.B. Dietary linoleic acid and risk of coronary heart disease: A systematic review and meta-analysis of prospective cohort studies. *Circulation* **2014**, *130*, 1568–1578. [CrossRef]
11. Siri-Tarino, P.W.; Sun, Q.; Hu, F.B.; Krauss, R.M. Meta-analysis of prospective cohort studies evaluating the association of saturated fat with cardiovascular disease. *Am. J. Clin. Nutr.* **2010**, *91*, 535–546. [CrossRef] [PubMed]
12. Chowdhury, R.; Warnakula, S.; Kunutsor, S.; Crowe, F.; Ward, H.A.; Johnson, L.; Franco, O.H.; Butterworth, A.S.; Forouhi, N.G.; Thompson, S.G. Association of dietary, circulating, and supplement fatty acids with coronary risk: A systematic review and meta-analysis. *Ann. Intern. Med.* **2014**, *160*, 398–406. [CrossRef] [PubMed]
13. Jakobsen, M.U.; O'Reilly, E.J.; Heitmann, B.L.; Pereira, M.A.; Bälter, K.; Fraser, G.E.; Goldbourt, U.; Hallmans, G.; Knekt, P.; Liu, S.; et al. Major types of dietary fat and risk of coronary heart disease: A pooled analysis of 11 cohort studies. *Am. J. Clin. Nutr.* **2009**, *89*, 1425–1432. [CrossRef] [PubMed]
14. De Souza, R.J.; Mente, A.; Maroleanu, A.; Cozma, A.I.; Ha, V.; Kishibe, T.; Uleryk, E.; Budylowski, P.; Schünemann, H.; Beyene, J. Intake of saturated and trans unsaturated fatty acids and risk of all cause mortality, cardiovascular disease, and type 2 diabetes: Systematic review and meta-analysis of observational studies. *BMJ* **2015**, *351*, h3978. [CrossRef]
15. Nettleton, J.A.; Brouwer, I.A.; Mensink, R.P.; Diekman, C.; Hornstra, G. Fats in Foods: Current Evidence for Dietary Advice. *Ann. Nutr. Metab.* **2018**, *72*, 248–254. [CrossRef]
16. Sacks, F.M.; Lichtenstein, A.H.; Wu, J.H.Y.; Appel, L.J.; Creager, M.A.; Kris-Etherton, P.M.; Miller, M.; Rimm, E.B.; Rudel, L.L.; Robinson, J.G.; et al. Dietary Fats and Cardiovascular Disease: A Presidential Advisory from the American Heart Association. *Circulation* **2017**, *136*, e1–e23. [CrossRef]
17. Zhu, Y.; Tsai, M.Y.; Sun, Q.; Hinkle, S.N.; Rawal, S.; Mendola, P.; Ferrara, A.; Albert, P.S.; Zhang, C. A prospective and longitudinal study of plasma phospholipid saturated fatty acid profile in relation to cardiometabolic biomarkers and the risk of gestational diabetes. *Am. J. Clin. Nutr.* **2018**, *107*, 1017–1026. [CrossRef]
18. Micha, R.; Mozaffarian, D. Saturated fat and cardiometabolic risk factors, coronary heart disease, stroke, and diabetes: A fresh look at the evidence. *Lipids* **2010**, *45*, 893–905. [CrossRef]
19. Boateng, L.; Ansong, R.; Owusu, W.B.; Steiner-Asiedu, M. Coconut oil and palm oil's role in nutrition, health and national development: A review. *Ghana Med. J.* **2016**, *50*, 189–196.
20. Barter, P.; Genest, J. HDL cholesterol and ASCVD risk stratification: A debate. *Atherosclerosis* **2019**, *283*, 7–12. [CrossRef]
21. Hewlings, S.J.; Medeiros, D.M. *Nutrition: Real People, Real Choices*; Pearson Prentice Hall: Upper Saddle River, NJ, USA, 2009.
22. Hu, F.B.; Stampfer, M.J.; Manson, J.E.; Ascherio, A.; Colditz, G.A.; Speizer, F.E.; Hennekens, C.H.; Willett, W.C. Dietary saturated fats and their food sources in relation to the risk of coronary heart disease in women. *Am. J. Clin. Nutr.* **1999**, *70*, 1001–1008. [CrossRef] [PubMed]
23. Li, Y.; Hruby, A.; Bernstein, A.M.; Ley, S.H.; Wang, D.D.; Chiuve, S.E.; Sampson, L.; Rexrode, K.M.; Rimm, E.B.; Willett, W.C.; et al. Saturated Fats Compared With Unsaturated Fats and Sources of Carbohydrates in Relation to Risk of Coronary Heart Disease: A Prospective Cohort Study. *J. Am. Coll. Cardiol.* **2015**, *66*, 1538–1548. [CrossRef] [PubMed]
24. Chan, E.; Elevitch, C.R. *Cocos nucifera* (coconut). *Species Profiles Pac. Isl. Agrofor.* **2006**, *2*, 1–27.
25. Krishna, A.G.; Gaurav, R.; Singh, B.A.; Kumar, P.P.; Preeti, C. Coconut oil: Chemistry, production and its applications—A review. *Indian Coconut J.* **2010**, *53*, 15–27.
26. Nevin, K.; Rajamohan, T. Virgin coconut oil supplemented diet increases the antioxidant status in rats. *Food Chem.* **2006**, *99*, 260–266. [CrossRef]
27. Nevin, K.; Rajamohan, T. Beneficial effects of virgin coconut oil on lipid parameters and in vitro LDL oxidation. *Clin. Biochem.* **2004**, *37*, 830–835. [CrossRef]
28. Lima, E.B.; Sousa, C.N.; Meneses, L.N.; Ximenes, N.C.; Santos Junior, M.A.; Vasconcelos, G.S.; Lima, N.B.; Patrocinio, M.C.; Macedo, D.; Vasconcelos, S.M. *Cocos nucifera* (L.) (Arecaceae): A phytochemical and pharmacological review. *Braz. J. Med. Biol. Res. Rev. Bras. Pesqui. Med. Biol.* **2015**, *48*, 953–964. [CrossRef]
29. Nair, D. Global Scenario on Sustainable Coconut Development. In Proceedings of the IOP Conference Series: Earth and Environmental Science, Padang, West Sumatra Province, Indonesia, 9–30 October 2018; p. 012006.

30. Fernando, W.M.A.D.B.; Martins, I.J.; Goozee, K.; Brennan, C.S.; Jayasena, V.; Martins, R.N. The role of dietary coconut for the prevention and treatment of Alzheimer's disease: Potential mechanisms of action. *Br. J. Nutr.* **2015**, *114*, 1–14. [CrossRef]
31. Bach, A.; Babayan, V. Medium-chain triglycerides: An update. *Am. J. Clin. Nutr.* **1982**, *36*, 950–962. [CrossRef]
32. Willett, W. *Nutritional Epidemiology*; Oxford University Press: Oxford, UK, 2012.
33. Dayrit, F.M. Lauric acid is a medium-chain fatty acid, coconut oil is a medium-chain triglyceride. *Philipp. J. Sci.* **2014**, *143*, 157–166.
34. Dayrit, F.M.; Buenafe, O.E.; Chainani, E.T.; de Vera, I.M. Analysis of monoglycerides, diglycerides, sterols, and free fatty acids in coconut (*Cocos nucifera* L.) oil by 31P NMR spectroscopy. *J. Agric. Food Chem.* **2008**, *56*, 5765–5769. [CrossRef] [PubMed]
35. Lockyer, S.; Stanner, S. Coconut oil—A nutty idea? *Nutr. Bull.* **2016**, *41*, 42–54. [CrossRef]
36. Kannaian, U.P.N.; Edwin, J.B.; Rajagopal, V.; Shankar, S.N.; Srinivasan, B. Phytochemical composition and antioxidant activity of coconut cotyledon. *Heliyon* **2020**, *6*, 03411.
37. Teng, M.; Zhao, Y.J.; Khoo, A.L.; Yeo, T.C.; Yong, Q.W.; Lim, B.P. Impact of coconut oil consumption on cardiovascular health: A systematic review and meta-analysis. *Nutr. Rev.* **2020**, *78*, 249–259. [CrossRef]
38. Eyres, L.; Eyres, M.F.; Chisholm, A.; Brown, R.C. Coconut oil consumption and cardiovascular risk factors in humans. *Nutr. Rev.* **2016**, *74*, 267–280. [CrossRef]
39. Bremer, J. Carnitine—metabolism and functions. *Physiol. Rev.* **1983**, *63*, 1420–1480. [CrossRef]
40. Swift, L.L.; Hill, J.; Peters, J.; Greene, H. Medium-chain fatty acids: Evidence for incorporation into chylomicron triglycerides in humans. *Am. J. Clin. Nutr.* **1990**, *52*, 834–836. [CrossRef]
41. Dehghan, M.; Mente, A.; Zhang, X.; Swaminathan, S.; Li, W.; Mohan, V.; Iqbal, R.; Kumar, R.; Wentzel-Viljoen, E.; Rosengren, A.; et al. Associations of fats and carbohydrate intake with cardiovascular disease and mortality in 18 countries from five continents (PURE): A prospective cohort study. *Lancet* **2017**, *390*, 2050–2062. [CrossRef]
42. Ascherio, A.; Rimm, E.B.; Giovannucci, E.L.; Spiegelman, D.; Stampfer, M.; Willett, W.C. Dietary fat and risk of coronary heart disease in men: Cohort follow up study in the United States. *BMJ* **1996**, *313*, 84–90. [CrossRef]
43. Praagman, J.; de Jonge, E.A.; Kiefte-de Jong, J.C.; Beulens, J.W.; Sluijs, I.; Schoufour, J.D.; Hofman, A.; van der Schouw, Y.T.; Franco, O.H. Dietary Saturated Fatty Acids and Coronary Heart Disease Risk in a Dutch Middle-Aged and Elderly Population. *Arterioscler. Thromb. Vasc. Biol.* **2016**, *36*, 2011–2018. [CrossRef]
44. Seidelmann, S.B.; Claggett, B.; Cheng, S.; Henglin, M.; Shah, A.; Steffen, L.M.; Folsom, A.R.; Rimm, E.B.; Willett, W.C.; Solomon, S.D. Dietary carbohydrate intake and mortality: A prospective cohort study and meta-analysis. *Lancet Public Health* **2018**, *3*, 419–428. [CrossRef]
45. Ho, F.K.; Gray, S.R.; Welsh, P.; Petermann-Rocha, F.; Foster, H.; Waddell, H.; Anderson, J.; Lyall, D.; Sattar, N.; Gill, J.M. Associations of fat and carbohydrate intake with cardiovascular disease and mortality: Prospective cohort study of UK Biobank participants. *BMJ* **2020**, *368*. [CrossRef] [PubMed]
46. Mensink, R.P.; World Health Organization. *Effects of Saturated Fatty Acids on Serum Lipids and Lipoproteins: A Systematic Review and Regression Analysis*; World Health Organization: Geneva, Switzerland, 2016.
47. Khaw, K.T.; Sharp, S.J.; Finikarides, L.; Afzal, I.; Lentjes, M.; Luben, R.; Forouhi, N.G. Randomised trial of coconut oil, olive oil or butter on blood lipids and other cardiovascular risk factors in healthy men and women. *BMJ Open* **2018**, *8*, 020167. [CrossRef] [PubMed]
48. Cardoso, D.A.; Moreira, A.S.; de Oliveira, G.M.; Raggio Luiz, R.; Rosa, G. A Coconut extra virgin oil rich diet increases HDL cholesterol and decrease waist circumference and body mass in coronary artery disease patients. *Nutr. Hosp.* **2015**, *32*, 2144–2152. [CrossRef] [PubMed]
49. Feranil, A.B.; Duazo, P.L.; Kuzawa, C.W.; Adair, L.S. Coconut oil is associated with a beneficial lipid profile in pre-menopausal women in the Philippines. *Asia Pac. J. Clin. Nutr.* **2011**, *20*, 190–195. [PubMed]
50. Cox, C.; Mann, J.; Sutherland, W.; Chisholm, A.; Skeaff, M. Effects of coconut oil, butter, and safflower oil on lipids and lipoproteins in persons with moderately elevated cholesterol levels. *J. Lipid Res.* **1995**, *36*, 1787–1795. [CrossRef]
51. Neelakantan, N.; Seah, J.Y.H.; van Dam, R.M. The Effect of Coconut Oil Consumption on Cardiovascular Risk Factors: A Systematic Review and Meta-Analysis of Clinical Trials. *Circulation* **2020**, *141*, 803–814. [CrossRef]

52. Schwingshackl, L.; Bogensberger, B.; Benčič, A.; Knüppel, S.; Boeing, H.; Hoffmann, G. Effects of oils and solid fats on blood lipids: A systematic review and network meta-analysis. *J. Lipid Res.* **2018**, *59*, 1771–1782. [CrossRef]
53. Patterson, C. *World Alzheimer Report 2018: The State of the Art of Dementia Research: New Frontiers*; Alzheimer's Disease International (ADI): London, UK, 2018; pp. 32–36.
54. Baumgart, M.; Snyder, H.M.; Carrillo, M.C.; Fazio, S.; Kim, H.; Johns, H. Summary of the evidence on modifiable risk factors for cognitive decline and dementia: A population-based perspective. *Alzheimer's Dement.* **2015**, *11*, 718–726. [CrossRef]
55. Chatterjee, P.; Fernando, M.; Fernando, B.; Dias, C.B.; Shah, T.; Silva, R.; Williams, S.; Pedrini, S.; Hillebrandt, H.; Goozee, K.; et al. Potential of coconut oil and medium chain triglycerides in the prevention and treatment of Alzheimer's disease. *Mech. Ageing Dev.* **2020**, *186*, 111209. [CrossRef]
56. Newport, M. *What If There Was a Cure for Alzheimer's Disease and No One Knew?—A Case Study by Dr. Mary Newport*; Foundation for Alternative and Integrative Medicine: Loveland, CO, USA, 2008.
57. De la Rubia Ortí, J.E.; García-Pardo, M.P.; Drehmer, E.; Sancho Cantus, D.; Julián Rochina, M.; Aguilar, M.A.; Hu Yang, I. Improvement of main cognitive functions in patients with alzheimer's disease after treatment with coconut oil enriched mediterranean diet: A pilot study. *J. Alzheimer's Dis.* **2018**, *65*, 577–587. [CrossRef] [PubMed]
58. Doty, L. Coconut oil for Alzheimer's disease. *Clin. Pract.* **2012**, *1*, 12–17.
59. Taylor, M.K.; Sullivan, D.K.; Mahnken, J.D.; Burns, J.M.; Swerdlow, R.H. Feasibility and efficacy data from a ketogenic diet intervention in Alzheimer's disease. *Alzheimer's Dement. Transl. Res. Clin. Interv.* **2018**, *4*, 28–36. [CrossRef] [PubMed]
60. Krikorian, R.; Shidler, M.D.; Dangelo, K.; Couch, S.C.; Benoit, S.C.; Clegg, D.J. Dietary ketosis enhances memory in mild cognitive impairment. *Neurobiol. Aging* **2012**, *33*, 425.e19–425.e427. [CrossRef]
61. DebMandal, M.; Mandal, S. Coconut (*Cocos nucifera* L.: Arecaceae): In health promotion and disease prevention. *Asian Pac. J. Trop. Med.* **2011**, *4*, 241–247. [CrossRef]
62. Kabara, J.J. *The Pharmacological Effect of Lipids III: Role of Lipids in Cancer Research*; The American Oil Chemists Society: Urbana, IL, USA, 1989; Volume 3.
63. Oyi, A.; Onaolapo, J.; Obi, R. Formulation and antimicrobial studies of coconut (*Cocos nucifera* Linne) oil. *Res. J. Appl. Sci. Eng. Technol.* **2010**, *2*, 133–137.
64. Verma, V.; Bhardwaj, A.; Rathi, S.; Raja, R. A potential antimicrobial agent from Cocos nucifera mesocarp extract; Development of a new generation antibiotic. *Int. Res. J. Biol. Sci.* **2012**, *1*, 48–54.
65. Akinyele, T.A.; Okoh, O.O.; Akinpelu, D.A.; Okoh, A.I. In-vitro antibacterial properties of crude aqueous and n-hexane extracts of the husk of *Cocos nucifera*. *Molecules* **2011**, *16*, 2135–2145. [CrossRef]
66. Tangwatcharin, P.; Khopaibool, P. Activity of virgin coconut oil, lauric acid or monolaurin in combination with lactic acid against *Staphylococcus aureus*. *Southeast Asian J. Trop. Med. Public Health* **2012**, *43*, 969–985.
67. Shilling, M.; Matt, L.; Rubin, E.; Visitacion, M.P.; Haller, N.A.; Grey, S.F.; Woolverton, C.J. Antimicrobial effects of virgin coconut oil and its medium-chain fatty acids on *Clostridium difficile*. *J. Med. Food* **2013**, *16*, 1079–1085. [CrossRef]
68. Yassen, L.T.; Khelkal, I.N. Effect of some fatty acids on virulence factors of *Proteus mirabilis*. *Int. J. Adv. Biol. Res.* **2015**, *5*, 108–117.
69. Kohli, D.; Hugar, S.M.; Bhat, K.G.; Shah, P.P.; Mundada, M.V.; Badakar, C.M. Comparative evaluation of the antimicrobial susceptibility and cytotoxicity of husk extract of *Cocos nucifera* and chlorhexidine as irrigating solutions against *Enterococcus faecalis*, *Prevotella intermedia* and *Porphyromonas gingivalis*—An in-vitro study. *J. Indian Soc. Pedod. Prev. Dent.* **2018**, *36*, 142–150. [CrossRef] [PubMed]
70. Projan, S.J.; Brown-Skrobot, S.; Schlievert, P.M.; Vandenesch, F.; Novick, R.P. Glycerol monolaurate inhibits the production of beta-lactamase, toxic shock toxin-1, and other staphylococcal exoproteins by interfering with signal transduction. *J. Bacteriol.* **1994**, *176*, 4204–4209. [CrossRef] [PubMed]

3

Dietary Adherence of Saudi Males to the Saudi Dietary Guidelines and its Relation to Cardiovascular Diseases

Areej Ali Alkhaldy [1,*], Reem Saleh Alamri [1], Rozana Khalid Magadmi [1], Nrvana Yasser Elshini [1], Rania Abd El Hamid Hussein [1,2] and Kamal Waheeb Alghalayini [3]

1 Clinical Nutrition Department, Faculty of Applied Medical Sciences, King Abdulaziz University, P.O. Box 80215, Jeddah 21589, Saudi Arabia; reemsalamri@gmail.com (R.S.A.); rozana-magadmi@hotmail.com (R.K.M.); nrvanaalshini@gmail.com (N.Y.E.); rahussein2002@yahoo.com (R.A.E.H.H.)

2 Internal Medicine Department, Gamal Abd El Nasser Hospital, Health Insurance Authority, Alexandria 21516, Egypt

3 Department of Medicine, Faculty of Medicine, King Abdulaziz University, P.O. Box 80215, Jeddah 21589, Saudi Arabia; kalghalayini@kau.edu.sa

* Correspondence: aalkhaldy@kau.edu.sa

Abstract: Cardiovascular disease (CVD) is a major public health problem in Saudi Arabia. Dietary intake plays a major role in CVD incidence; however, the dietary intake status in Saudi nationals with CVD is unknown. We aimed to investigate whether the dietary patterns of Saudi males, using the Saudi dietary guidelines adherence score, in parallel with the measurement of a selective number of cardiovascular disease-related biomarkers, are contributing factors to CVD risk. Demographics, dietary adherence score, and blood biomarker levels were collected for 40 CVD patients and forty non-CVD patients. Fasting blood glucose ($p = 0.006$) and high-density lipoprotein levels ($p = 0.03$) were significantly higher in CVD patients. The adherence score to the Saudi dietary guidelines was not significantly different between the CVD and non-CVD patients; however, the specific adherence scores of fruit ($p = 0.02$), olive oil ($p = 0.01$), and non-alcoholic beer ($p = 0.02$) were significantly higher in the non-CVD patients. The differences in CVD family history ($p = 0.02$) and adherence scores to specific groups/foods between the CVD and non-CVD patients may contribute to CVD risk in Saudi males. However, as the sample size of this study was small, further research is required to validate these findings.

Keywords: dietary intake; nutrition; cardiovascular disease

1. Introduction

Cardiovascular disease (CVD) is considered a major public health problem in Saudi Arabia [1,2]. with an estimated 46% of all deaths attributed to CVD, and a 36% higher death rate in men compared to women [1]. The risk factors of CVD are characterized as modifiable factors such as diet, physical activity, obesity, and smoking, or non-modifiable factors such as aging, family history, and ethnicity [3–5]. The most important modifiable risk factor for CVD is diet [6–9]. Studies showed that a diet high in fruits, vegetables, whole grains as the major source of carbohydrates, and non-hydrogenated unsaturated fats as the main form of dietary fat, with adequate omega-3 fatty acids (monounsaturated fatty acid and polyunsaturated fatty acid), may reduce the risk of CVD [9–13]. Vitamins, minerals, fiber, and phenolic compounds are the main protective components found in fruit, vegetables, and whole grains with a functional role in reducing oxidative stress, inflammation, blood pressure, and improving insulin sensitivity and the lipoprotein profile [14–16]. In contrast, a diet containing a high intake of saturated fats, and refined and processed carbohydrates is linked with an increased CVD risk as a result of raised levels of blood glucose, total cholesterol, and low-density lipoprotein (LDL) cholesterol [17–22].

However, it is important to note that most of these nutritional studies evaluated the intake of a single nutrient, or small number of nutrients or food items in relation to risk of CVD. As individuals do not eat a single food or isolated nutrient, many researchers argued the importance of considering a holistic approach, investigating dietary patterns (combination of nutrients) rather than nutrient-based studies, when assessing health consequences [23–25]. Moreover, diet has a synergistic effect as it is a complex mixture of nutrients (within-food or across-food combinations), which could induce antagonistic effects on optimal health [23–25].

Dietary guidelines are a useful tool in public health policy, which can help reduce risk and prevent non-communicable diseases. Studies on dietary guideline adherence demonstrated their effectiveness in reducing the risk of disease, including CVD in multiple countries [24,26,27].

Current CVD research is dominated by studies that were conducted on Western populations with a paucity of research investigating the link between CVD and diet in Saudi Arabia [28,29]. Furthermore, to our knowledge no study used a holistic approach to consider the association of adherence to Saudi dietary guidelines with risk of CVD. We hypothesized that the non-adherence to the Saudi dietary guidelines could increase the risk of CVD in Saudi males.

2. Material and Methods

2.1. Study Design and Participants

A cross-sectional design study was performed at King Abdulaziz University Hospital (KAUH) in Jeddah, Saudi Arabia. Patients were recruited from the medical ward, surgical ward, and coronary care unit at KAUH. The inclusion criteria for CVD patients consisted of male cardiac patients, aged between 30–80 years old, as the prevalence of CVD among Saudi population increases after 30 years old [30]. The inclusion criteria for the non-CVD patients included male patients, in the same age range, who were free of CVD and had been admitted to the hospital for minor clinical conditions, including abdominal pain, eye surgery, and fever. Patients with liver, kidney, or respiratory disease, or any type of cancer diagnosis were excluded from recruitment to either group. Ethical approvals were obtained from the Faculty of Medicine Research Committee at King Abdulaziz University (Reference no. 307-14). All patients gave informed written consent.

2.2. The Saudi Dietary Guidelines

The message of the Saudi dietary guidelines is to follow a healthy diet including variety, balance, and moderation [31]. The main goals of these guidelines are (1) to improve health by promoting healthy eating options and encouraging physical activities; (2) to promote valuable food that high in nutrients such as foods rich in protein, fiber, vitamins, and minerals, and reduce foods of poor nutritional value such as foods high in salt, sugars, saturated fats, and hydrogenated fat; (3) to support the normal growth and development of infants, children, and adolescents; (4) to decrease the diseases related to diet in the Saudi community; and (5) to support physical activity.

To communicate the recommended food groups and serving sizes, the Saudi dietary guidelines are graphically represented in the form of a palm tree with the food groups distributed in the trunk and leaves of the palm in proportion to their recommended level of intake. The largest food group of bread and cereals was placed in the bottom big leaf of the palm and represents the most important source of carbohydrates (6–11 servings/day). Vegetables (3–5 servings/day) and fruits (2–4 servings/day) come next as they are high in vitamins and minerals. Milk and its products (2–4 servings/day) are the third largest group, which are essential sources of protein and calcium. The smallest group constitutes meat and beans (2–4 servings/day), and they are considered as sources of protein. Fat and sugar were in the smallest upper leaves of the palm (representing lower quantities); this shows the need to minimize their intake. Water was also added to the healthy food palm, due to the hot weather of

Saudi Arabia. As regular physical activity is essential, together with a balanced diet, the healthy food palm also recommends individuals to exercise for 30–60 min daily according to the individual's health status [31].

2.3. The Saudi Dietary Guideline Score

The score of adherence was given according to the Saudi dietary guidelines [31]. The ratings of the consumption of each food group (from 0 to 5 or the reverse) was adapted from Panagiotakos et al. (2006) [24]. The dietary adherence score included non-refined cereals and bread (whole bread, rice, pasta, and other grains), fruit, vegetables, legumes, fish, olive oil, non-alcoholic beer, meat and meat products, poultry, full-fat dairy products, sweets, and oils.

For the intake of food items assumed to be close to the Saudi dietary guidelines or higher (non-refined cereals, fruits, vegetables), we allocated a score of 0 when the individual stated no consumption, a score of 1 when they stated consumption of 1–4 servings/month, a score of 2 for 5–8 servings/month, a score of 3 for 9–12 servings/month, a score of 4 for 13–18 servings/month, and a score of 5 for more than 18 servings/month. Moreover, we included legumes, fish, and olive oil in this group after separating them from the meat and oil groups. Originally excluded from the Saudi guidelines, non-alcoholic beer was also added due to its health benefits for heart disease [32]. In contrast, for the intake of food items assumed to be limited in Saudi dietary guidelines (i.e., rare or monthly intake; meat and meat products, poultry, and full-fat dairy products), we allocated the scores on a reverse scale (i.e., 5, when individuals stated no intake, to 0, when they stated almost daily intake). Hence, the scores ranged from 0 to 60. Higher values of score show better adherence to the Saudi dietary guidelines (Table 1).

Table 1. The Saudi dietary guideline score.

No.	Food Groups	Frequency of Consumption (Servings/Month)					
		Never	1–4	5–8	9–12	13–18	>18
1	Non-refined cereals and bread [a]	0	1	2	3	4	5
2	Fruit [b]	0	1	2	3	4	5
3	Vegetable	0	1	2	3	4	5
4	Legumes	0	1	2	3	4	5
5	Fish	0	1	2	3	4	5
6	Olive oil	0	1	2	3	4	5
7	Non-alcoholic beer	0	1	2	3	4	5
8	Meat and meat products	5	4	3	2	1	0
9	Poultry	5	4	3	2	1	0
10	Full-fat dairy products	5	4	3	2	1	0
11	Sweets	5	4	3	2	1	0
12	Oils	5	4	3	2	1	0

[a] Whole-grain bread, rice, pasta etc. [b] Fresh (e.g., apple, oranges, banana, grapes, etc.) and dried fruit, including dates.

2.4. Procedure and Data Collection

An interview-administered survey consisting of four sections (demographics, anthropometrics, medical history, and a dietary assessment by food frequency questionnaire (FFQ)) was completed for each patient.

2.5. Demographics and Medical History

Personal information, including date of birth, gender, marital status, any medical diagnoses, and family history of cardiovascular diseases (whether at least one first-degree relative had CVD) was collected from the hospital electronic system at KAUH. Data regarding the education level, employment status, and tobacco use was collected during the interview process.

2.6. Anthropometric Measurements

The anthropometric measurements, including height, weight, waist circumference (WC), and body mass index (BMI) were performed according to standard procedures and carried out in the patient's ward. Patients were weighed in light clothing, without shoes, using a calibrated scale to the nearest 0.1 kg measured in kilograms. Height was measured to the nearest 0.1 cm. The BMI was computed as the fraction of weight to the squared height, with consideration for the cut-off for older adults (65 years old and older). The WC was taken at the level of the narrowest point between the lowest costal border and the iliac crest by the research team.

2.7. Estimation of Habitual Dietary Intake

The dietary intake was assessed using a 60-item food frequency questionnaire (FFQ). For each food item, patients were asked how frequently it was consumed during the last year on a daily, weekly, or monthly basis, along with the portion sizes. Food intake was grouped into food groups (milk and dairy products, fruits, vegetables, meats, rice, breads, beverages, legumes, and sweets). The average servings of each item consumed per week were calculated using Microsoft Excel version 1808 (Redmond, WA, USA).

2.8. Assessment of Blood Variables

Blood data were collected from the patients' records for the lipid profile (high-density lipoprotein (HDL), low-density lipoprotein (HDL), total cholesterol (TC), and triglycerides (TG)); blood glucose (fasting blood glucose (FBG) and glycated hemoglobin (HbA1c)); hemoglobin (HGB) and hematocrit (HCT); cardiac enzymes (aspartate aminotransferase (AST), creatine kinase (CK), lactate dehydrogenase (LDH), and cardiac troponin I (CTN-I)); and electrolytes (sodium (Na), potassium (K), and chloride (Cl)), according to the hospital policy.

2.9. Sample Size Calculation

This is a preliminary study to identify factors of interest and to develop a study protocol for a larger-scale study. No power calculation was conducted in this study due to the absence in Saudi literature of endpoints similar to the hypothesis proposed in this study. The data of this study serve as preliminary data to determine the needed sample size to achieve the aim of the study. We aimed to include 80 patients (40 with CVD and 40 without CVD disease).

2.10. Statistical Analysis

The statistical analysis was carried out using SPSS (version 23, SPSS, Inc, Chicago, IL, USA, 2015). A normality test was run on all data to determine if each dataset was well modeled by a normal distribution. Descriptive statistics are presented as medians and inter-quartile ranges (IQRs).

Linear regression models were performed using the diet score as an independent variable, with age, smoking history, educational level, diabetic history, and family history of CVD as covariates. Systolic blood pressure, serum total cholesterol, LDL, HDL, triglycerides, waist circumference, and body mass index were utilized as outcome variables. The results were presented as *b*-coefficients and standard error of the coefficient. Bonferroni correction was used due to multiple comparisons.

In addition, comparisons between the non-CVD patients and CVD patients were performed using a Mann–Whitney test for non-normally distributed data, and by paired *t*-test or two-sample *t*-test for normally distributed data. A chi-square test was used to compare the employment status and education level between the groups.

3. Results

3.1. Subject Characteristics

Eighty male patients were recruited for the study, aged between 30 and 80 years old. The demographic data for all individuals are presented in Table 2. There were no significant differences between non-CVD and CVD patients in terms of their age, education, or employment. However, there was a difference between non-CVD and CVD patients in terms of their family history, with significantly more CVD patients having at least one first-degree relative with CVD ($p = 0.02$; Table 3). The anthropometric characteristics, including blood pressure, weight, and BMI, were not significantly different between non-CVD and CVD patients (Table 4). The median BMI for both non-CVD and CVD patients was within the overweight cut-off range, with a value of 27.2 kg/m^2 (IQR 23.4–31.1) for the non-CVD patients and 25.7 kg/m^2 (IQR 23.4–27.7) for the CVD patients. The median waist circumference was within the normal range (< 102 cm) for both non-CVD (95.0 cm; IQR 85.8–100.0) and CVD patients (94.0 cm; IQR 90.0–98.3).

Table 2. Demographic data of the study participants.

Demographic Variable		All Patients (n = 80)		Non-CVD Patients (n = 40)		CVD Patients (n = 40)		p-Value *
		n	%	n	%	n	%	
Age (years)	30–55	36.0	45.0	21.0	52.5	15.0	37.5	0.09
	56–80	44.0	55.0	19.0	47.5	25.0	62.5	
Marital Status	Married	73.0	91.3	34.0	85.0	39.0	97.5	0.05
	Single	7.0	8.8	6.0	15.0	1.0	2.5	
Education	None	6.0	7.5	1.0	2.5	5.0	12.5	0.13
	Elementary	12.0	15.0	7.0	17.5	5.0	12.5	
	Intermediate	8.0	10.0	2.0	5.0	6.0	15.0	
	High School	32.0	40.0	20.0	50.0	12.0	30.0	
	University	22.0	27.5	10.0	25.0	12.0	30.0	
Employment	Employed	34.0	42.5	13.0	32.5	21.0	52.5	0.07
	Non-Employed	46.0	57.5	27.0	67.5	19.0	47.5	

n: number of patients; CVD: cardiovascular disease. * p-value between non-CVD and CVD patients.

Table 3. Family and smoking history of the study participants.

Variables		All Patients (n = 80)		Non-CVD Patients (n = 40)		CVD Patients (n = 40)		p-Value *
		n	%	n	%	n	%	
Family History	Negative	54.0	67.5	32.0	80.0	22.0	55.0	0.02
	Positive	26.0	32.5	8.0	20.0	18.0	45.0	
Diabetic	Yes	36.0	45.0	9	22.5	27	67.5	0.06
	No	44.0	55.0	31	77.5	13	32.5	
Smoking	Never	29.0	36.3	18.0	45.0	11.0	27.5	0.2
	Former >3 years	28.0	35.0	11.0	27.5	17.0	42.5	
	Former <3 years	7.0	8.8	2.0	5.0	5.0	12.5	
	Current	16.0	20.0	9.0	22.5	7.0	17.5	

n: number of patients; CVD: cardiovascular disease. * p-value between non-CVD and CVD patients.

Table 4. Anthropometric measurements of the study participants.

Variables	All Patients		Non-CVD Patients		CVD Patients		p-Value *
	Median	IQR	Median	IQR	Median	IQR	
Height (cm)	168.0 (n = 80)	160.0–172.2	165.0 (n = 40)	160.0–170.8	170.0 (n = 40)	160.0–170.8	0.6
Weight (kg)	70.0 (n = 80)	68.0–84.0	75.0 (n = 40)	67.5–86.0	70.0 (n = 40)	68.8–80.0	0.4
BMI (kg/m^2)	26.6 (n = 80)	23.4–29.4	27.2 (n = 40)	23.4–31.1	25.7 (n = 40)	23.4–27.7	0.3
WC (cm)	94.5 (n = 80)	88.2–99.7	95.0 (n = 40)	85.8–100.0	94.0 (n = 40)	90.0–98.3	0.5
Systolic BP	128.0 (n = 45)	117.5–140.0	128.0 (n = 26)	120.0–139.3	131.0 (n = 19)	119.5–142.0	0.1
Diastolic BP	76.0 (n = 45)	70.0–85.5	81.7 (n = 26)	75.0–87.8	70.0 (n = 19)	64.0–78.5	0.03
	n	%	n	%	n	%	
Underweight	7.0	8.8	2.0	5.0	5.0	12.5	
Normal weight	36.0	45.0	17.0	42.5	19.0	47.5	
Overweight	26.0	32.5	13.0	32.5	13.0	32.5	
Obese	11.0	13.8	8.0	20.0	3.0	7.5	

n: number of patients; CVD: cardiovascular disease; BMI: body mass index; BP: blood pressure; WC: waist circumference. * *p*-value between non-CVD and CVD patients.

3.2. Habitual Dietary Intake

The score of total adherence to the Saudi dietary guidelines was not significantly different between the non-CVD and CVD patients (Table 5); however, there were differences in adherence to dietary intake of some individual food groups. The specific adherence scores of fruit ($p = 0.02$), olive oil ($p = 0.01$), and non-alcoholic beer ($p = 0.02$) groups were significantly higher in the non-CVD patients (Table 5).

Table 5. The score of the adherence to the Saudi dietary guidelines.

	All Patients ($n = 80$)		Non-CVD Patients ($n = 40$)		CVD Patients ($n = 40$)		*p*-Value *
	Mean	SD	Mean	SD	Mean	SD	
Non-refined cereals and bread	1.2	2.1	1.5	2.3	1.0	1.9	0.29
Fruit	4.9	0.4	5.0	0.0	4.8	0.5	0.02
Vegetable	4.9	0.5	5.0	0.0	4.9	0.7	0.15
Legumes	3.6	1.6	3.6	1.6	3.6	1.7	0.98
Fish	2.8	1.6	2.7	1.6	3.0	1.5	0.37
Olive oil	2.7	2.1	3.2	2.1	2.1	2.0	0.01
Non-alcoholic beer	0.8	1.5	1.3	1.8	0.4	0.9	0.01
Meat and meat products	1.5	1.4	1.5	1.4	1.5	1.5	0.93
Poultry	1.5	1.6	1.2	1.5	1.8	1.6	0.06
Full-fat dairy products	0.1	0.6	0.1	0.3	0.2	0.7	0.17
Sweets	2.5	2.1	2.4	2.2	2.7	2.1	0.76
Oils	0.7	1.7	0.7	1.8	0.7	1.7	0.80
Total adherence to Saudi dietary guidelines	27.3	6.0	28.1	6.6	26.5	5.4	0.23

CVD: cardiovascular disease. * *p*-value between non-CVD and CVD patients.

Moreover, we evaluated the effect of the Saudi diet on various health outcomes such as systolic blood pressure, serum cholesterol, low-density lipoprotein, high-density lipoprotein, triglycerides, waist circumference, and body mass index. Table 6 shows the results of multiple linear regression after adjusting for age, smoking history, educational level, diabetic history, and family history of CVD. There were only significant associations found between the total adherence to Saudi dietary guideline score and serum total cholesterol and LDL.

Table 6. The association between different clinical and anthropometric factors (dependent) and total adherence to Saudi dietary guideline score (independent). Results of multiple linear regression analysis.

	β-Coefficient $\pm$ SE	*p*-Value
Model 1: Systolic blood pressure	-0.284 ± 0.508	0.579
Model 2: Serum cholesterol	-0.071 ± 0.023	0.004
Model 3: Low-density lipoprotein	-0.072 ± 0.028	0.012
Model 4: High-density lipoprotein	-0.021 ± 0.011	0.074
Model 5: Triglycerides	-0.032 ± 0.018	0.077
Model 6: Waist circumference	-0.308 ± 0.229	0.183
Model 7: Body mass index	-0.087 ± 0.102	0.399

All models were adjusted for age, smoking history, educational level, diabetic history, and family history of CVD. SE: Standard error.

3.3. Blood Variables

There were no significant differences in the lipid profile measurements of total cholesterol, triglycerides, or LDL between the non-CVD and CVD patients (Table 7). However, the HDL was significantly higher in the CVD patients compared to the non-CVD patients ($p = 0.03$). The HDL was 1.1 mmol/L (IQR 1.0–1.5) in the CVD patients and 1.0 mmol/L (IQR 0.6–1.1) in the non-CVD patients. There was no difference in hematological profile, with the exception of the median fasting blood glucose level, which was raised in all patients (normal range <5.6 mmol/L), but significantly higher ($p = 0.006$) in the CVD patients (7.5 mmol/L; IQR 6.2–11.7) than the non-CVD patients (6.1 mmol/L; IQR 5.1–7.2). In terms of the electrolyte and cardiac enzyme levels (Table 7), all biomarkers were non-significant between the non-CVD and CVD patients, with the exception of the potassium level ($p = 0.03$), which was within normal range (3.6–5.2 mmol/L) for all patients, but significantly higher in the CVD patients 4.1 mmol/L (IQR 3.5–4.4) than the non-CVD patients 3.7 mmol/L (IQR 3.5–4.0). In contrast, the chloride level was also within the normal range for all patients (98–106 mmol/L) but significantly lower ($p = 0.05$) in the CVD patients (99.0 mmol/L; IQR 94.8–102.0) compared to the non-CVD patients (101.0 mmol/L; IQR 98.0–104.0).

Table 7. Cardiovascular-related biomarkers.

Biomarkers	All patients		Non-CVD Patients		CVD Patients		*p*-Value *
	Median	**IQR**	**Median**	**IQR**	**Median**	**IQR**	
Lipids							
TC (mmol/L)	4.0 (n = 80)	3.0–4.6	4.0 (n = 40)	3.4–4.6	3.7 (n = 40)	3.0–4.6	0.7
TG (mmol/L)	1.3 (n = 80)	0.8–1.7	1.3 (n = 40)	0.8–1.9	1.2 (n = 40)	0.9–1.6	0.5
LDL (mmol/L)	2.7 (n = 46)	1.9–3.4	3.0 (n = 18)	2.3-3.6	2.6 (n = 28)	1.9-3.2	0.2
HDL (mmol/L)	1.1 (n = 42)	0.8–1.3	1.0 (n = 17)	0.6–1.1	1.1 (n = 25)	1.0–1.5	0.03
Hematological							
FBG (mmol/L)	6.5 (n = 80)	5.5–9.6	6.1 (n = 40)	5.1–7.2	7.5 (n = 40)	6.2–11.7	0.006
HbA1c (mmol/L)	7.4 (n = 80)	5.8–8.9	6.3 (n = 40)	5.4–7.4	8.2 (n = 40)	6.1–9.0	0.1
HGB (g/dl)	12.0 (n = 80)	10.0–13.6	12.3 (n = 40)	9.0–14.0	12.0 (n = 40)	10.3–13.1	0.7
HCT (%)	35.4 (n = 80)	30.1–40.5	36.5 (n = 40)	27.5–41.0	35.2 (n = 40)	31.8–39.3	0.8
Electrolytes							
Na (mmol/L)	137.0 (n = 80)	134.0–139.0	138.0 (n = 40)	135.0–140.0	137.0 (n = 40)	131.0–139.0	0.9
K (mmol/L)	3.9 (n = 80)	3.5–4.2	3.7 (n = 40)	3.5–4.0	4.1 (n = 40)	3.5–4.4	0.03
Cl (mmol/L)	99.5 (n = 80)	97.0–103.0	101.0 (n = 40)	98.0–104.0	99.0 (n = 40)	94.8–102.0	0.05
Cardiac Enzymes							
AST (U/L)	27.0 (n = 69)	19.0–41.3	26.0 (n = 29)	19.0–45.0	28.5 (n = 40)	19.0–40.5	0.12
CK (IU/L)	109.0 (n = 52)	52.0–214.0	95.5 (n = 12)	49.5–171.8	116.0 (n = 40)	63.0–249.0	0.4
LDH (U/L)	244.5 (n = 51)	191.8–304.0	215.0 (n = 11)	176.5–250.0	255.0 (n = 40)	212.0–310.0	0.1
CTN–I (ug/L)	0.1 (n = 49)	0.0–0.6	0.1 (n = 09)	0.0–0.3	0.1 (n = 40)	0.0–0.6	0.4

TC = total cholesterol; TG = triglycerides; LDL = low-density lipoprotein; HDL = high-density lipoprotein; FBG = fasting blood glucose; HbA1 = glycated hemoglobin; HGB = hemoglobin; HCT = hematocrit; Na = sodium; K = potassium; Cl = chloride; AST = aspartate aminotransferase; CK = creatine kinase; LDH = lactate dehydrogenase; CTN-I = cardiac troponin I. * *p*-value between non-CVD and CVD patients.

4. Discussion

This study was performed to test the hypothesis that the dietary patterns of Saudis may play a role in increasing the risk of CVD. To our knowledge, this is the first study that assesses the dietary intake using the adherence score to the Saudi dietary guidelines and its relationship to CVD in Saudi males living in Jeddah. As such, the data obtained from this study may be considered an important preliminary step in gaining an increased understanding of variables in the Saudi population that may affect their risk of CVD.

This study found a number of significant differences between the non-CVD and CVD patients that align with previously published studies. Firstly, the present study found that a family history of CVD was significantly higher in the CVD patients. This indicates the strong effect of genetics as a factor that could increase the risk of CVD. Studies showed that a family history is associated with an increase in CVD mortality across long-term follow-up [33].

Secondly, the evaluation of dietary habits using the adherence score to the Saudi dietary guidelines revealed that fruit, olive oil, and non-alcoholic beer were more highly consumed in the non-CVD patients than in the CVD patients. These food items are rich in polyphenols and dietary fiber, nutrients for which high levels of intake were previously associated with a decreased risk of developing CVD [34]. Moreover, we found that the consumption of non-refined cereals and breads was particularly low relative to recommendation. The high intake of refined carbohydrate is reported to increase the risk of type 2 diabetes and CVD [35]. The Saudi dietary guidelines are well publicized; however, more effort may be needed on education and promotion of the guidelines to reduce the risk of diseases including CVD.

Olive oil is the main source of fat in the Mediterranean diet and is linked with a lower mortality for CVD [18]. An olive-oil-rich diet is associated with enhanced lipoprotein metabolism and a reduction in oxidative damage, inflammation, blood pressure, endothelial dysfunction, and thrombosis [36]. A study by Guasch-Ferre et al, demonstrated that olive-oil intake, in particular the extra-virgin variety, decreased the risk of mortality and cardiovascular disease for individuals from Spain who were at high CVD risk [37]. Furthermore, a study by Carnevale et al. reported that olive oil advanced the post-prandial glucose and lipid profile in patients with impaired fasting glucose [38].

A study carried out by Woodside et al. found a strong correlation between the intake of fruits and vegetables and a reduction in the risk of developing coronary heart disease (CHD) [22]. Vegetables and fruits are a good source of nutrients, including vitamins, minerals, dietary fiber, and other biologically active compounds. These compounds have important mechanisms of action, including enhancing the immune system, reducing platelet aggregation, modulating cholesterol synthesis, reduction of blood pressure, and antioxidant, antibacterial, and antiviral effects [39].

The higher non-alcoholic beer consumption among the non-CVD patients may indicate that non-alcoholic beer could have a positive effect on heart health. It was reported that non-alcoholic beer can inhibit blood coagulation and platelet activation, which benefits the cardiovascular system without the negative effects of alcohol [32]. Despite the differences between non-CVD and CVD patients in their dietary habits, the lipid profile biomarkers, including total cholesterol, triglycerides, and LDL, were not significantly different. This is in contrast with the reported study by Rossouw, who showed that cholesterol levels are correlated with the risk of CHD, even at "normal" levels of cholesterol, in both men and women of all ages [40]. In addition, unpredictably, the levels of HDL were significantly higher in the CVD patients. The reason underlying this association is unknown, but one plausible explanation could be due to medications that were prescribed to CVD patients to control blood pressure, hyperlipidemia, and cardiac disease. These types of medications, such as niacin and atorvastatin, are known to enhance the lipid profile, and they were reported to increase HDL [41]. The current study also did not detect any significant differences between the non-CVD and CVD patients in the anthropometric measurements of weight, waist circumference, and BMI. This is in contrast with Alissa et al., who reported a strong significant relationship between BMI and the CVD risk in Saudi participants [29]. The inconsistency between these results could be due to differences in the sample size, which was smaller in this preliminary study. This study is the first to assess the adherence to the Saudi dietary guidelines among CVD male patients in Saudi Arabia. Currently, there is no validated food frequency questionnaire available specifically for the Saudi population; therefore, in this study, efforts were made to include food items that are more representative of the typical components of the Saudi diet. Furthermore, the analysis of adherence to the Saudi dietary guidelines was performed in parallel with the collection of blood biomarkers. As such, the data generated by this pilot study offer a unique insight into Saudi CVD populations, which may help in the planning and design of future studies to validate these findings. Further studies are now recommended to assess the association between the adherence to the Saudi dietary guidelines and the risk of CVD on a larger population sample. Moreover, as not all biomarker data of all for our patients were found in the patients' electronic system, the sample size calculation for future studies needs to consider the missing biomarker data of patients in the hospital electronic records when determining the power of their studies to allow for examining a more complete dataset of biomarkers.

5. Conclusions

The data from this preliminary study report a number of significant differences between non-CVD and CVD patients in terms of intake of particular food groups and CVD family history. These factors could be important contributors to the CVD risk in the Saudi population. Further research is now needed, using a larger sample size, in order to validate these findings and increase insight into the risk factors of the Saudi lifestyle that are associated with CVD.

Author Contributions: All authors made substantial contributions to the conception and study design. R.S.A, R.K.M, N.Y.E, and K.W.A carried out the data collation. A.A.A, R.S.A, R.K.M, and N.Y.E performed data analysis. R.S.A, R.K.M, and N.Y.E prepared the first draft of the manuscript. A.A.A, R.A.E.H.H, and K.W.A reviewed and edited the manuscript. All authors approved the final version of the manuscript.

Acknowledgments: We would like to thank all our participants for their time and contribution in this study.

References

1. World Health Organization. Global Health Observatory: Cardiovascular Diseases-Country Statistics. Available online: https://www.who.int/cardiovascular_diseases/en/ (accessed on 04 August 2018).
2. Ahmed, A.M.; Hersi, A.; Mashhoud, W.; Arafah, M.R.; Abreu, P.C.; Al Rowaily, M.A.; Al-Mallah, M.H. Cardiovascular risk factors burden in Saudi Arabia: The Africa Middle East Cardiovascular Epidemiological (ACE) study. *J. Saudi Heart Assoc.* **2017**, *29*, 235–243. [CrossRef]
3. Petersen, S.E.; Sanghvi, M.M.; Aung, N.; Cooper, J.A.; Paiva, J.M.; Zemrak, F.; Fung, K.; Lukaschuk, E.; Lee, A.M.; Carapella, V.; et al. The impact of cardiovascular risk factors on cardiac structure and function: Insights from the UK Biobank imaging enhancement study. *PLoS ONE* **2017**, *12*, e0185114. [CrossRef]
4. Stamler, J.; Vaccaro, O.; Neaton, J.D.; Wentworth, D. Diabetes, other Risk-Factors, and 12-Yr Cardiovascular Mortality For Men Screened in The Multiple Risk Factor Intervention Trial. *Diabetes Care* **1993**, *16*, 434–444. [CrossRef] [PubMed]
5. Wong, N.D. Epidemiological studies of CHD and the evolution of preventive cardiology. *Nat. Rev. Cardiol.* **2014**, *11*, 276–289. [CrossRef]
6. Yusuf, S.; Hawken, S.; Ounpuu, S. Effect of potentially modifiable risk factors associated with myocardial infarction in 52 countries (the INTERHEART study): Case-control study. *Lancet* **2004**, *364*, 937–952. [CrossRef]
7. Hu, F.B.; Willett, W.C. Optimal diets for prevention of coronary heart disease. *JAMA* **2002**, *288*, 2569–2578. [CrossRef] [PubMed]
8. Hu, F. Optimal diet and lifestyle for prevention of coronary heart disease. *Atheroscler. Suppl.* **2003**, *4*, 6. [CrossRef]
9. Waskiewicz, A.; Szczesniewska, D.; Szostak-Wegierek, D.; Kwasniewska, M.; Pajak, A.; Stepaniak, U.; Kozakiewicz, K.; Tykarski, A.; Zdrojewski, T.; Zujko, M.E.; et al. Are dietary habits of the Polish population consistent with the recommendations for prevention of cardiovascular disease?—WOBASZ II project. *Kardiol. Pol.* **2016**, *74*, 969–977.
10. Panagiotakos, D.B.; Notara, V.; Kouvari, M.; Pitsavos, C. The Mediterranean and other Dietary Patterns in Secondary Cardiovascular Disease Prevention: A Review. *Curr. Vasc. Pharmacol.* **2016**, *14*, 442–451. [CrossRef] [PubMed]
11. Mahmood, D.; Jahan, K.; Habibullah, K. Primary prevention with statins in cardiovascular diseases: A Saudi Arabian perspective. *J. Saudi Heart Assoc.* **2015**, *27*, 179–191. [CrossRef] [PubMed]
12. Aljefree, N.; Ahmed, F. Association between dietary pattern and risk of cardiovascular disease among adults in the Middle East and North Africa region: A systematic review. *Food Nutr. Res.* **2015**, *59*, 27486. [CrossRef] [PubMed]
13. Vasilopoulou, A.; Galitsianos, I.; Fotiou, M.; Menexes, G.; Tsakoumaki, F.; Tsitlakidou, P.; Psirropoulos, D.; Michaelidou, A.M. An exploratory study of dietary intake patterns among adults diagnosed with cardiovascular risk factors. *Int. J. Food Sci. Nutr.* **2015**, *66*, 458–465. [CrossRef]
14. Conrad, Z.; Raatz, S.; Jahns, L. Greater vegetable variety and amount are associated with lower prevalence of coronary heart disease: National Health and Nutrition Examination Survey, 1999–2014. *Nutr. J.* **2018**, *17*, 67. [CrossRef]
15. Li, B.R.; Li, F.; Wang, L.F.; Zhang, D.F. Fruit and Vegetables Consumption and Risk of Hypertension: A Meta-Analysis. *J. Clin. Hypertens.* **2016**, *18*, 468–476. [CrossRef] [PubMed]
16. Aune, D.; Giovannucci, E.; Boffetta, P.; Fadnes, L.T.; Keum, N.; Norat, T.; Greenwood, D.C.; Riboli, E.; Vatten, L.J.; Tonstad, S. Fruit and vegetable intake and the risk of cardiovascular disease, total cancer and all-cause mortality-a systematic review and dose-response meta-analysis of prospective studies. *Int. J. Epidemiol.* **2017**, *46*, 1029–1056. [CrossRef] [PubMed]

17. Wang, X.; Ouyang, Y.; Liu, J.; Zhu, M.; Zhao, G.; Bao, W.; Hu, F.B. Fruit and vegetable consumption and mortality from all causes, cardiovascular disease, and cancer: Systematic review and dose-response meta-analysis of prospective cohort studies. *BMJ (Clin. Res. Ed.)* **2014**, *349*, g4490. [CrossRef] [PubMed]
18. Estruch, R.; Ros, E.; Salas-Salvado, J.; Covas, M.I.; Corella, D.; Aros, F.; Gomez-Gracia, E.; Ruiz-Gutierrez, V.; Fiol, M.; Lapetra, J.; et al. Primary Prevention of Cardiovascular Disease with a Mediterranean Diet Supplemented with Extra-Virgin Olive Oil or Nuts. *N. Engl. J. Med.* **2018**, *378*, e34. [CrossRef]
19. Menezes, R.; Rodriguez-Mateos, A.; Kaltsatou, A.; González-Sarrías, A.; Greyling, A.; Giannaki, C.; Andres-Lacueva, C.; Milenkovic, D.; Gibney, E.R.; Dumont, J.; et al. Impact of Flavonols on Cardiometabolic Biomarkers: A MetaAnalysis of Randomized Controlled Human Trials to Explore the Role of Inter-Individual Variability. *Nutrients* **2017**, *9*, 117. [CrossRef]
20. Trinity, J.D.; Pahnke, M.D.; Trombold, J.R.; Coyle, E.F. Impact of Polyphenol Antioxidants on Cycling Performance and Cardiovascular Function. *Nutrients* **2014**, *6*, 1273–1292. [CrossRef]
21. Zamora-Ros, R.; Knaze, V.; Lujan-Barroso, L.; Romieu, I.; Scalbert, A.; Slimani, N.; Hjartaker, A.; Engeset, D.; Skeie, G.; Overvad, K.; et al. Differences in dietary intakes, food sources and determinants of total flavonoids between Mediterranean and non-Mediterranean countries participating in the European Prospective Investigation into Cancer and Nutrition (EPIC) study. *Br. J. Nutr.* **2013**, *109*, 1498–1507. [CrossRef]
22. Woodside, J.; Young, I.S.; McKinley, M.C. Fruit and vegetable intake and risk of cardiovascular disease. *Proc. Nutr. Soc.* **2013**, *72*, 399–406. [CrossRef] [PubMed]
23. Tapsell, L.C.; Neale, E.P.; Satija, A.; Hu, F.B. Foods, Nutrients, and Dietary Patterns: Interconnections and Implications for Dietary Guidelines. *Adv. Nutr.* **2016**, *7*, 445–454. [CrossRef] [PubMed]
24. Panagiotakos, D.B.; Pitsavos, C.; Stefanadis, C. Dietary patterns: A Mediterranean diet score and its relation to clinical and biological markers of cardiovascular disease risk. *Nutr. Metab. Cardiovasc. Dis.* **2006**, *16*, 559–568. [CrossRef] [PubMed]
25. Martinez-Gonzalez, M.A.; Sanchez-Villegas, A. The emerging role of Mediterranean diets in cardiovascular epidemiology: Monounsaturated fats, olive oil, red wine or the whole pattern? *Eur. J. Epidemiol.* **2004**, *19*, 9–13. [CrossRef]
26. Reedy, J.; Krebs-Smith, S.M.; Miller, P.E.; Liese, A.D.; Kahle, L.L.; Park, Y.; Subar, A.F. Higher Diet Quality Is Associated with Decreased Risk of All-Cause, Cardiovascular Disease, and Cancer Mortality among Older Adults. *J. Nutr.* **2014**, *144*, 881–889. [CrossRef] [PubMed]
27. Russell, J.; Flood, V.; Rochtchina, E.; Gopinath, B.; Allman-Farinelli, M.; Bauman, A.; Mitchell, P. Adherence to dietary guidelines and 15-year risk of all-cause mortality. *Br. J. Nutr.* **2013**, *109*, 547–555. [CrossRef] [PubMed]
28. Alissa, E.M.; Bahjri, S.M.; Al-Ama, N.; Ahmed, W.H.; Starkey, B.; Ferns, G.A.A. Dietary vitamin A may be a cardiovascular risk factor in a Saudi population. *Asia Pac. J. Clin. Nutr.* **2005**, *14*, 137–144. [PubMed]
29. Eman, A.; Nabeel, A. Nutritional Intake and Cardiovascular Risk Factors in Saudi Subjects with Different Degrees of Atherosclerosis: A Case Control Study. *J. Nutr. Med. Diet. Care* **2015**, *1*, 008.
30. Rahman Al-Nuaim, A. High prevalence of metabolic risk factors for cardiovascular diseases among Saudi population, aged 30–64 years. *Int. J. Cardiol.* **1997**, *62*, 227–235. [CrossRef]
31. Ministry of Health. The Dietary Guidelines for Saudis. Available online: https://www.moh.gov.sa/en/HealthAwareness/Pages/SaudihealthFoodGuide.aspx (accessed on 16 March 2019).
32. Bassus, S.; Mahnel, R.; Scholz, T.; Wegert, W.; Westrup, D.; Kirchmaier, C.M. Effect of dealcoholized beer (Bitburger Drive) consumption on hemostasis in humans. *Alcohol. Clin. Exp. Res.* **2004**, *28*, 786–791. [CrossRef] [PubMed]
33. Bachmann, J.M.; Willis, B.L.; Ayers, C.R.; Khera, A.; Berry, J.D. Association Between Family History and Coronary Heart Disease Death Across Long-Term Follow-Up in Men The Cooper Center Longitudinal Study. *Circulation* **2012**, *125*, 3092–3098. [CrossRef] [PubMed]
34. Michalska, M.; Gluba, A.; Mikhailidis, D.P.; Nowak, P.; Bielecka-Dabrowa, A.; Rysz, J.; Banach, M. The role of polyphenols in cardiovascular disease. *Med. Sci. Monit.* **2010**, *16*, Ra110–Ra119. [PubMed]
35. Liu, S. Intake of refined carbohydrates and whole grain foods in relation to risk of type 2 diabetes mellitus and coronary heart disease. *J. Am. Coll. Nutr.* **2002**, *21*, 298–306. [CrossRef]
36. Covas, M.-I. Olive oil and the cardiovascular system. *Pharmacol. Res.* **2007**, *55*, 175–186. [CrossRef] [PubMed]

37. Guasch-Ferre, M.; Hu, F.B.; Martinez-Gonzalez, M.A.; Fito, M.; Bullo, M.; Estruch, R.; Ros, E.; Corella, D.; Recondo, J.; Gomez-Gracia, E.; et al. Olive oil intake and risk of cardiovascular disease and mortality in the PREDIMED Study. *BMC Med.* **2014**, *12*, 78. [CrossRef] [PubMed]
38. Carnevale, R.; Loffredo, L.; Del Ben, M.; Angelico, F.; Nocella, C.; Petruccioli, A.; Bartimoccia, S.; Monticolo, R.; Cava, E.; Violi, F. Extra virgin olive oil improves post-prandial glycemic and lipid profile in patients with impaired fasting glucose. *Clin. Nutr.* **2017**, *36*, 782–787. [CrossRef] [PubMed]
39. Lampe, J.W. Health effects of vegetables and fruit: Assessing mechanisms of action in human experimental studies. *Am. J. Clin. Nutr.* **1999**, *70* (Suppl. 3), 475s–490s. [CrossRef] [PubMed]
40. Rossouw, J.E. Serum cholesterol as a risk factor for coronary heart disease revisited. *S. Afr. J. Clin. Nutr.* **2015**, *28*, 34–37. [CrossRef]
41. Mani, P.; Rohatgi, A. Niacin Therapy, HDL Cholesterol, and Cardiovascular Disease: Is the HDL Hypothesis Defunct? *Curr. Atheroscler. Rep.* **2015**, *17*, 43. [CrossRef]

4

Role of Magnesium Deficiency in Promoting Atherosclerosis, Endothelial Dysfunction and Arterial Stiffening as Risk Factors for Hypertension

Krasimir Kostov [1,*] and Lyudmila Halacheva [2]

[1] Department of Pathophysiology, Medical University-Pleven, 1 Kliment Ohridski Str., 5800 Pleven, Bulgaria
[2] Department of Physiology, Medical University-Pleven, 1 Kliment Ohridski Str., 5800 Pleven, Bulgaria; l_halacheva@abv.bg
* Correspondence: dr.krasi_kostov@abv.bg

Abstract: Arterial hypertension is a disease with a complex pathogenesis. Despite considerable knowledge about this socially significant disease, the role of magnesium deficiency (MgD) as a risk factor is not fully understood. Magnesium is a natural calcium antagonist. It potentiates the production of local vasodilator mediators (prostacyclin and nitric oxide) and alters vascular responses to a variety of vasoactive substances (endothelin-1, angiotensin II, and catecholamines). MgD stimulates the production of aldosterone and potentiates vascular inflammatory response, while expression/activity of various antioxidant enzymes (glutathione peroxidase, superoxide dismutase, and catalase) and the levels of important antioxidants (vitamin C, vitamin E, and selenium) are decreased. Magnesium balances the effects of catecholamines in acute and chronic stress. MgD may be associated with the development of insulin resistance, hyperglycemia, and changes in lipid metabolism, which enhance atherosclerotic changes and arterial stiffness. Magnesium regulates collagen and elastin turnover in the vascular wall and matrix metalloproteinase activity. Magnesium helps to protect the elastic fibers from calcium deposition and maintains the elasticity of the vessels. Considering the numerous positive effects on a number of mechanisms related to arterial hypertension, consuming a healthy diet that provides the recommended amount of magnesium can be an appropriate strategy for helping control blood pressure.

Keywords: magnesium deficiency; arterial hypertension; vascular tone; arterial stiffness; vascular remodeling; insulin resistance; magnesium supplementation; dietary magnesium intake

1. Introduction

Magnesium (Mg^{2+}) is the fourth most common mineral in the human body after calcium (Ca^{2+}), potassium (K^+), and sodium (Na^+), and should be continuously replenished by food and water intake [1]. Mg^{2+} is the second richest intracellular cation after K^+ and is a cofactor in more than 325 enzyme systems in cells [2]. Mg^{2+} is abundant in all green leafy vegetables, cereal, nuts, and legumes. Chocolate products, fruits, meat, and fish contain moderate amounts of Mg^{2+}, and dairy products are low in Mg^{2+}. Drinking water can be an important source of Mg^{2+} when it contains up to 30 mg/L of Mg^{2+} [3]. Chronic inadequate intake of Mg^{2+} over a long period of time can manifest as latent magnesium deficiency (MgD) [1]. Chronic MgD is associated with an increased risk of multiple preclinical and clinical manifestations including hypertension (HTN), atherosclerosis, cardiac arrhythmias, stroke, changes in lipid metabolism, insulin resistance, metabolic syndrome (MetS), type 2 diabetes (T2D), osteoporosis, depression, and other neuropsychiatric disorders [4] (Table 1). The assessment of Mg^{2+} status in the body is difficult because most is found in the cells or in the bones. Only 1% of the total Mg^{2+} in the body is present in extracellular fluids, and only 0.3% is found in the serum. The normal reference range for Mg^{2+} in the serum is 0.76–1.15 mmol/L [4]. In order to maintain these levels, the Recommended Dietary Allowance (RDA) for Mg^{2+} is 420 mg/day for men and 320 mg/day for women [5]. The hypomagnesaemia is defined as a condition where the serum concentration of Mg^{2+} in the body is <0.75 mmol/L [4]. When the Mg^{2+} intake is poor, the kidney can compensate by increasing reabsorption to >99% of the filtered amount, mainly in Henle's loop and further in the distal tubules [1]. Signs and symptoms of hypomagnesemia usually occur when serum Mg^{2+} is decreased below 0.5 mmol/L. Many patients with hypomagnesemia remain asymptomatic [6,7].

Table 1. Negative effects of MgD on the body and organs.

General: anxiety, agitation, irritability, headache, loss of appetite, nausea.
Musculature: muscle spasm and tetany.
CNS/Nerves: nervousness, migraine, depression, poor memory, low stress tolerance, paraesthesia, tremor, and seizures.
Cardiovascular system: HTN, risk of arrhythmias, coronary spasm, atherosclerosis, endothelial dysfunction, low-grade vascular inflammation, arterial stiffness, vascular ECM remodeling, arterial calcification, vascular aging, increased platelet aggregation, potentiates Ca^{2+}-mediated vasoconstriction, potentiates the vasoconstrictor effects of ATII, ET-1, NA, Adr, and TxA_2.
Electrolytes: sodium retention, hypokalemia, and hypocalcemia.
Metabolism: dyslipoproteinemia, insulin resistance, pancreatic β-cell dysfunction, decreased glucose tolerance, increased risk of MetS and T2D, disorders of vitamin D metabolism, resistance to PTH, and osteoporosis.
Pregnancy: pregnancy complications (e.g., eclampsia).
Gastrointestinal tract: constipation.

Over the last eight decades, nutritional and serum Mg^{2+} levels have received more attention and have been the subject of comprehensive cardiovascular health studies. MgD is considered an important risk factor for various types of cardiovascular diseases (CVD) [8] (Table 1). Dietary studies in Europe and the United States of America (USA) reveal that Mg^{2+} intake is lower than recommended [4]. The often recommended daily intake for adults is 320–400 mg/day (or 6 mg/kg/bodyweight for both sexes) [1]. Epidemiological studies in Europe and North America show that people who consume Western-style diets have low Mg^{2+} content, <30–50% of the RDA for Mg^{2+}. It is assumed that the Mg^{2+} intake in the USA has decreased over the past 100 years from about 500 mg/day to 175–225 mg/day. This is probably the result of the increasing use of fertilizers and processed foods [4]. Refining or processing of food may deplete Mg^{2+} content by nearly 85%. Especially boiling of Mg^{2+}-rich foods can result in a significant loss of Mg^{2+} [3]. Furthermore, the incidence rate of MgD can vary considerably in different regions due to the large differences of Mg^{2+} content in drinking water, which can provide up to 30% of daily needs [1].

Therefore, it seems reasonable to assume that MgD is mainly related to the low intake of Mg^{2+} in food and drinking water, including the use of purified salt to cook, which may lead to a negative balance over time [1]. The processing and cooking of food may therefore explain the apparently high prevalence of low Mg^{2+} intake in many populations [3]. In the USA, the prevalence of insufficient Mg^{2+} intake in adults is about 64% among men and 67% among women. Among people over 71 years of age, the figure increases to 81% for men and 82% for women respectively [8]. In the USA the RDA, set at 320 and 420 mg/day for females and males respectively, is higher than the Reference Nutrient Intake of the United Kingdom (UK). Reported data for Mg^{2+} intake in UK compared to the USA RDA are significantly lower than recommended for all population groups. The UK general population's mean intake is 270 mg and 221.4 mg for males and females respectively, representing only 64% and 69% of the US RDA [9]. Dietary intake of Mg^{2+} has also been shown to be insufficient in middle aged French adults, as 77% of women and 72% of men consume less than the recommended levels [10]. Furthermore, MgD may be potentiated by malabsorption or medication intake, such as diuretics (loop and thiazide), proton pump inhibitors, some antibiotics, and chemotherapeutic agents. With age, the absorption of Mg^{2+} from the intestine is reduced and its loss from the body in the urine increases in both sexes [1].

A number of literature reviews and editorials have focused on the importance of Mg^{2+} for the occurrence of CVD. These examinations have shown that the prevalence of cardiovascular disease events caused by an inadequate intake of Mg^{2+} and low serum concentrations of Mg^{2+}, have been underestimated and cardiovascular health may be associated with the intake of Mg^{2+}. A significant association was found between dietary Mg^{2+} intake and total cardiovascular disease risk. The greatest risk reduction was observed when dietary Mg^{2+} intake increased from 150 mg/day to 400 mg/day. Higher serum Mg^{2+} concentrations with 0.1 mmol/L were associated with a 9% lower risk for total cardiovascular events [8].

A significant part of the experimental studies link MgD and CVD, such as HTN, and atherosclerosis [4]. Given the increasing incidence of HTN, the identification of effective and safe preventative measures that offer even modest lowering of blood pressure (BP), could have a significant public health impact. In this regard, Mg^{2+} may have beneficial health effects for the primary prevention of HTN [11]. HTN is the largest contributor to the global burden of cardiovascular disease. The World Health Organization (WHO) estimates that the number of adults with high BP will increase from 1 billion to 1.5 billion worldwide by 2020 [12]. HTN is a major risk factor for heart disease and stroke [4]. According to WHO, 62% of all strokes and 49% of coronary heart disease events are attributable to high BP. Furthermore, experimental and epidemiological studies considered that HTN may serve as an effect modifier of the Mg^{2+} and CVD association [8].

2. Mechanisms Connecting MgD and Arterial Hypertension

Mg^{2+} is involved in BP regulation. Every modification of the endogenous Mg^{2+} status leads to changes in vascular tonus, and as a consequence, changes in arterial BP [4]. Mg^{2+} plays an important role in BP regulation by modulating vascular tone and reactivity [13]. Small changes in both extracellular and intracellular Mg^{2+} concentrations have significant effects on vascular tone, contractility, reactivity, and growth [14,15]. MgD can increase BP by affecting multiple molecular and cellular mechanisms [16] (Figure 1).

2.1. Disturbances of Mg^{2+} Transport and Its Endocrine Control

Mg^{2+} transport occurs through two main pathways—transcellular and paracellular [5]. Transcellular transport includes influx and efflux transport systems. Mg^{2+} influx is controlled by a number of transporters such as mitochondrial RNA splicing 2 protein (Mrs2p), human solute carrier family 41, members 1 and 2 (SLC41A1 and SLC41A2), ancient conserved domain protein 2 (ACDP2), and Mg^{2+} transporter 1 (MagT1), as well as specialized cationic channels—transient receptor potential melastatin-6 and -7 (TRPM6 and TRPM7) cation channels [17]. TRPM6 channels are predominantly expressed in the kidneys and caecum, where they regulate Mg^{2+} reabsorption. TRPM7 channels are ubiquitously expressed and their absence is lethal [18]. Mg^{2+} efflux is accomplished by Na^+-dependent and Na^+-independent pathways [17]. Na^+-dependent transport involves Na^+/Mg^{2+} pump. The following participate in Na^+-independent transport. The Mg^{2+}/Ca^{2+} pump and Mn^{2+}/Mg^{2+} antiporter Cl^-/Mg^{2+} co-transporter. Paracellular Mg^{2+} transport is a passive process and takes place through dense intercellular contacts of the epithelial cells in the intestinal tract and the kidneys and depends on the specific structural proteins—claudins. Intestinal Mg^{2+} absorption is connected with the relatively low expression of 'tightening' claudins 1, 3, 4, 5, and 8. In the kidney paracellular Mg^{2+} transport depends mainly of claudin 16 (paracellin-1) and claudin 19 [5]. Disturbances of Mg^{2+} transport may predispose to the development of HTN and subsequent CVD [17].

The data reported up to now indicates the potential regulatory role of cation TRPM7 channels in maintenance of vascular integrity [19]. In vascular cells Mg^{2+} influx is mainly determined by the TRPM7 channels and disturbances in vascular smooth muscle cells (VSMCs) function in HTN can be partially linked to defective TRPM7 expression or activity [18]. TRPM7, implicated as a signaling kinase, is involved in a number of processes affecting VSMCs—growth, apoptosis, adhesion, cohesion, contraction, cytoskeletal organization, and migration. TRPM7 channels expressed in vasculature are regulated by vasoactive agents such as bradykinin, aldosterone (ALDO), endothelin-1 (ET-1), and angiotensin II (ATII) and different effects on the vascular wall such as pressure, tension, and osmotic changes. Thus these channels alter intracellular Mg^{2+} concentration by influencing the influx and efflux and may be associated with the onset and maintenance of HTN [17,18,20]. Experimental studies with Spontaneously Hypertensive (SHR) and Wistar-Kyoto (WKY) rats showed that TRPM6 and TRPM7 are differently regulated in their VSMCs. Inhibition of TRPM7, but not of TRPM6, may play a role in the altered Mg^{2+} homeostasis in VSMCs of SHR rats [21]. TRPM6 and TRPM7 are expressed in the endothelium, where they play an important role in intracellular Mg^{2+} homeostasis [22]. Because these channels have different effects on cell endothelial function it is suggested that they have potential importance, especially TRPM7, in the regulation of angiogenesis and vascular remodeling [23]. Mechanisms regulating vascular Mg^{2+} in health and disease remain unclear but TRPM7 could be important in HTN [20]. TRPM7 channels modulate endothelial behavior and any condition that leads to their increased expression, e.g., MgD or oxidative stress can damage endothelial function [19]. TRPM7 plays an important role in modulating VSMCs Mg^{2+} homeostasis, a major determinant of VSMCs function and vascular tone. Antunes et al. showed that in heterozygous TRPM7 kinase-deficient mice, ATII induces an exaggerated hypertensive response. These observations indicate that TRPM7 kinase differentially regulates vascular function in HTN. TRPM7 kinase is a modulator of BP regulation, which, when downregulated, promotes severe HTN and worsening of cardiovascular function. Moreover, ATII is a negative regulator of TRPM7. The study defines a novel TRPM7 kinase-sensitive mechanism involved in ATII-induced HTN. Based on these results, it can be concluded that aberrant TRPM7 expression/activity may contribute to impaired intracellular-free Mg^{2+} concentration and VSMCs contraction, proliferation, inflammation, and fibrosis, important determinants of vascular dysfunction and remodeling in HTN [20].

It has been proven that estrogens and epidermal growth factor (EGF) are magnesiotropic hormones [24–27]. Estrogens stimulate TRPM6 activity in short-term treatment and have long-term regulatory effects on TRPM6 transcription. The stimulation of a specific EGF receptor (EGFR) promotes TRPM6 trafficking to the plasma membrane. Long-term treatment with EGF regulates TRPM6 expression [28]. Considering the role of TRPM6 channels for changes of intracellular Mg^{2+} concentrations could be assumed that they are related to the modifications of the electrical and mechanical activity of cardiac myocytes or VSMCs and hence to CVD such as cardiac arrhythmias or HTN [29]. Thus, estrogen deficiency and the lack of their regulatory effects on Mg^{2+} exchange may be directly linked to increased loss of Mg^{2+} in postmenopausal women, which can lead to the development of HTN, cardiac arrhythmias, increased neuro-muscular excitability, and osteoporosis.

It is known that 1,25-dihydroxyvitamin D [$1,25(OH)_2D$] can stimulate intestinal Mg^{2+} absorption [30]. In addition, conversion of vitamin D by hepatic 25-hydroxylation and renal 1α-hydroxylation into the active form and the vitamin D-binding protein are Mg^{2+}-dependent. MgD leads to reduced $1,25(OH)_2D$ and impaired parathyroid hormone (PTH) response. Absorption of Mg^{2+} and Ca^{2+} is inter-related. MgD impairs hypocalcemic-induced PTH release, which can be corrected after infusion of Mg^{2+}. Mg^{2+} is also an important factor for the sensitivity of the target tissues to PTH. On the other hand, PTH has significant effects on Mg^{2+} homeostasis. For example, PTH release enhances Mg^{2+} reabsorption in the kidneys and absorption in the gut. PTH influences Mg^{2+} absorption, however, hypercalcemia antagonizes this effect [4]. The findings indicate a possible link between the vasculature and mineral metabolism. Epidemiological studies have shown that both PTH and Ca^{2+} are associated with high BP [31], which may be due to Mg^{2+} homeostasis disturbances.

2.2. Mg^{2+} as a Regulator of Vascular Tone and Reactivity

Mg^{2+} is one of the important physiological regulators of blood vessel tone. It improves vascular relaxation responses and attenuates agonist-induced vasoconstriction, thus mitigating the increased peripheral vascular resistance. The effects of Mg^{2+} as a regulator of vascular tone are most often the result of a competitive relationship with Ca^{2+}. MgD increases the contractile response to various agonists and changes vascular responses to a number of vasoactive substances (Figure 1).

2.2.1. Mg^{2+} as a Natural Calcium Antagonist

In the dissolved state, Mg^{2+} binds hydration water tighter than Ca^{2+}. Thus, the hydrated Mg^{2+} is more difficult to dehydrate. The radius of hydrated Mg^{2+} is ~400 times larger than its dehydrated radius. This difference explains a lot of the biological properties of Mg^{2+}, including its often antagonistic behavior to Ca^{2+}, despite similar chemical reactivity and charge. For example, it is almost impossible for Mg^{2+} to pass through narrow channels in biological membranes, compared to Ca^{2+}, because it cannot easily lose its hydration shell [32]. Because of its unique chemical properties, Mg^{2+} is linked to the modulation of intracellular Ca^{2+} homeostasis and decreased extracellular or intracellular Mg^{2+} can be combined with an increase in Ca^{2+} levels [16]. Ca^{2+} concentration in the cytosol is one of the principal factors determining the contractile properties of the VSMCs. Mg^{2+} counteracts Ca^{2+} and functions as physiological Ca^{2+} blocker, like synthetic Ca^{2+} antagonists [33–35]. Both extracellular and intracellular free Mg^{2+} can modulate VSMCs tone by voltage-dependent L-type Ca^{2+} channels. Extracellular Mg^{2+} inhibits Ca^{2+} current in VSMCs by two main mechanisms. First, extracellular Mg^{2+} effectively neutralizes the fixed negative charges on the external surface of the cell membrane. This stabilizes the excitable membranes and raises the excitation threshold which diminishes current via the voltage-gated Ca^{2+} channels. Second, some evidence suggests that extracellular Mg^{2+} can decrease Ca^{2+} current by directly binding to the Ca^{2+} channels. Binding of Mg^{2+} may either mechanically block the channel pore or may cause an allosteric modulation of the channel gating, resulting in its closure [36]. Elevated levels of extracellular Mg^{2+} inhibit Ca^{2+} influx, while decreased extracellular Mg^{2+} activates Ca^{2+} influx through Ca^{2+} channels [37]. Intracellular Mg^{2+} concentrations modulate VSMCs tone via its effects on ion channels and signal transduction pathways, especially those involving Ca^{2+}. Changes in intracellular Mg^{2+} are known to influence these channels by affecting its amplitude, its activation/inactivation kinetics, and its modulation by factors such as phosphorylation, ultimately leading to decreased Ca^{2+} entry. Intracellular Mg^{2+} activates sarcoplasmic/endoplasmic reticular Ca^{2+} ATPase pump that sequesters intracellular Ca^{2+} into the sarcoplasmic reticulum. Elevated intracellular Mg^{2+} stimulates inositol-1,4,5-trisphosphate (IP3) breakdown, inhibits IP3-induced Ca^{2+} release from the sarcoplasmic reticulum, and competes with intracellular Ca^{2+} for cytoplasmic and reticular binding sites [36]. Low intracellular Mg^{2+} stimulates IP3 mediated mobilization of Ca^{2+} from the sarcoplasmic reticulum and reduces Ca^{2+} ATPase activity, decreasing Ca^{2+} efflux and reuptake by the sarcoplasmic reticulum. This leads to accumulation of cytosolic Ca^{2+}, increased intracellular Ca^{2+} concentration, which is a crucial factor for vasoconstriction [37]. Mg^{2+} can also block Ca^{2+} release from the sarcoplasmic reticulum via the ryanodine receptor [17]. An important property of Mg^{2+} is to compete with Ca^{2+} for binding sites on regulatory molecule troponin C. Thus, Mg^{2+} regulates the activity of contractile proteins and their dynamics [16]. Lastly, intracellular Mg^{2+} regulates activity of the G-protein-coupled receptors as AT1 (ATII), ETA (ET-1), V1a (vasopressin), and α_1-adrenoceptors (norepinephrine and epinephrine) on VSMCs and intracellular Ca^{2+} signal transduction pathways as translocation of phospholipase C (PLC) and protein kinase C (PKC) activation [36].

Besides the direct effects of Mg^{2+} on VSMCs, Mg^{2+} also modulates endothelial function, which in turn contributes to its vasodilatory actions. Normal endothelium plays a fundamental role in regulating vasomotor tone by synthesizing vasodilatory prostacyclin (PGI_2) and nitric oxide (NO). Mg^{2+} has been shown to increase endothelial release of PGI_2 in cultured human endothelial cells and in healthy human volunteers [17,36].

2.2.2. MgD and Vascular Reactivity

Other Mg^{2+} effects could be due to altered binding of agonists to their specific cell membrane receptors and/or the production of vasoactive peptides, such as ATII and ET-1, which are powerful vasoconstrictors [38]. ATII, ET-1, vasopressin, and epinephrine/norepinephrine exert their vasoconstrictor effect via stimulation of AT1, ETA, V1a, and α_1 receptors, respectively, on VSMCs. Activation of these Gq–protein-coupled receptors initiates the PLC, IP3, diacylglycerol, Ca^{2+}, and PKC signal transduction pathway. Evidence suggests that following receptor–ligand interaction intracellular Mg^{2+} is also altered and that it too functions as a second messenger to modulate signal transduction [36]. For example, elevated levels of Mg^{2+} decrease ET-1 induced contraction, whereas decreased Mg^{2+} levels increase it [38]. Kharitonova et al. have explored the role of various Mg^{2+} compounds for the development of systemic inflammation and endothelial dysfunction in rats fed on a low Mg^{2+} diet for 74 days. Low Mg^{2+} diet reduces Mg^{2+} concentration in the plasma and red blood cells (RBCs), which is accompanied by a decreased concentration of endothelial NO synthase (eNOS), elevated levels of ET-1 in serum and impaired endothelial-dependent vasodilation. ET-1 produces multiple effects in the blood vessels: causes significant vasoconstriction, has proinflammatory effects, possesses mitogenic and proliferative properties, stimulates the formation of free radicals, and activates platelets. The analysis of the activity of the inorganic Mg^{2+} salts showed that supplementation with Mg-sulfate did not significantly reduce pathologically elevated levels of ET-1, but Mg-chloride completely restored the concentration of ET-1 to a normal value. Tested Mg-organic compounds Mg-oxybutyrate and Mg-*L*-aspartate reduce the concentration of ET-1 to a normal level, whereas treatment with Mg-*N*-acetyltaurate leads only to partial reduction of ET-1 in MgD groups [39]. Mg^{2+} is an essential cofactor of the enzyme δ-6-desaturase, which is the rate determining conversion of linoleic acid to gamma-linolenic, which in turn is converted to dihomo-γ-linoleic acid. The latter is a precursor of prostaglandin E_1 (PGE_1), which is both a vasodilator and inhibitor of platelet aggregation. MgD disrupts production of PGE_1, which leads to vasoconstriction and increase in BP [17].

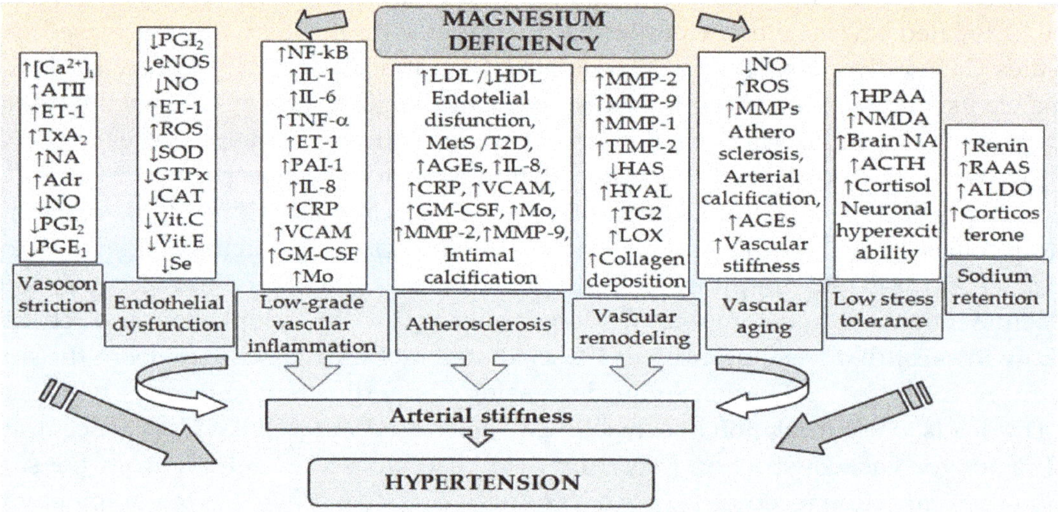

Figure 1. Pathogenetic relationships between MgD and arterial hypertension. (Abbreviations: ↑: increased; ↓: decreased; $[Ca^{2+}]_i$: intracellular calcium in VSMCs; ATII: angiotensin II; ET-1: endothelin-1; TxA_2: thromboxane A_2; NO: nitric oxide; PGE_1: prostaglandin E_1; PGI_2: prostaglandin I_2; ROS: reactive oxygen species; NF-kB: nuclear factor kappa B; TNF-α: tumor necrosis factor-α; IL-1: interleukin-1; IL-6: interleukin-1; IL-8: interleukin-8; PAI-1: plasminogen activator inhibitor-1; VCAM: vascular cell adhesion molecule-1; GM-CSF: granulocyte-macrophage colony-stimulating factor; Mo: monocytes; CRP: C-reactive protein; SOD: superoxide dismutase; GTPx: glutathione peroxidase; CAT: catalase; Vit.C: vitamin C; Vit.E: vitamin E; Se: selenium; LDL: low-density lipoproteins; HDL: high-density lipoproteins; MetS: metabolic syndrome; T2D: type 2 diabetes; AGEs: advanced glycation end products; MMPs: matrix metalloproteinases; MMP-1: matrix metalloproteinase-1; MMP-2: matrix metalloproteinase-2; MMP-9: matrix metalloproteinase-9; TIMP-2: tissue inhibitor of metalloprotease-2; HAS: hyaluronan synthases; HYAL: hyaluronidase; TG2: transglutaminase; LOX: lysyl oxidase; HPAA: hypothalamic pituitary adrenal axis; NMDA: N-methyl-D-aspartate receptor; NA: noradrenaline; Adr: adrenaline; ACTH: adrenocorticotropic hormone; RAAS: renin-angiotensin-aldosterone system; ALDO: aldosterone).

2.2.3. MgD and the Renin-Angiotensin-Aldosterone System (RAAS)

Few studies have investigated the effects of MgD on the hormonal systems which control BP. The RAAS plays an essential role in humoral and hemodynamic regulation [40]. It was established, that in hypertensive patients with high plasma renin activity, serum Mg^{2+} was much lower than in normotensive persons [16]. MgD increases the ATII-induced plasma concentration of ALDO, as well as the production of thromboxane A_2 and vasoconstrictor prostaglandins [3]. Mg^{2+} has some direct effects on ALDO synthesis rather than indirect effects via the RAAS. ALDO secretion from the zona glomerulosa of the adrenal gland is Ca^{2+} dependent process. Mg^{2+} infusion in humans decreases the production of ALDO, by inhibiting the cellular Ca^{2+} influx. MgD facilitates cellular Ca^{2+} influx, which may stimulate the production and release of ALDO [40]. It was proved that MgD rats have increased plasma renin activity and circulating levels of ALDO and corticosterone. Additionally, other authors indicate that Mg^{2+} supplementation decreases ATII stimulated production and release of ALDO from the adrenal cortex of normotensive subjects [16]. Rats fed with an MgD diet showed a continuous increment of the juxtaglomerular granulation index and width of the zona glomerulosa of the adrenal cortex, whereas the thickness of the inner zones diminished slightly. In Mg^{2+}-recovering rats juxtaglomerular granulation index the width of the zona glomerulosa returned to normal [41]. Thus, one could suggest that MgD, by facilitating cellular Ca^{2+} entry, may promote ALDO production and release. Experimental studies have reported that MgD-induced HTN in rats is associated with increased vascular total Ca^{2+} content, and increased vasoconstrictor activity to endogenous agonists such as ATII and noradrenaline (NA) [40]. Mg^{2+} supplementation can reduce the pressor effect of ATII and stimulate the production of the vasodilator PGI_2 [3].

2.2.4. MgD and Catecholamines (CA)

Ca^{2+} exerts a major role in CA release from the adrenal gland and adrenergic nerve terminals in response to sympathetic stimulation. Because Mg^{2+} competes with Ca^{2+} for membrane channels, it can modify these types of Ca^{2+}-mediated responses. The ability of Mg^{2+} to inhibit the release of CA from both the adrenal gland and peripheral adrenergic nerve terminals is well established in laboratory experiments. On the basis of these effects, Mg^{2+} can be used in patients where an excess of CA is prevalent, such as in phaeochromocytoma [42]. Acetylcholine (ACh) evoked CA release from adrenal glands. Ca^{2+} stimulates the secretion of ACh and there exists a direct relationship between Ca^{2+} concentration and the rate of CA release. Mg^{2+} antagonizes the stimulant effects of ACh on adrenal chromaffin cells; this effect can be overcome by the addition of Ca^{2+} [43]. Mg^{2+} is required for the catalytic action of adenylate cyclase (ADCY). For example, the decreased activity of the ADCY9 in the absence of Mg^{2+} results in increased secretion of ACh from preganglionic nerves, which in turn stimulates further release of CA from the adrenal glands [44]. On the other hand, Mg^{2+} together with ATP can greatly stimulate the release of CA from adrenal medullary granules. Neither ATP nor Mg^{2+} alone may have any effect on the release of CA. The effects of Ca^{2+}, which cause the release of CA from the granules, are inhibited in the presence of ATP and Mg^{2+}. The uptake of ^{14}C-adrenaline (Adr) into the granules can also be stimulated by ATP and Mg^{2+} [45].

There are evidences that high concentrations of Mg^{2+} prevent the release of NA in some arteries by blocking *N*-type Ca^{2+} channels of nerve endings, which counteracts the rise in BP. Also rats fed with a MgD diet showed an increase in CA excretion [16]. The effects of Ca^{2+} and Mg^{2+} concentrations on responses to periarterial nervous sympathetic stimulation, NA, and tyramine have been investigated on the isolated rabbit central ear artery. An increase in Ca^{2+} concentrations potentiates responses to sympathetic stimulation until complete removal of Ca^{2+} inhibits these responses. The addition of the Mg^{2+} solution greatly reduced the responses to sympathetic stimulation, NA, and tyramine. These actions of Mg^{2+} on sympathetic transmission are important in determining the responsiveness of arterial smooth muscle to direct and indirectly acting sympathomimetic amines [46]. The effects of Adr infusion, sufficient to achieve its pathophysiological levels, and of therapeutic intravenous infusion of salbutamol, a β_2-agonist, on plasma Mg^{2+} levels, were studied in a placebo-controlled design in healthy subjects. Plasma Mg^{2+} levels fell significantly during the Adr infusion and also during the salbutamol infusion, though more slowly. It is propose that intracellular shifts of Mg^{2+} occur as a result of β-adrenergic stimulation [47]. In another study, infusion of Adr in man significantly reduced the plasma Mg^{2+} levels in healthy males. This effect was abolished by simultaneous infusion of propranolol. NA had no such effect. These results suggest that the β-adrenergic system affect Mg^{2+} homeostasis [48]. On the other hand, dose-dependent increase in circulating Mg^{2+} was observed in rats infused with isoproterenol (ISO). Pretreatment with butoxamine or propranolol has prevented the ISO-induced increase in serum Mg^{2+} levels, whereas administration of atenolol has minimal effects. This evidence demonstrates the existence of a pool of Mg^{2+} that is mobilized into the circulation in response to selective β_2-adrenergic stimulation [49].

2.3. MgD and Arterial Stiffness

Normally conduit arteries adapt pressure and blood flow during cardiac systole to facilitate perfusion to tissues during diastole. This is determined in large part by the elasticity, distensibility, and compliance of the arterial system. Loss of elasticity and increased stiffness demand greater force to accommodate blood flow, leading to increased systolic BP and consequent increased cardiac work load. Multiple interacting factors at the systemic (BP, hemodynamics), vascular (vascular contraction/dilatation, extracellular matrix remodeling), cellular (cytoskeletal organization and inflammatory responses), and molecular (oxidative stress, intracellular signaling, and mechanotransduction) levels contribute to arterial stiffness in HTN. Dysregulation of endothelial cells, VSMCs, and adaptive immune responses are also implicated in HTN [12]. Changes in Mg^{2+} concentrations play an important role in many of these processes.

2.3.1. MgD, Low-Grade Inflammation, and Oxidative Stress at the Vascular Wall

A number of immunopathological mechanisms may be at the basis of HTN. There are evidence in animal models and humans that link HTN with changes in both humoral and cellular immunity, and in particular with the key role of low-grade vascular inflammation [50]. One study showed that the total intracellular Mg^{2+} is considerably lower in lymphocytes of the hypertensive patients, compared with healthy subjects, whereas serum Mg^{2+}, erythrocyte Mg^{2+} and ionized platelet Mg^{2+} were not significantly different [51]. MgD leads to inflammation and increased production of free radicals [52] in the vascular wall, and they in turn contribute to the development of endothelial dysfunction and vascular remodeling. Low Mg^{2+} intake is associated with a higher probability of increased serum C-reactive protein (CRP) levels in children [53]. There is also an association between the dietary intake of Mg^{2+} and elevated CRP levels in the adult population. Insufficient dietary intake of Mg^{2+} may be associated with an increased inflammatory response resulting in more frequent occurrence of cardiovascular accidents [54]. Intake of Mg^{2+} is also inversely related to the level of hs-CRP, interleukin 6 (IL-6), and fibrinogen [55]. MgD significantly increases production of various proinflammatory molecules such as, interleukin 1 (IL-1), IL-6, tumor necrosis factor α (TNF-α), vascular cell adhesion molecule-1 (VCAM), plasminogen activator inhibitor-1 (PAI-1), and decreases expression and activity of the antioxidant enzymes such as glutathione peroxidase, superoxide dismutase, and catalase. Cellular and tissue levels of important antioxidants such as glutathione, vitamin C, vitamin E and selenium are also reduced [16]. This shows that MgD can increase cytotoxicity of the free radicals to endothelial cells [56]. For example Mg^{2+} deficit, in rats leads to an increase in the inflammatory mediators, such as histamine, IL-1, IL-6, TNF-α, and ET-1, which is associated with leukocytosis and generation of free radicals [34] (Figure 1).

2.3.2. MgD, Vascular Structure and Remodeling

Vascular remodeling is a permanent process of structural changes in the vessel wall in response to a number of hemodynamic stimulus [57]. In HTN, resistance arteries undergo an inward remodeling, while larger arteries show outward hypertrophic remodeling [58–60]. The vascular extracellular matrix (ECM) comprises multiple structural proteins, including collagens, elastin, fibronectin, and proteoglycans.

The absolute and relative quantities of collagen and elastin determine biomechanical properties of vessels. Excessive ECM protein deposition, in particular collagen and fibronectin, contributes to increased intima–media thickening, vascular fibrosis, and stiffening leading to the development of HTN [12]. Mg^{2+} regulates collagen and elastin turnover and the structure of the ECM. MgD leads to a delay in the synthesis of all structural molecules (collagen, elastin, proteoglycans and glycosaminoglycans) (Figure 1). Hyaluronan synthases (HAS)—HAS1, HAS2 and HAS3, contain Mg^{2+} ion in their active centers. On the other hand it is known that inhibitors of the hyaluronidase (HYAL) depend on the concentration of Mg^{2+} ions. Thus, low levels of Mg^{2+} could lead to decreased activity of HAS, and at the same time to an increased activity of HYAL. Tissue transglutaminase (TG2) is an enzyme of the transglutaminase superfamily that is ubiquitously expressed in the vasculature [61]. TG2 is associated with a wide range of CVD and processes, including the development of HTN, and the progression of atherosclerosis, regulating vascular permeability, and angiogenesis. TG2 activity is associated with arterial stiffening in humans and rats. TG2 forms glutamine-lysine cross-links between variety of extracellular proteins, including collagen and elastin [62]. TG2 is secreted through a Golgi-independent mechanism to the ECM, where it can be activated to a Ca^{2+}-bound open conformation to catalyze the formation of isopeptide bonds [61]. Thus, Ca^{2+} may be limiting TG2 activity in the ECM [62]. TG2 is activated by Ca^{2+}, and inhibited by Mg^{2+} [63]. A disturbance in lysyl oxidase (LOX) expression has also been reported in CVD, and an increase in vascular LOX activity has been described in experimental models of HTN. Mg^{2+} can inhibit LOX, which is also associated with crosslinking of chains of elastin and/or collagen [63,64]. Additionally, MgD could lead to the production of defective collagen, elastin, and fibronectin by fibroblasts [65].

Fundamental to many of the processes underlying ECM reorganization and fibrosis in HTN is activation of matrix metalloproteinases (MMPs) and tissue inhibitors of metalloproteinases (TIMPs). ECM MMPs and TIMPs may contribute to the profibrotic phenotype in HTN. Activated MMPs degrade collagen, elastin, and other ECM proteins, resulting in a modified ECM, often associated with a proinflammatory microenvironment that triggers a shift of endothelial and VSMCs to a more secretory, migratory, and proliferative phenotype, which contributes to fibrosis, calcification, endothelial dysfunction, and increased intima–media thickness, further impacting on vascular remodeling and arterial stiffness [12]. In endothelial cells cultured in MgD medium, a significant increase in expression and activity of MMP-2 and MMP-9 has been reported. Also, MMP-2 and MMP-9 have been associated with alterations of the vascular wall in Mg^{2+}-deficient rats [66]. In addition, there is evidence that the addition of Mg-sulfate effectively attenuated MMP-9 activity in a human umbilical cord vein endothelial cell line [67]. These data are confirmed by K. Kostov et al. who find that in patients with essential HTN there was a moderate negative correlation of serum Mg^{2+} with MMP-2 ($r = -0.318$, $p = 0.013$). There was a similar correlation of Mg^{2+} with MMP-9 in patients with HTN and T2D ($r = -0.376$, $p = 0.003$). The results show that lower and higher serum Mg^{2+} levels correlate inversely with MMP-2 and MMP-9 levels in HTN [68]. It is noteworthy that in Mg^{2+}-deficient endothelial cells, MMP-2 and MMP-9 activity overrides the inhibitory effect of TIMP-2, which probably is induced as an attempt to counterbalance the effects of the proteases [66]. A nuclear factor (NF)-κB-binding site is present in the promoter of the MMP-9 gene. It is therefore possible that low Mg^{2+} availability might directly increase MMP-9 expression via NF-κB [66,69]. In cultured rat VSMCs, Mg^{2+} significantly reduced the production of MMP-2 under basal and platelet-derived growth factor-stimulated conditions in a dose-dependent manner, while neither verapamil nor nifedipine showed any effect under the same conditions. These data suggest that the beneficial effect of Mg^{2+} supplementation on vascular disease processes may be due, at least in part, to the inhibitory effect of Mg^{2+} on the production of MMP-2 in VSMCs [70]. Evidence supporting this data is that in cultured rat cardiac fibroblasts, Mg^{2+} significantly reduced the production of MMP-2 in a dose-dependent manner [71]. MgD may increase the activity of MMPs, including collagenases, which begin to degrade the extracellular vascular matrix and primarily collagen with an increased speed. The degradation of elastin fibers can significantly increase (up to 2–3 times) in the presence of Mg^{2+}. MgD is associated with low elastase activity and an increased number of elastic fibers [63]. Altura et al. describe and other possible mechanisms by which MgD can affect vascular remodeling processes. They present new evidence for effects on platelet-activating factor, proto-oncogenes, and sphingolipids, e.g., ceramide and sphingosine with upstream regulation in both VSMCs and cardiac muscle cells. These findings will be helpful in explaining many of the known cardiovascular manifestations of MgD, especially vascular remodeling seen in atherosclerosis and HTN [72].

2.3.3. MgD, Endothelial Dysfunction and Atherosclerosis

MgD may potentiate the development of endothelial dysfunction via activation of NF-κB, which includes the transcriptional program leading to development of the proinflammatory phenotype [69]. Low extracellular Mg^{2+} slows endothelial cell proliferation, stimulates the adhesion of monocytes, and affect the synthesis of vasoactive molecules, such as NO and PGI_2. Endothelial function is significantly impaired in a model of familial hypomagnesemia in mice. Compared to controls, in the aortas of these animals were found reduced amounts of eNOS and increased expression of proinflammatory molecules, such as VCAM, PAI-1, as well as of the TRPM7 channel [19]. Endothelial dysfunction is an early event in the process of atherogenesis and precedes the angiographic and ultrasound evidences of damage to the arterial wall [66]. The pathogenesis of atherosclerotic changes and disturbances in endothelial function are complex and multifactorial. In this context, Mg^{2+} deficit is too important [73]. This mineral is especially important because of its antiatherosclerotic effects [74]. Endothelial function correlates to the levels of Mg^{2+} and results of Mg^{2+} supplementation have showed significantly improved endothelial function in patients with ischemic heart disease and diabetes. These results in humans have also been observed in different experimental models in which Mg^{2+} deficit affects vascular structure and function. Low levels of extracellular Mg^{2+} favor and increase endothelial permeability. More specifically, MgD enhance the transport of low-density lipoproteins (LDL) through the endothelial layer [66]. Several studies have reported beneficial effects of Mg^{2+} supplementation on plasma LDL levels, as well as on high-density lipoproteins (HDL) levels, which are increased [75]. Another possibility by which Mg^{2+} contributes to the development of atherogenesis is through the effect on triglyceride levels which are increased in MgD. Accumulation of triglyceride-rich lipoproteins is accompanied by decreased concentration of HDL and increased plasma concentration of apolipoprotein B. Since the oxidation of lipoproteins play a key role in the development of atherosclerosis, it could be another mechanism by which Mg^{2+} influences. It is also possible proatherogenic lipoprotein changes found in MgD to be a consequence of the inflammatory response [76]. A central role for Mg^{2+} mediated effects on endothelial cells has IL-1α, which is regulated by NF-κB and may be inducer of the NF-κB. IL-1α increases significantly in the environment of low Mg^{2+} content. IL-1α also induces the production of various chemokines and adhesion molecules in vascular endothelial cells by activation of NF-κB, and thus favors aggregation, adhesion, and diapedesis of monocytes. In particular, low concentrations of Mg^{2+} stimulate the secretion of interleukin 8 (IL-8), and chemokines, which are overexpressed in human atherosclerotic lesions. IL-8 is essential for chemotaxis and adhesion of monocytes to endothelial cells, which is a fundamental event in the initiation of atherogenesis and also stimulates proliferation and migration of VSMCs. By induction of IL-1α, low serum Mg^{2+} may also stimulate overexpression of VCAM-1 on the surface of endothelial cells which assists in the migration of leukocytes. In addition, the secretion of granulocyte-macrophage colony-stimulating factor is significantly higher in endothelial cells with Mg^{2+} deficit [66]. All these date indicate that the MgD is a potential factor for accumulation of monocytes/macrophages in the arterial wall during the early stages of atherosclerosis (Figure 1).

2.3.4. MgD, MetS, and T2D

The presence of MetS is also associated with altered Mg^{2+} metabolism [77]. Usually, the triad consisting of obesity, HTN, and impaired glucose tolerance/insulin resistance is denoted as MetS [78]. Furthermore, HTN is present in a high proportion of patients with T2D [79,80]. A common feature in patients with T2D, HTN, and low levels of HDL is MgD (Table 1).

Currently, there is little data on serum Mg^{2+} levels in people with MetS. The relationship between the intake of Mg^{2+} and MetS was investigated prospectively in 5115 young Americans (aged 18–30 years), initially without MetS and diabetes, which were enrolled in Coronary Artery Risk Development in Young Adults (CARDIA) study from 1985 to 1986. The total number of participants included in the analysis was 4637, and 74% were evaluated at the 15-year period in 2000–2001. During this interval 608 cases of MetS were diagnosed. The findings showed that young people with a high Mg^{2+} intake had a lower risk of developing MetS and that risk was dose-dependent [78]. Guerrero-Romero et al. found a link between Mg^{2+} levels, inflammation, and oxidative stress, as risk factors for the development of MetS. Mg^{2+} intake is inversely proportional to the components of MetS and fasting insulin levels, suggesting that higher Mg^{2+} intake may have a protective role against the risk of developing MetS [77]. The results of several clinical studies have shown that increased synthesis and release of proinflammatory cytokines trigger the process of chronic inflammation, which may be the link between obesity and MetS. On the other hand hypomagnesemia triggers low-grade chronic inflammation and Mg^{2+} deficit may be associated with the development of MetS. These findings support the hypothesis that MgD can play an important role in the pathophysiology of MetS, and the actuation of the inflammatory reaction caused by the shortage of Mg^{2+} could be the link between MgD and MetS [81]. Some studies linked decreased Mg^{2+} levels with chronic inflammatory stress in obese people. Obesity affects over 35% of the adult population of the USA and is a main risk factor for chronic diseases, associated with a lower Mg^{2+} status, such as atherosclerosis and T2D. MgD is often found in people with MetS and T2D, which are connected with higher plasma concentrations of CRP [82].

Mg^{2+} plays a very important role in the development of T2D [83]. Corica et al. have recently shown that patients with T2D having lipid profile with high risk, high BP, and abdominal obesity, have lower levels of Mg^{2+}, compared with patients without metabolic risk factors. Furthermore, plasma triglycerides and waist circumference were independently associated with hypomagnesaemia [77]. T2D is often linked with hypomagnesaemia, as has been reported at an occurrence rate of 13.5–47.7% [78]. The relationship between insulin and Mg^{2+} is bipartite. Insulin regulates Mg^{2+} homeostasis, but on the other hand Mg^{2+} is a major factor determining insulin and glucose metabolism. Extracellular Mg^{2+} acts as Ca^{2+} antagonist and inhibits Ca^{2+} influx, required for insulin secretion. Thus a decreased concentration of extracellular free Mg^{2+} results in an increased Ca^{2+} influx and increased concentration of intracellular free Ca^{2+}. The increased intracellular Ca^{2+} stimulates insulin secretion by beta-cells, as was demonstrated in experiments with an insulinoma cell line [84]. The effect of extracellular Mg^{2+} on insulin secretion was found in healthy human subjects. In subjects with 0.79 mmol/L plasma Mg^{2+}, fasting plasma insulin was 23 μU/mL, while in those with plasma Mg^{2+} 0.87 or 1.00 mmol/L, fasting plasma insulin amounted to 11 μU/mL [85].

There are growing evidences that highlight the clinical significance of altered Mg^{2+} metabolism for the occurrence of peripheral insulin resistance. MgD can lead to disturbances of the tyrosine kinase activity of the insulin receptor (IR), associated with the development of post receptor insulin resistance and reduced cellular glucose utilization, as a lower Mg^{2+} concentration, requires a greater amount of insulin for glucose metabolism [77]. The effects of MgD on glucose-stimulated insulin secretion and insulin action on skeletal muscle were studied in experimental animals. The hypothesis that changes in Mg^{2+} metabolism induce insulin resistance is confirmed by data showing that lower dietary intake of Mg^{2+} is associated with insulin resistance. Rats fed on a low Mg^{2+} diet showed a significant increase of blood glucose and triglycerides. The insulin resistance, observed in the skeletal muscle of rats with MgD is partially associated with a defect of tyrosine kinase activity of the IR [86–88]. Insulin action begins with the binding of insulin to an IR on the cell membrane of the target cells. The IR is a transmembrane glycoprotein with tyrosine kinase activity [89]. Activation of the receptor is an important step in transmembrane signaling for insulin action. The activated kinase promotes autophosphorylation of receptor tyrosine residues. The insulin–receptor complex is internalized and phosphorylates IR substrates 1–6 (IRS 1–6) and other kinases in the insulin signaling cascade [90]. When the intrinsic tyrosine kinase activity of the receptor is triggered by insulin binding, two major signaling pathways have been activated: (1) Ras-mitogen-activated protein kinase (MAPK) pathway, which controls cell growth and differentiation; (2) Phosphoinositide 3-kinase/Akt (PI3K/Akt) pathway. Binding of IRS to the regulatory subunit of phosphoinositide 3-kinase (PI3K) results in activation of PI3K, which phosphorylates membrane phospholipids and phosphatidylinositol 4,5-bisphosphate (PIP2). This complex activates the 3-phosphoinositide-dependent protein kinases (PDK-1 and PDK-2) resulting in activation of Akt/protein kinase B and atypical protein kinase [91,92]. Activated Akt phosphorylates its 160 kDa substrate, which stimulates the translocation of insulin-mediated glucose transporter type 4 (GLUT4) from intracellular vesicles to the plasma membrane [93]. The PI3K/Akt pathway is a key component of the insulin signaling cascade, which is necessary for the metabolic effects of insulin and GLUT4 translocation [94]. Since Mg^{2+} is a necessary cofactor in all ATP transfer reactions, intracellular Mg^{2+} concentration is critical in the phosphorylation of the IR and other kinases [95]. In all these reactions Mg^{2+} operates together with ATP as a kinase substrate. Additionally Mg^{2+} is bound to a regulatory site of the IR tyrosine kinase (IRTK). The apparent affinity of the IRTK for Mg^{2+}-ATP increased as the concentration of free Mg^{2+} increased, and the apparent affinity of the IRTK for free Mg^{2+} increased as the concentration of Mg^{2+}-ATP increased [84]. There are evidences that show a link between decreased Mg^{2+} concentration and reduction of tyrosine-kinase activity at the IR level, which results in the impairment of insulin action and development of insulin resistance [96]. Studies in multiple insulin resistant cell models have demonstrated that an impaired response of the tyrosine kinase to insulin stimulation is one potential mechanism causing insulin-resistant state in T2D [97]. Nadler et al. have reported that insulin sensitivity decreases even in nondiabetic individuals after induction of MgD [98]. Finally, Mg^{2+} can also be a limiting factor in carbohydrate metabolism, since many of the enzymes in this process require Mg^{2+} as a cofactor during reactions that utilize the phosphorus bond [99].

Inadequate dietary intake of Mg^{2+} is an independent risk factor for the development of T2D. Lopez-Ridaura et al., evaluating 37,309 participants free of cardiovascular disease and T2D, found a significant inverse association between Mg^{2+} intake and diabetes risk [100]. Van Dam et al. reported a similar relationship. Their findings indicated that a diet high in Mg^{2+}-rich foods, particularly whole grains, is associated with a substantially lower risk of T2D [101]. Benefits of Mg^{2+} supplementation in diabetic subjects have been found in some clinical studies. Rodriguez-Moran et al. reported that Mg^{2+} supplementation improves insulin sensitivity and secretion as well as metabolic control in patients with T2D [96]. Mooren et al. have shown beneficial effect of oral Mg^{2+} supplementation on insulin sensitivity in overweight, nondiabetic subjects [102].

2.3.5. MgD and Vascular Calcification

Vascular calcification is the extracellular deposition of Ca^{2+} in the arterial wall and is intimately linked with the HTN. On the other hand, HTN was considered a risk factor for atherosclerosis and associated calcification. Two types of extracellular vascular calcification are recognized, intimal and medial. Intimal calcification is exclusively associated with atherosclerosis. Medial calcification may contribute to increasing BP by decreasing the elasticity of the media. Decreased elasticity results in arterial stiffening which accelerates pulse wave velocity and widening the pulse pressure, leading ultimately to HTN. Intimal and, especially, medial vascular calcification are associated with arterial stiffening, the major cause of isolated systolic HTN in the elderly [103]. The first in vitro evidence in human aortic VSMCs for a protective role of Mg^{2+} on vascular calcification was based on the observation that living cells are necessary for Mg^{2+} ions to exert its protective effect. These studies suggested a potentially active intracellular role for Mg^{2+} ions in attenuating the vascular calcification process [33,35,104]. In confirmation of this, Hruby et al. reported on favorable associations between dietary and supplemental Mg^{2+} intake and lower calcification of the coronary arteries [105]. Furthermore, it was found that higher Mg^{2+} levels prevented calcification of bovine VSMCs, and further progression of the already established calcification. Inhibition of the Wnt/β -catenin signaling pathway was identified as one of the possible intracellular mechanisms by which Mg^{2+} achieved its anti-calcifying effect [104].

2.3.6. MgD and Vascular Aging

Aging represents a major risk factor for MgD. The total body Mg^{2+} content and intracellular Mg^{2+} tend to decrease with age. Aging is often associated with a Mg^{2+} deficiency due to reduced intake and/or absorption, increased renal wasting and/or reduced tubular reabsorption, as well as age-related illnesses and their treatment with certain drugs [106]. The aging process is associated with alterations in the properties of all the elements of the vascular wall, including endothelium, VSMCs, and ECM. This increases vascular stiffness and leads to the development of isolated systolic HTN. "Aging"-associated arterial changes and those associated with HTN (and early atherosclerosis and diabetes) are fundamentally intertwined at the cellular and molecular levels [107]. At the molecular and cellular levels, arterial aging and HTN-associated vascular changes are characterized by reduced NO production, increased generation of reactive oxygen species (oxidative stress), activation of transcription factors, induction of "aging" genes, stimulation of proinflammatory and profibrotic signaling pathways, reduced collagen turnover, calcification, VSMCs proliferation, and ECM remodeling. These processes contribute to increased fibrosis, which is further promoted by prohypertensive vasoactive agents, such as ATII, ET-1, and ALDO [12]. The cellular and molecular proinflammatory mechanisms that underlie arterial aging are novel putative candidates to be targeted by interventions aimed at attenuating arterial aging, and thus possibly attenuating the major risk factors for HTN and atherosclerosis [107]. Targeted interventions aimed at correcting MgD and maintaining an optimal Mg^{2+} balance may prove to be an appropriate strategy against arterial aging due to its positive effects on low-grade inflammation and oxidative stress associated with aging process (Figure 1).

2.4. MgD and Stress Response

Stress is among the potential psychological risk factors for HTN. Acute stressful events have no consistent association with the HTN. Chronic stress on the other hand, particularly the non-adaptive response to stress, may be a more likely cause of sustained elevation of BP. The mechanisms underlying the association between psychosocial stress and HTN can be divided into behavioral, psychological and pathophysiological. The latter involves neuro-endocrine activation mediated by the hypothalamic pituitary adrenal axis (HPAA) [108]. Mg^{2+} plays a key role in the activity of psychoneuroendocrine systems. For example, all elements of the limbic-HPAA are sensitive to the action of Mg^{2+}. Mg^{2+} modulates activity of the HPAA which is a central substrate of the stress response system. Activation of the HPAA instigates adaptive autonomic, neuroendocrine, and behavioral responses to cope with the demands of the stressor [10]. MgD induced an increase in the transcription of the corticotropin releasing hormone in the paraventricular hypothalamic nucleus, and elevated adrenocorticotropic hormone (ACTH) plasma levels, indicating an enhanced set-point of the HPAA [109]. MgD results in a stressor effect and increases susceptibility to the physiological damage produced by stress (Figure 1). Mg^{2+} supply has been shown to attenuate the development of adverse stress reactions. Stress activates the HPAA and the sympathetic nervous system. The innervation of the kidney may result in the overproduction of renin, which in turn activates the production of ATII, a powerful vasoconstrictor that elevates the BP [110]. Additionally, Mg^{2+} deficient mice are more sensitive to anxiety-provoking situations. Dysregulation of the HPAA evoked by MgD is normalizes by chronic desipramine or diazepam treatment. These data indicate that dysregulation in the HPAA may contribute to hyper-emotionality in response to dietary induced hypomagnesaemia [109].

Mg^{2+} ions also have a key role in the modulation of neurotransmission. Numerous studies have confirmed that the function of the native *N*-methyl-D-aspartate (NMDA) receptor is the result of equilibrium between extracellular and intracellular concentration of Mg^{2+}. The blockade of the ion channel of the NMDA receptor is the most well-known and established way in which Mg^{2+} affects the functioning of the central nervous system (CNS) [109]. Mg^{2+} reduces neuronal hyperexcitability by inhibiting NMDA receptor activity and also is essential for the activity of metabotropic glutamate receptors (mGluRs) in the brain. The mGluRs play a key modulatory role in glutamatergic activity, secretion, and presynaptic release of glutamate, activity of the gamma-aminobutyric acid (GABA)-ergic system, and regulation of the neuroendocrine system. Mg^{2+} may additionally modulate anxiety via increasing GABA availability by decreasing presynaptic glutamate release. GABA is a primary inhibitory transmitter in the CNS that counterbalances the excitatory action of glutamate [111]. The state of acute and chronic stress leads to depletion of intracellular Mg^{2+} and its loss in the urine, because in stressful situations secreted elevated amounts of Adr and NA help to remove Mg^{2+} from the cells. Intracellular RBCs Mg^{2+} depletion is found in patients with HTN. MgD affects the balance of monoamines, such as CA and serotonin in the brain. CA released into the blood is rapidly inactivated by the enzyme catechol-*O*-methyl transferase (COMT). The latter is activated by Mg^{2+} and is inhibited by Ca^{2+}. MgD leads to decreased activity of COMT, which in turn increases the concentration of circulating CA [44]. Brain NA was determined in adult male mice with genetically low (MGL) or high (MGH) blood Mg^{2+} levels. NA levels were significantly higher in MGL than in MGH mice. These data together with the higher urinary NA excretion observed in the MGL line might account for the higher sensitivity and/or reactivity of MGL animals to stress [112]. Moreover, in stressful conditions, MGL mice displayed a more aggressive behavior than the control MGH strain. Altogether, MGL mice showed a more restless behavior, and much higher brain and urine NA levels than the MGH animals [113]. An analysis of the literature suggests the possible role of MgD in the susceptibility to CVD, observed among subjects displaying a type A behavior pattern. Type A subjects are more sensitive to stress and produce more CA than type B subjects. This, in turn, seems to induce an intracellular Mg^{2+} loss. In the long run, type A individuals would develop a state of MgD, which may promote a greater sensitivity to stress, and ultimately to the development of CVD [114], including HTN. Hypomagnesemia usually involves cellular Mg^{2+} depletion, but acute stress that increase serum concentrations of CA may lower serum Mg^{2+} concentration, which does not always imply depleted tissue Mg^{2+} stores [115].

The potential effect of Mg^{2+} in attenuating psychological response to stress merits further investigation since stress is a ubiquitous feature of modern life. The modulation of HPAA by Mg^{2+}, which has been shown to reduce central (ACTH), peripheral (cortisol) endocrine responses [111], and reduces neuronal hyperexcitability by NMDA, mGluRs and GABA-effects suggests that behavioral responses to stress exposure may be attenuated by Mg^{2+} supplementation in patients with HTN.

3. MgD, Groups at Risk, Replacement Therapy and Prevention

3.1. Mg^{2+} Supplements in Hypertensive Subjects

HTN is a complex, heterogeneous disorder whose etiology, pathogenesis, and treatment still raises some unresolved questions. Maintenance of optimal Mg^{2+} status in the human body may help prevent or treat HTN. Although most epidemiological and experimental studies support a role of MgD in the pathophysiology of HTN, data from clinical studies have been less convincing [38]. In some studies the inverse association between Mg^{2+} and BP remained inconclusive, but not in others [116]. Ultimately, the view is that MgD in patients with HTN is linking with significant adverse effects on BP. In the Atherosclerosis Risk in Communities (ARIC) study, serum Mg^{2+} level in hypertensive patients was inversely proportional to the systolic BP. The study examined a cohort of 15248 participants aged 45–64 years [117]. In another meta-analysis of 34 randomized, double-blind, placebo-controlled trials involving a total of 2028 subjects, it was found that oral administration of Mg^{2+} resulted in a significant reduction in both systolic and diastolic BP (2.00 mmHg and 1.78 mmHg respectively) [118]. An analytical review of 44 studies in humans have shown that low doses of Mg^{2+} supplementation, for example 243 mg/day can significantly lower BP in patients with uncomplicated HTN, treated six months or longer with antihypertensive drugs [119]. Moreover, the researchers reported that patients with MgD require higher doses of antihypertensive drugs compared to those with normal Mg^{2+} concentration [118]. The evidence supporting the cause–consequence antihypertensive effect of Mg^{2+} in adults suggest that oral Mg^{2+} supplements may be recommended for the prevention of arterial HTN or as adjuvant antihypertensive therapy [11]. It should be noted that MgD is not found in all patients with HTN. On the other hand, not all people with hypomagnesemia have high BP. These differences are probably due to the fact that patients with high BP do not constitute a homogenous group [78]. This may be one of the possible causes for the discrepancy between epidemiological and clinical data. Despite these discrepancies concerning Mg^{2+} status and high BP, some hypertensive patients constantly demonstrate hypomagnesemia. Among them are patients with obesity, insulin resistance, hypertriglyceridemia, severe forms of HTN, hyperaldosteronism (volume-dependent HTN), pregnancy induced HTN, and patients of African-American origin [120]. In view of the still ill-defined role of Mg^{2+} in clinical HTN, Mg^{2+} supplementation is advised in those hypertensive patients who are receiving diuretics, who have resistant or secondary HTN or who have frank MgD [121]. In the USA, the Estimated Average Requirement (EAR) and RDA of Mg^{2+} for adult women are set at 255–265 mg and 310–320 mg/day, respectively. The EAR and RDA of Mg^{2+} for adult men are set at 330–350 mg and 410–420 mg/day, respectively. These dietary reference intakes are based on data from 16 men and 18 women who have consumed self-selected diets and have had a decreased Mg^{2+} intake during the balance periods, which could have affected balance values [122,123]. The current RDA for Mg^{2+} ranges from 80 mg/day for children 1–3 years of age to 130 mg/day for children 4–8 years of age. For older males, the RDA for Mg^{2+} ranges from as low as 240 mg/day (range, 9–13 years of age) and increases to 420 mg/day for males 31–70 years of age and older. For females, the RDA ranges from 240 mg/day (9–13 years of age) to 360 mg/day for females 14–18 years of age. The RDA for females 31–70 years of age and older is 320 mg/day. Many nutritional experts feel the ideal intake for Mg^{2+} should be based on the body weight (e.g., 4–6 mg per kg/day) [4]. Intravenous Mg^{2+} supplementation may be more effective, but this treatment has the disadvantage that it requires regular hospital visits. The treatment regimen of intravenous Mg^{2+} supplementation normally consists of 8–12 g of Mg-sulfate in the first 24 h followed by 4–6 g/day for 3 or 4 days. When serum Mg^{2+} levels are extremely low or are accompanied by hypokalemia, Mg^{2+} supplementation may not be sufficient to restore normal Mg^{2+} levels. In that case, patients are often cosupplemented with K^+ or receive amiloride to prevent K^+ secretion [124]. Recent reports indicate that individuals with serum Mg^{2+} concentrations >0.75 mmol/L, or high as 0.85 mmol/L, could be Mg^{2+}-deficient. Thus, to assess Mg^{2+} status of an individual with a serum Mg^{2+} concentration between 0.75 and 0.85 mmol/L is requires additional measures of status. A urinary excretion of <80 mg (3.29 mmol)/day and/or dietary intake history showing a Mg^{2+} intake of <250 mg/day would support the presence of MgD [122]. In the treatment of MgD are recommended organic bound Mg^{2+} salts, such as Mg^{2+} citrate, gluconate, orotate, or aspartate, because of their high bioavailability [4,125].

Hypermagnesemia is a rare condition and is seen most often in patients with renal impairment who take medicines containing Mg^{2+}. Excessive intake of supplemental Mg^{2+} can result in adverse effects, especially in impaired renal function. Serum concentrations >8 mmol/L cause drowsiness, vasodilation, slowing of atrioventricular conduction, and hypotension [126–128].

3.2. *Food and Water Sources of Mg^{2+}*

3.2.1. Mg^{2+} Intake from Food

In the Western World, dietary intake of Mg^{2+} is subnormal, with shortfalls of between 65 and 225 mg of Mg^{2+}/day, depending upon geographic region. Several epidemiologic studies in North America and Europe have shown that children and adults, some which are pregnant women, consuming Western-type diets are low in Mg^{2+} content (i.e., 30–50% of the RDA for these populations) [129]. Epidemiological observations suggest a negative correlation between dietary Mg^{2+} intake and BP [11]. Overall, the current evidence supports the importance of adequate dietary Mg^{2+} intake for the reduction of BP and total CVD risk. These findings support the importance of increasing the consumption of Mg^{2+}-rich foods, including fruits, vegetables, nuts, and whole grains in the treatment and prevention of high BP [125].

A Mg^{2+}-rich diet should be encouraged in hypertensive subjects as well as in predisposed communities because of the advantages of such a diet in the prevention of HTN [121]. The Dietary Approaches to Stop HTN (DASH) diet (originally termed the "combination diet"4) contains larger amounts of Mg^{2+}, K^+, Ca^{2+}, dietary fiber, and protein and smaller amounts of total and saturated fat and cholesterol than the typical diet [130]. The Mediterranean diet is also rich in Mg^{2+}, dietary fiber, antioxidant capacity, and polyphenolic compounds [131]. In trials of vegetarian diets, replacing animal products with vegetable products reduced BP in normotensive and hypertensive people. Aspects of vegetarian diets believed to reduce BP include their high levels of fiber and minerals (such as Mg^{2+} and K^+) and their reduced fat content. In observational studies, significant inverse associations of BP with intake of Mg^{2+}, K^+, Ca^{2+}, and fiber have also been reported [132].

3.2.2. Mg^{2+} Intake from Water

Water is a variable source of Mg^{2+} intake. Typically, water with increased "hardness" has a higher concentration of Mg^{2+} salts. Since this varies depending on the area from which water comes, Mg^{2+} intake from water is usually not estimated to a sufficient extent. This omission may lead to impaired assessment and underestimation of total intake of Mg^{2+} in certain regions [123]. The modern processed food diet, which is low in Mg^{2+} and is spreading globally, makes this well-researched potential of drinking-water Mg^{2+} worth serious consideration, especially in areas where insufficient dietary intake of Mg^{2+} is prevalent. It would be wise and forward-thinking for public health officials to consider how high-Mg^{2+} drinking water might be made available to communities, i.e., water with Mg^{2+} levels of at least 10 mg/L and ideally 25–100 mg/L [133].

4. Conclusions

The enhancing effect of MgD on BP should be considered in the context of total intake and loss of Mg^{2+} in each individual patient with HTN. Special attention should be given to the risk groups in which serum Mg^{2+} levels should be monitored periodically. Considering the numerous positive effects of Mg^{2+} on a number of mechanisms related to HTN, consuming a healthy diet that provides the recommended amount of Mg^{2+} can be an appropriate strategy for helping control BP.

Author Contributions: K.K. designed the review, interpreted the data, and wrote the manuscript; K.K. and L.H. performed the literature research. The authors approved the final version of the manuscript.

Acknowledgments: This review was accomplished with the financial support from the Medical University-Pleven, Bulgaria.

Abbreviations

MgD	Magnesium deficiency
Mg^{2+}	Magnesium
Ca^{2+}	Calcium
K^+	Potassium
Na^+	Sodium
HTN	Hypertension
MetS	Metabolic syndrome
T2D	Type 2 diabetes
RDA	Recommended Dietary Allowance
EAR	Estimated Average Requirement
CVD	Cardiovascular diseases
BP	Blood pressure
WHO	World Health Organization
TRPM6	Transient receptor potential melastatin-6 channel
TRPM7	Transient receptor potential melastatin-7 channel

VSMCs	Vascular smooth muscle cells
ET-1	Endothelin-1
ATII	Angiotensin II
ALDO	Aldosterone
SHR	Spontaneously hypertensive rats
WKY	Wistar-Kyoto rats
EGF	Epidermal growth factor
PTH	Parathyroid hormone
IP3	Inositol-1,4,5-trisphosphate
PIP2	Phosphatidylinositol 4,5-bisphosphate
AT1	Angiotensin II receptor type 1
ETA	Endothelin A receptor
V1a	Vasopressin receptor 1a
PLC	Phospholipase C
PKC	Protein kinase C
PGI_2	Prostacyclin
NO	Nitric oxide
RBCs	Red blood cells
eNOS	Endothelial nitric oxide synthase
PGE_1	Prostaglandin E_1
RAAS	Renin-Angiotensin-Aldosterone System
NA	Noradrenaline
Adr	Adrenaline
CA	Catecholamines
ACh	Acetylcholine
ADCY	Adenylate cyclase
ISO	Isoproterenol
CRP	C-reactive protein
IL	Interleukin
TNF-α	Tumor necrosis factor-α
VCAM	Vascular cell adhesion molecule-1
PAI-1	Plasminogen activator inhibitor-1
ECM	Extracellular matrix
HAS	Hyaluronan synthases
HYAL	Hyaluronidase
TG2	Transglutaminase
LOX	Lysyl oxidase
MMPs	Matrix metalloproteinases
TIMPs	Tissue inhibitors of metalloproteinases
NF-κB	Nuclear factor kappa B
LDL	Low-density lipoproteins
HDL	High-density lipoproteins
IR	Insulin receptor
MAPK	Mitogen-activated protein kinase
PI3K	Phosphoinositide 3-kinase
PIP2	Phosphatidylinositol 4,5-bisphosphate
GLUT4	Glucose transporter type 4
IRTK	Insulin receptor tyrosine kinase
CNS	Central nervous system
HPAA	Hypothalamic Pituitary Adrenal Axis
ACTH	Adrenocorticotropic hormone
NMDA	*N*-methyl-D-aspartate receptor
mGluRs	Metabotropic glutamate receptors
GABA	Gamma-aminobutyric acid
COMT	Catechol-*O*-methyl transferase
MGL	Magnesium low blood levels
MGH	Magnesium high blood levels

References

1. Ismail, A.A.; Ismail, N.A. Magnesium: A mineral essential for health yet generally underestimated or even ignored. *J. Nutr. Food Sci.* **2016**, *6*, 2. [CrossRef]
2. Choi, M.K.; Bae, Y.J. Association of magnesium intake with high blood pressure in Korean adults: Korea national health and nutrition examination survey 2007–2009. *PLoS ONE* **2015**, *10*, e0130405. [CrossRef] [PubMed]
3. Swaminathan, R. Magnesium metabolism and its disorders. *Clin. Biochem. Rev.* **2003**, *24*, 47. [PubMed]
4. Gröber, U.; Schmidt, J.; Kisters, K. Magnesium in prevention and therapy. *Nutrients* **2015**, *7*, 8199–8226. [CrossRef] [PubMed]
5. De Baaij, J.H.; Hoenderop, J.G.; Bindels, R.J. Regulation of magnesium balance: Lessons learned from human genetic disease. *Clin. Kidney J.* **2012**, *5*, i15–i24. [CrossRef] [PubMed]
6. Seo, J.W.; Park, T.J. Magnesium metabolism. *Electrolyte Blood Press.* **2008**, *6*, 86–95. [CrossRef] [PubMed]
7. Anand, G.; Konrad, M.; Heuss, L.T.; Schorn, R. A Case of Severe Hypomagnesaemia. *Open J. Nephrol.* **2013**, *3*, 66. [CrossRef]
8. Qu, X.; Jin, F.; Hao, Y.; Li, H.; Tang, T.; Wang, H.; Yan, W.; Dai, K. Magnesium and the risk of cardiovascular events: A meta-analysis of prospective cohort studies. *PLoS ONE* **2013**, *8*, e57720. [CrossRef] [PubMed]
9. Kass, L.; Sullivan, K.R. Low Dietary Magnesium Intake and Hypertension. *World J. Cardiovasc. Dis.* **2016**, *6*, 447. [CrossRef]
10. Galan, P.; Preziosi, P.; Durlach, V.; Valeix, P.; Ribas, L.; Bouzid, D.; Favier, A.; Hercberg, S. Dietary magnesium intake in a French adult population. *Magnes. Res.* **1997**, *10*, 321–328. [PubMed]
11. Zhang, X.; Li, Y.; Del Gobbo, L.C.; Rosanoff, A.; Wang, J.; Zhang, W.; Song, Y. Effects of magnesium supplementation on blood pressure: A meta-analysis of randomized double-blind placebo-controlled trials. *Hypertension* **2016**, *68*, 324–333. [CrossRef] [PubMed]
12. Harvey, A.; Montezano, A.C.; Lopes, R.A.; Rios, F.; Touyz, R.M. Vascular fibrosis in aging and hypertension: Molecular mechanisms and clinical implications. *Can. J. Cardiol.* **2016**, *32*, 659–668. [CrossRef] [PubMed]
13. Landau, R.; Scott, J.A.; Smiley, R.M. Magnesium-induced vasodilation in the dorsal hand vein. *BJOG* **2004**, *111*, 446–451. [CrossRef] [PubMed]
14. Cunha, A.R.; Medeiros, F.; Umbelino, B.; Oigman, W.; Touyz, R.M.; Neves, M.F. Altered vascular structure and wave reflection in hypertensive women with low magnesium levels. *J. Am. Soc. Hypertens.* **2013**, *7*, 344–352. [CrossRef] [PubMed]
15. Touyz, R.M.; Yao, G. Modulation of vascular smooth muscle cell growth by magnesium-role of mitogen-activated protein kinases. *J. Cell. Physiol.* **2003**, *197*, 326–335. [CrossRef] [PubMed]
16. Belin, R.J.; He, K. Magnesium physiology and pathogenic mechanisms that contribute to the development of the metabolic syndrome. *Magnes. Res.* **2007**, *20*, 107–129. [PubMed]
17. Houston, M. The role of magnesium in hypertension and cardiovascular disease. *J. Clin. Hypertens. (Greenwich)* **2011**, *13*, 843–847. [CrossRef] [PubMed]
18. Paravicini, T.M.; Chubanov, V.; Gudermann, T. TRPM7: A unique channel involved in magnesium homeostasis. *Int. J. Biochem. Cell Biol.* **2012**, *44*, 1381–1384. [CrossRef] [PubMed]
19. Baldoli, E.; Castiglioni, S.; Maier, J.A. Regulation and function of TRPM7 in human endothelial cells: TRPM7 as a potential novel regulator of endothelial function. *PLoS ONE* **2013**, *8*, e59891. [CrossRef] [PubMed]
20. Antunes, T.T.; Callera, G.E.; He, Y.; Yogi, A.; Ryazanov, A.G.; Ryazanova, L.V.; Zhai, A.; Stewart, D.J.; Shrier, A.; Touyz, R.M. Transient receptor potential melastatin 7 cation channel kinase: New player in angiotensin II-induced hypertension. *Hypertension* **2016**, *67*, 763–773. [CrossRef] [PubMed]
21. Touyz, R.M.; He, Y.; Montezano, A.C.; Yao, G.; Chubanov, V.; Gudermann, T.; Callera, G.E. Differential regulation of transient receptor potential melastatin 6 and 7 cation channels by ANG II in vascular smooth muscle cells from spontaneously hypertensive rats. *Am. J. Physiol. Regul. Integr. Comp. Physiol.* **2006**, *290*, R73–R78. [CrossRef] [PubMed]
22. Baldoli, E.; Maier, J.A. Silencing TRPM7 mimics the effects of magnesium deficiency in human microvascular endothelial cells. *Angiogenesis* **2012**, *15*, 47–57. [CrossRef] [PubMed]
23. Di, A.; Malik, A.B. TRP channels and the control of vascular function. *Curr. Opin. Pharmacol.* **2010**, *10*, 127–132. [CrossRef] [PubMed]

24. Groenestege, W.M.T.; Thébault, S.; van der Wijst, J.; van den Berg, D.; Janssen, R.; Tejpar, S.; van den Heuvel, L.P.; van Cutsem, E.; Hoenderop, J.G.; Knoers, N.V.; et al. Impaired basolateral sorting of pro-EGF causes isolated recessive renal hypomagnesemia. *J. Clin. Investig.* **2007**, *117*, 2260–2267. [CrossRef] [PubMed]
25. Thebault, S.; Alexander, R.T.; Groenestege, W.M.T.; Hoenderop, J.G.; Bindels, R.J. EGF increases TRPM6 activity and surface expression. *J. Am. Soc. Nephrol.* **2009**, *20*, 78–85. [CrossRef] [PubMed]
26. Groenestege, W.M.T.; Hoenderop, J.G.; van den Heuvel, L.; Knoers, N.; Bindels, R.J. The epithelial Mg^{2+} channel transient receptor potential melastatin 6 is regulated by dietary Mg^{2+} content and estrogens. *J. Am. Soc. Nephrol.* **2006**, *17*, 1035–1043. [CrossRef] [PubMed]
27. Cao, G.; van der Wijst, J.; van der Kemp, A.; van Zeeland, F.; Bindels, R.J.; Hoenderop, J.G. Regulation of the epithelial Mg^{2+} channel TRPM6 by estrogen and the associated repressor protein of estrogen receptor activity (REA). *J. Biol. Chem.* **2009**, *284*, 14788–14795. [CrossRef] [PubMed]
28. Van Der Wijst, J.; Hoenderop, J.G.; Bindels, R.J. Epithelial Mg^{2+} channel TRPM6: Insight into the molecular regulation. *Magnes. Res.* **2009**, *22*, 127–132. [PubMed]
29. Mubagwa, K.; Gwanyanya, A.; Zakharov, S.; Macianskiene, R. Regulation of cation channels in cardiac and smooth muscle cells by intracellular magnesium. *Arch. Biochem. Biophys.* **2007**, *458*, 73–89. [CrossRef] [PubMed]
30. Ritchie, G.; Kerstan, D.; Dai, L.J.; Kang, H.S.; Canaff, L.; Hendy, G.N.; Quamme, G.A. $1,25(OH)_2D3$ stimulates Mg^{2+} uptake into MDCT cells: Modulation by extracellular Ca^{2+} and Mg^{2+}. *Am. J. Physiol. Ren. Physiol.* **2001**, *280*, F868–F878. [CrossRef] [PubMed]
31. Hagström, E.; Ahlström, T.; Ärnlöv, J.; Larsson, A.; Melhus, H.; Hellman, P.; Lind, L. Parathyroid hormone and calcium are independently associated with subclinical vascular disease in a community-based cohort. *Atherosclerosis* **2015**, *238*, 420–426. [CrossRef] [PubMed]
32. Jahnen-Dechent, W.; Ketteler, M. Magnesium basics. *Clin. Kidney J.* **2012**, *5*, i3–i14. [CrossRef] [PubMed]
33. Louvet, L.; Bazin, D.; Büchel, J.; Steppan, S.; Passlick-Deetjen, J.; Massy, Z.A. Characterisation of calcium phosphate crystals on calcified human aortic vascular smooth muscle cells and potential role of magnesium. *PLoS ONE* **2015**, *10*, e0115342. [CrossRef] [PubMed]
34. Chakraborti, S.; Chakraborti, T.; Mandal, M.; Mandal, A.; Das, S.; Ghosh, S. Protective role of magnesium in cardiovascular diseases: A review. *Mol. Cell. Biochem.* **2002**, *238*, 163–179. [CrossRef] [PubMed]
35. Villa-Bellosta, R. Impact of magnesium: Calcium ratio on calcification of the aortic wall. *PLoS ONE* **2017**, *12*, e0178872. [CrossRef] [PubMed]
36. Kolte, D.; Vijayaraghavan, K.; Khera, S.; Sica, D.A.; Frishman, W.H. Role of magnesium in cardiovascular diseases. *Cardiol. Rev.* **2014**, *22*, 182–192. [CrossRef] [PubMed]
37. Cunha, A.R.; Umbelino, B.; Correia, M.L.; Neves, M.F. Magnesium and vascular changes in hypertension. *Int. J. Hypertens.* **2012**, *2012*, 754250. [CrossRef] [PubMed]
38. Sontia, B.; Touyz, R.M. Role of magnesium in hypertension. *Arch. Biochem. Biophys.* **2007**, *458*, 33–39. [CrossRef] [PubMed]
39. Kharitonova, M.; Iezhitsa, I.; Zheltova, A.; Ozerov, A.; Spasov, A.; Skalny, A. Comparative angioprotective effects of magnesium compounds. *J. Trace Elem. Med. Biol.* **2015**, *29*, 227–234. [CrossRef] [PubMed]
40. Laurant, P.; Dalle, M.; Berthelot, A.; Rayssiguier, Y. Time-course of the change in blood pressure level in magnesium-deficient Wistar rats. *Br. J. Nutr.* **1999**, *82*, 243–251. [PubMed]
41. Cantin, M. Relationship of juxtaglomerular apparatus and adrenal cortex to biochemical and extracellular fluid volume changes in magnesium deficiency. *Lab. Investig.* **1970**, *22*, 558–568. [PubMed]
42. James, M.F.; Beer, R.E.; Esser, J.D. Intravenous magnesium sulfate inhibits catecholamine release associated with tracheal intubation. *Anesth. Analg.* **1989**, *68*, 772–776. [CrossRef] [PubMed]
43. Douglas, W.W.; Rubin, R.P. The mechanism of catecholamine release from the adrenal medulla and the role of calcium in stimulus-secretion coupling. *J. Physiol.* **1963**, *167*, 288–310. [CrossRef] [PubMed]
44. Torshin, I.Y.; Gromova, O.A.; Gusev, E.I. Mechanisms of antistress and antidepressant action of magnesium and pyridoxine. *Korsakov's J. Neurol. Psychiatry* **2009**, *109*, 107–111.
45. Oka, M.; Ohuchi, T.; Yoshida, H.; Imaizumi, R. Stimulatory effect of adenosine triphosphate and magnesium on the release of catecholamines from adrenal medullary granules. *Jpn. J. Pharmacol.* **1967**, *17*, 199–207. [CrossRef] [PubMed]
46. Farmer, J.B.; Campbell, I.K. Calcium and magnesium ions: Influence on the response of an isolated artery to sympathetic nerve stimulation, noradrenaline and tyramine. *Br. J. Pharmacol.* **1967**, *29*, 319–328. [CrossRef]

47. Whyte, K.F.; Addis, G.J.; Whitesmith, R.; Reid, J.L. Adrenergic control of plasma magnesium in man. *Clin. Sci.* **1987**, *72*, 135–138. [CrossRef] [PubMed]
48. Joborn, H.; Akerström, G.; Ljunghall, S. Effects of exogenous catecholamines and exercise on plasma magnesium concentrations. *Clin. Endocrinol.* **1985**, *23*, 219–226. [CrossRef]
49. Keenan, D.; Romani, A.; Scarpa, A. Differential regulation of circulating Mg^{2+} in the rat by β_1-and β_2-adrenergic receptor stimulation. *Circ. Res.* **1995**, *77*, 973–983. [CrossRef] [PubMed]
50. Boos, C.J.; Lip, G.Y. Is hypertension an inflammatory process? *Curr. Pharm. Des.* **2006**, *12*, 1623–1635. [CrossRef] [PubMed]
51. Arnaud, M.J. Update on the assessment of magnesium status. *Br. J. Nutr.* **2008**, *99*, S24–S36. [CrossRef] [PubMed]
52. Barbagallo, M.; Belvedere, M.; Dominguez, L.J. Magnesium homeostasis and aging. *Magnes. Res.* **2009**, *22*, 235–246. [PubMed]
53. King, D.E.; Mainous, A.G., III; Geesey, M.E.; Ellis, T. Magnesium intake and serum C-reactive protein levels in children. *Magnes. Res.* **2007**, *20*, 32–36. [PubMed]
54. King, D.E.; Mainous, A.G., III; Geesey, M.E.; Woolson, R.F. Dietary magnesium and C-reactive protein levels. *J. Am. Coll. Nutr.* **2005**, *24*, 166–171. [CrossRef] [PubMed]
55. Kim, D.J.; Xun, P.; Liu, K.; Loria, C.; Yokota, K.; Jacobs, D.R.; He, K. Magnesium intake in relation to systemic inflammation, insulin resistance, and the incidence of diabetes. *Diabetes Care* **2010**, *33*, 2604–2610. [CrossRef] [PubMed]
56. Maier, J.A.; Malpuech-Brugère, C.; Zimowska, W.; Rayssiguier, Y.; Mazur, A. Low magnesium promotes endothelial cell dysfunction: Implications for atherosclerosis, inflammation and thrombosis. *Biochim. Biophys. Acta Mol. Basis Dis.* **2004**, *1689*, 13–21. [CrossRef] [PubMed]
57. Friese, R.S.; Rao, F.; Khandrika, S.; Thomas, B.; Ziegler, M.G.; Schmid-Schönbein, G.W.; O'Connor, D.T. Matrix metalloproteinases: Discrete elevations in essential hypertension and hypertensive end-stage renal disease. *Clin. Exp. Hypertens.* **2009**, *31*, 521–533. [CrossRef] [PubMed]
58. Heagerty, A.M.; Aalkjaer, C.; Bund, S.J.; Korsgaard, N.; Mulvany, M.J. Small artery structure in hypertension. Dual processes of remodeling and growth. *Hypertension* **1993**, *21*, 391–397. [CrossRef] [PubMed]
59. Mulvany, M.J.; Baumbach, G.L.; Aalkjaer, C.; Heagerty, A.M.; Korsgaard, N.; Schiffrin, E.L.; Heistad, D.D. Vascular remodeling. *Hypertension* **1996**, *28*, 505–506. [PubMed]
60. Mulvany, M.J. Small artery remodeling and significance in the development of hypertension. *Physiology* **2002**, *17*, 105–109. [CrossRef]
61. Steppan, J.; Bergman, Y.; Viegas, K.; Armstrong, D.; Tan, S.; Wang, H.; Melucci, S.; Hori, D.; Park, S.Y.; Barreto, S.F.; et al. Tissue transglutaminase modulates vascular stiffness and function through crosslinking-dependent and crosslinking-independent functions. *J. Am. Heart. Assoc.* **2017**, *6*, e004161. [CrossRef] [PubMed]
62. Bains, W. Transglutaminse 2 and EGGL, the protein cross-link formed by transglutaminse 2, as therapeutic targets for disabilities of old age. *Rejuvenation Res.* **2013**, *16*, 495–517. [CrossRef] [PubMed]
63. Torshin, I.Y.; Gromova, O.A. Connective tissue dysplasia, cell biology and molecular mechanisms of magnesium exposure. *RMZh* **2008**, *16*, 230–238.
64. Martínez-Revelles, S.; García-Redondo, A.B.; Avendaño, M.S.; Varona, S.; Palao, T.; Orriols, M.; Roque, F.R.; Fortuño, A.; Touyz, R.M.; Martínez-González, J.; et al. Lysyl oxidase induces vascular oxidative stress and contributes to arterial stiffness and abnormal elastin structure in hypertension: Role of p38MAPK. *Antioxid. Redox Signal.* **2017**, *27*, 379–397. [CrossRef] [PubMed]
65. Avtandilov, A.G.; Pukhaeva, A.A.; Manizer, E.D. Magnesium and mitral valve prolapse. Efficiency and application points. *Ration. Pharmacother. Card.* **2010**, *6*, 677–684. [CrossRef]
66. Maier, J.A. Endothelial cells and magnesium: Implications in atherosclerosis. *Clin. Sci.* **2012**, *122*, 397–407. [CrossRef] [PubMed]
67. Dolinsky, B.M.; Ippolito, D.L.; Tinnemore, D.; Stallings, J.D.; Zelig, C.M.; Napolitano, P.G. The effect of magnesium sulfate on the activity of matrix metalloproteinase-9 in fetal cord plasma and human umbilical vein endothelial cells. *Am. J. Obstet. Gynecol.* **2010**, *203*, 371e1–371e5. [CrossRef] [PubMed]
68. Kostov, K. Pathophysiological Role of Endothelin-1, Matrix Metalloproteinases-2, -9 and Magnesium in the Development and Dynamics of Vascular Changes at Various Degrees of Arterial Hypertension. Doctoral Disertation, Medical University of Pleven, Pleven, Bulgaria, 2 December 2016. Available online: http://www.mu-pleven.bg/procedures/59/Avtoreferat.pdf (accessed on 1 December 2016).

69. Ferrè, S.; Baldoli, E.; Leidi, M.; Maier, J.A. Magnesium deficiency promotes a pro-atherogenic phenotype in cultured human endothelial cells via activation of NFkB. *Biochim. Biophys. Acta Mol. Basis Dis.* **2010**, *1802*, 952–958. [CrossRef] [PubMed]
70. Yue, H.; Lee, J.D.; Shimizu, H.; Uzui, H.; Mitsuke, Y.; Ueda, T. Effects of magnesium on the production of extracellular matrix metalloproteinases in cultured rat vascular smooth muscle cells. *Atherosclerosis* **2003**, *166*, 271–277. [CrossRef]
71. Yue, H.; Uzui, H.; Lee, J.D.; Shimizu, H.; Ueda, T. Effects of magnesium on matrix metalloproteinase-2 production in cultured rat cardiac fibroblasts. *Basic Res. Cardiol.* **2004**, *99*, 257–263. [CrossRef] [PubMed]
72. Altura, B.M. Insights into the possible mechanisms by which platelet-activating factor and PAF-receptors function in vascular smooth muscle in magnesium deficiency and vascular remodeling: Possible links to atherogenesis, hypertension and cardiac failure. *Int. J. Cardiol. Res.* **2016**, *3*, 1–3.
73. Kisters, K.; Gröber, U. Magnesium in health and disease. *Plant Soil* **2013**, *368*, 155–165. [CrossRef]
74. Sakaguchi, Y.; Fujii, N.; Shoji, T.; Hayashi, T.; Rakugi, H.; Isaka, Y. Hypomagnesemia is a significant predictor of cardiovascular and non-cardiovascular mortality in patients undergoing hemodialysis. *Kidney Int.* **2014**, *85*, 174–181. [CrossRef] [PubMed]
75. Mishra, S.; Padmanaban, P.; Deepti, G.N.; Sarkar, G.; Sumathi, S.; Toora, B.D. Serum magnesium and dyslipidemia in type 2 diabetes mellitus. *Biomed. Res.* **2012**, *23*, 295–300.
76. King, D.E. Inflammation and elevation of C-reactive protein: Does magnesium play a key role? *Magnes. Res.* **2009**, *22*, 57–59. [PubMed]
77. Barbagallo, M.; Dominguez, L.J. Magnesium metabolism in type 2 diabetes mellitus, metabolic syndrome and insulin resistance. *Arch. Biochem. Biophys.* **2007**, *458*, 40–47. [CrossRef] [PubMed]
78. Geiger, H.; Wanner, C. Magnesium in disease. *Clin. Kidney J.* **2012**, *5*, i25–i38. [CrossRef] [PubMed]
79. Kostov, K.; Blazhev, A.; Atanasova, M.; Dimitrova, A. Serum concentrations of endothelin-1 and matrix metalloproteinases-2,-9 in pre-hypertensive and hypertensive patients with type 2 diabetes. *Int. J. Mol. Sci.* **2016**, *17*, 1182. [CrossRef] [PubMed]
80. De Boer, I.H.; Bangalore, S.; Benetos, A.; Davis, A.M.; Michos, E.D.; Muntner, P.; Rossing, P.; Zoungas, S.; Bakris, G. Diabetes and hypertension: A position statement by the American Diabetes Association. *Diabetes Care* **2017**, *40*, 1273–1284. [CrossRef] [PubMed]
81. Guerrero-Romero, F.; Bermudez-Peña, C.; Rodríguez-Morán, M. Severe hypomagnesemia and low-grade inflammation in metabolic syndrome. *Magnes. Res.* **2011**, *24*, 45–53. [PubMed]
82. Nielsen, F.H. Magnesium, inflammation, and obesity in chronic disease. *Nutr. Rev.* **2010**, *68*, 333–340. [CrossRef] [PubMed]
83. Chaudhary, D.P.; Sharma, R.; Bansal, D.D. Implications of magnesium deficiency in type 2 diabetes: A review. *Biol. Trace Elem. Res.* **2010**, *134*, 119–129. [CrossRef] [PubMed]
84. Günther, T. The biochemical function of Mg^{2+} in insulin secretion, insulin signal transduction and insulin resistance. *Magnes. Res.* **2010**, *23*, 5–18. [PubMed]
85. Rosolova, H.; Mayer, O., Jr.; Reaven, G.M. Insulin-mediated glucose disposal is decreased in normal subjects with relatively low plasma magnesium concentrations. *Metabolism* **2000**, *49*, 418–420. [CrossRef]
86. Venu, L.; Padmavathi, I.J.; Kishore, Y.D.; Bhanu, N.V.; Rao, K.R.; Sainath, P.B.; Ganeshan, M.; Raghunath, M. Long-term effects of maternal magnesium restriction on adiposity and insulin resistance in rat pups. *Obesity* **2008**, *16*, 1270–1276. [CrossRef] [PubMed]
87. Suarez, A.; Pulido, N.; Casla, A.; Casanova, B.; Arrieta, F.J.; Rovira, A. Impaired tyrosine-kinase activity of muscle insulin receptors from hypomagnesaemic rats. *Diabetologia* **1995**, *38*, 1262–1270. [CrossRef] [PubMed]
88. Barbagallo, M.; Dominguez, L.J. Magnesium and the cardiometabolic syndrome. *Curr. Nutr. Rep.* **2012**, *1*, 100–108. [CrossRef]
89. Ward, C.W.; Lawrence, M.C. Ligand-induced activation of the insulin receptor: A multi-step process involving structural changes in both the ligand and the receptor. *Bioessays* **2009**, *31*, 422–434. [CrossRef] [PubMed]
90. Jensen, M.; Hansen, B.; De Meyts, P.; Schäffer, L.; Ursø, B. Activation of the insulin receptor by insulin and a synthetic peptide leads to divergent metabolic and mitogenic signaling and responses. *J. Biol. Chem.* **2007**, *282*, 35179–35186. [CrossRef] [PubMed]
91. Farese, R.V.; Sajan, M.P.; Standaert, M.L. Insulin-sensitive protein kinases (atypical protein kinase C and protein kinase B/Akt): Actions and defects in obesity and type II diabetes. *Exp. Biol. Med.* **2005**, *230*, 593–605. [CrossRef]

92. Sale, E.M.; Sale, G.J. Protein kinase B: Signalling roles and therapeutic targeting. *Cell. Mol. Life Sci.* **2008**, *65*, 113–127. [CrossRef] [PubMed]
93. Sano, H.; Kane, S.; Sano, E.; Mîinea, C.P.; Asara, J.M.; Lane, W.S.; Garner, C.W.; Lienhard, G.E. Insulin-stimulated phosphorylation of a Rab GTPase-activating protein regulates GLUT4 translocation. *J. Biol. Chem.* **2003**, *278*, 14599–14602. [CrossRef] [PubMed]
94. Siddle, K. Signalling by insulin and IGF receptors: Supporting acts and new players. *J. Mol. Endocrinol.* **2011**, *47*, R1–R10. [CrossRef] [PubMed]
95. Barbagallo, M.; Gupta, R.K.; Bardicef, O.; Bardicef, M.; Resnick, L.M. Altered ionic effects of insulin in hypertension: Role of basal ion levels in determining cellular responsiveness. *J. Clin. Endocrinol. Metab.* **1997**, *82*, 1761–1765. [CrossRef] [PubMed]
96. Rodríguez-Morán, M.; Guerrero-Romero, F. Oral magnesium supplementation improves insulin sensitivity and metabolic control in type 2 diabetic subjects: A randomized double-blind controlled trial. *Diabetes Care* **2003**, *26*, 1147–1152. [CrossRef] [PubMed]
97. Häring, H.U. The insulin receptor: Signalling mechanism and contribution to the pathogenesis of insulin resistance. *Diabetologia* **1991**, *34*, 848–861. [CrossRef] [PubMed]
98. Nadler, J.L.; Rude, R.K. Disorders of magnesium metabolism. *Endocrinol. Metab. Clin. N. Am.* **1995**, *24*, 623–641.
99. Chaudhary, D.P.; Boparai, R.K.; Sharma, R.; Bansal, D.D. Studies on the development of an insulin resistant rat model by chronic feeding of low magnesium high sucrose diet. *Magnes. Res.* **2004**, *17*, 293–300. [PubMed]
100. Lopez-Ridaura, R.; Willett, W.C.; Rimm, E.B.; Liu, S.; Stampfer, M.J.; Manson, J.E.; Hu, F.B. Magnesium intake and risk of type 2 diabetes in men and women. *Diabetes Care* **2004**, *27*, 134–140. [CrossRef] [PubMed]
101. Van Dam, R.M.; Hu, F.B.; Rosenberg, L.; Krishnan, S.; Palmer, J.R. Dietary calcium and magnesium, major food sources, and risk of type 2 diabetes in US black women. *Diabetes Care* **2006**, *29*, 2238–2243. [CrossRef] [PubMed]
102. Mooren, F.C.; Krüger, K.; Völker, K.; Golf, S.W.; Wadepuhl, M.; Kraus, A. Oral magnesium supplementation reduces insulin resistance in non-diabetic subjects—A double-blind, placebo-controlled, randomized trial. *Diabetes Obes. Metab.* **2011**, *13*, 281–284. [CrossRef] [PubMed]
103. Kalra, S.S.; Shanahan, C.M. Vascular calcification and hypertension: Cause and effect. *Ann. Med.* **2012**, *44*, S85–S92. [CrossRef] [PubMed]
104. Floege, J. Magnesium in CKD: More than a calcification inhibitor? *J. Neurol.* **2015**, *28*, 269–277. [CrossRef] [PubMed]
105. Hruby, A.; O'Donnell, C.J.; Jacques, P.F.; Meigs, J.B.; Hoffmann, U.; McKeown, N.M. Magnesium intake is inversely associated with coronary artery calcification: The Framingham Heart Study. *JACC Cardiovasc. Imaging* **2014**, *7*, 59–69. [CrossRef] [PubMed]
106. Barbagallo, M.; Dominguez, L.J. Magnesium, oxidative stress, and aging muscle. *Aging* **2014**, 157–166. [CrossRef]
107. Lakatta, E.G. The reality of aging viewed from the arterial wall. *Artery Res.* **2013**, *7*, 73–80. [CrossRef] [PubMed]
108. Agyei, B.; Nicolaou, M.; Boateng, L.; Dijkshoorn, H.; Agyemang, C. Relationship between psychosocial stress and hypertension among Ghanaians in Amsterdam, the Netherlands–the GHAIA study. *BMC Public Health* **2014**, *14*, 692. [CrossRef] [PubMed]
109. Pochwat, B.; Szewczyk, B.; Sowa-Kucma, M.; Siwek, A.; Doboszewska, U.; Piekoszewski, W.; Gruca, P.; Papp, M.; Nowak, G. Antidepressant-like activity of magnesium in the chronic mild stress model in rats: Alterations in the NMDA receptor subunits. *Int. J. Neuropsychopharmacol.* **2014**, *17*, 393–405. [CrossRef] [PubMed]
110. Rayssiguier, Y.; Libako, P.; Nowacki, W.; Rock, E. Magnesium deficiency and metabolic syndrome: Stress and inflammation may reflect calcium activation. *Magnes. Res.* **2010**, *23*, 73–80. [PubMed]
111. Boyle, N.B.; Lawton, C.; Dye, L. The effects of magnesium supplementation on subjective anxiety and stress–a systematic review. *Nutrients* **2017**, *9*, 429. [CrossRef] [PubMed]
112. Amyard, N.; Leyris, A.; Monier, C.; Frances, H.; Boulu, R.G.; Henrotte, J.G. Brain catecholamines, serotonin and their metabolites in mice selected for low (MGL) and high (MGH) blood magnesium levels. *Magnes. Res.* **1995**, *8*, 5–9. [PubMed]
113. Henrotte, J.G.; Franck, G.; Santarromana, M.; Francès, H.; Mouton, D.; Motta, R. Mice selected for low and high blood magnesium levels: A new model for stress studies. *Physiol. Behav.* **1997**, *61*, 653–658. [CrossRef]
114. Henrotte, J.G. Type A behavior and magnesium metabolism. *Magnesium* **1986**, *5*, 201–210. [PubMed]
115. Ryzen, E.; Servis, K.L.; Rude, R.K. Effect of intravenous epinephrine on serum magnesium and free intracellular red blood cell magnesium concentrations measured by nuclear magnetic resonance. *J. Am. Coll. Nutr.* **1990**, *9*, 114–119. [CrossRef] [PubMed]

116. Han, H.; Fang, X.; Wei, X.; Liu, Y.; Jin, Z.; Chen, Q.; Fan, Z.; Aaseth, J.; Hiyoshi, A.; He, J.; et al. Dose-response relationship between dietary magnesium intake, serum magnesium concentration and risk of hypertension: A systematic review and meta-analysis of prospective cohort studies. *Nutr. J.* **2017**, *16*, 26. [CrossRef] [PubMed]
117. Ma, J.; Folsom, A.R.; Melnick, S.L.; Eckfeldt, J.H.; Sharrett, A.R.; Nabulsi, A.A.; Hutchinson, R.G.; Metcalf, P.A. Associations of serum and dietary magnesium with cardiovascular disease, hypertension, diabetes, insulin, and carotid arterial wall thickness: The ARIC study. *J. Clin. Epidemiol.* **1995**, *48*, 927–940. [CrossRef]
118. Whang, R.; Chrysant, S.; Dillard, B.; Smith, W.; Fryer, A. Hypomagnesemia and hypokalemia in 1,000 treated ambulatory hypertensive patients. *J. Am. Coll. Nutr.* **1982**, *1*, 317–322. [CrossRef] [PubMed]
119. Rosanoff, A. Magnesium supplements may enhance the effect of antihypertensive medications in stage 1 hypertensive subjects. *Magnes. Res.* **2010**, *23*, 27–40. [PubMed]
120. Touyz, R.M. Magnesium in clinical medicine. *Front. Biosci.* **2004**, *9*, 1278–1293. [CrossRef] [PubMed]
121. Touyz, R.M. Role of magnesium in the pathogenesis of hypertension. *Mol. Aspects Med.* **2003**, *24*, 107–136. [CrossRef]
122. Nielsen, F.H. Guidance for the determination of status indicators and dietary requirements for magnesium. *Magnes. Res.* **2016**, *29*, 154–160. [PubMed]
123. Standing Committee on the Scientific Evaluation of Dietary Reference Intakes; Food and Nutrition Board; Institute of Medicine (IOM). *Dietary Reference Intakes for Calcium, Phosphorus, Magnesium, Vitamin D, and Fluoride*; National Academies Press: Washington, DC, USA, 1997.
124. De Baaij, J.H.; Hoenderop, J.G.; Bindels, R.J. Magnesium in man: Implications for health and disease. *Physiol. Rev.* **2015**, *95*, 1–46. [CrossRef] [PubMed]
125. Rosique-Esteban, N.; Guasch-Ferré, M.; Hernández-Alonso, P.; Salas-Salvadó, J. Dietary Magnesium and Cardiovascular Disease: A Review with Emphasis in Epidemiological Studies. *Nutrients* **2018**, *10*, 168. [CrossRef] [PubMed]
126. Crosby, V.; Elin, R.J.; Twycross, R.; Mihalyo, M.; Wilcock, A. Magnesium. *J. Pain Symptom Manag.* **2013**, *45*, 137–144. [CrossRef] [PubMed]
127. Nishikawa, M.; Shimada, N.; Kanzaki, M.; Ikegami, T.; Fukuoka, T.; Fukushima, M.; Asano, K. The characteristics of patients with hypermagnesemia who underwent emergency hemodialysis. *Acute Med. Surg.* **2018**, *5*, 1–2. [CrossRef]
128. Celi, L.A.; Scott, D.J.; Lee, J.; Nelson, R.; Alper, S.L.; Mukamal, K.J.; Mark, R.G.; Danziger, J. Association of hypermagnesemia and blood pressure in the critically ill. *J. Hypertens.* **2013**, *31*, 2136. [CrossRef] [PubMed]
129. Altura, B.M.; Li, W.; Zhang, A.; Zheng, T.; Shah, N.C. Sudden cardiac death in infants, children and young adults: Possible roles of dietary magnesium intake and generation of platelet-activating factor in coronary arteries. *J. Heart Health* **2016**, *2*, 1–5.
130. Sacks, F.M.; Svetkey, L.P.; Vollmer, W.M.; Appel, L.J.; Bray, G.A.; Harsha, D.; Obarzanek, E.; Conlin, P.R.; Miller, E.R., 3rd; Simons-Morton, D.G.; et al. Effects on blood pressure of reduced dietary sodium and the Dietary Approaches to Stop Hypertension (DASH) diet. *N. Engl. J. Med.* **2001**, *344*, 3–10. [CrossRef] [PubMed]
131. Park, Y.M.; Steck, S.E.; Fung, T.T.; Zhang, J.; Hazlett, L.J.; Han, K.; Lee, S.H.; Kwon, H.S.; Merchant, A.T. Mediterranean diet, Dietary Approaches to Stop Hypertension (DASH) style diet, and metabolic health in US adults. *Clin. Nutr.* **2017**, *36*, 1301–1309. [CrossRef] [PubMed]
132. Appel, L.J.; Moore, T.J.; Obarzanek, E.; Vollmer, W.M.; Svetkey, L.P.; Sacks, F.M.; Bray, G.A.; Vogt, T.M.; Cutler, J.A.; Windhauser, M.M.; et al. A clinical trial of the effects of dietary patterns on blood pressure. *N. Engl. J. Med.* **1997**, *336*, 1117–1124. [CrossRef] [PubMed]
133. Rosanoff, A. The high heart health value of drinking-water magnesium. *Med. Hypotheses* **2013**, *81*, 1063–1065. [CrossRef] [PubMed]

5

Correlation of Vitamin D with Inflammatory Cytokines, Atherosclerotic Parameters and Lifestyle Factors in the Setting of Heart Failure: A 12-Month Follow-Up Study

Daniel N. Roffe-Vazquez [1], Anna S. Huerta-Delgado [1], Elena C. Castillo [2], José R. Villarreal-Calderón [1], Adrian M. Gonzalez-Gil [1], Cecilio Enriquez [2], Gerardo Garcia-Rivas [2,3,*] and Leticia Elizondo-Montemayor [1,3,*]

[1] Tecnologico de Monterrey, Center for Research in Clinical Nutrition, Escuela de Medicina, Monterrey 64710, N.L., Mexico; daniel.roffe@hotmail.com (D.N.R.-V.); anna.sofy@hotmail.com (A.S.H.-D.); joser.villarreal@udem.edu (J.R.V.-C.); amgonzalezgil@hotmail.com (A.M.G.-G.)

[2] Tecnologico de Monterrey, Centro de Investigacion Biomedica, Hospital Zambrano Hellion, San Pedro Garza-Garcia 66278, N.L., Mexico; ecgonzalez@tec.mx (E.C.C.); dr.cecilioenriquez@medicos.tecsalud.mx (C.E.)

[3] Tecnologico de Monterrey, Cardiovascular and Metabolomics Research Group, Escuela de Medicina, San Pedro Garza-Garcia 66278, N.L., Mexico

* Correspondence: gdejesus@tec.mx (G.G.-R.); lelizond@tec.mx (L.E.-M.)

Abstract: Vitamin D deficiency is highly prevalent worldwide. It has been associated with heart failure (HF) given its immunoregulatory functions. In-vitro and animal models have shown protective roles through mechanisms involving procollagen-1, JNK2, calcineurin/NFAT, NF-κB, MAPK, Th1, Th2, Th17, cytokines, cholesterol-efflux, oxLDL, and GLUT4, among others. A 12-month follow-up in HF patients showed a high prevalence of vitamin D deficiency, with no seasonal variation (64.7–82.4%). A positive correlation between serum 25(OH)D concentration and dietary intake of vitamin D-rich foods was found. A significant inverse correlation with IL-1β ($R = -0.78$), TNF-α ($R = -0.53$), IL-6 ($R = -0.42$), IL-8 (R = −0.41), IL-17A ($R = -0.31$), LDL-cholesterol ($R = -0.51$), Apo-B ($R = -0.57$), total-cholesterol ($R = -0.48$), and triglycerides ($R = -0.32$) was shown. Cluster analysis demonstrated that patients from cluster three, with the lowest 25(OH)D levels, presented the lowermost vitamin D intake, IL-10 (1.0 ± 0.9 pg/mL), and IL-12p70 (0.5 ± 0.4 pg/mL), but the highest TNF-α (9.1 ± 3.5 pg/mL), IL-8 (55.6 ± 117.1 pg/mL), IL-17A (3.5 ± 2.0 pg/mL), total-cholesterol (193.9 ± 61.4 mg/dL), LDL-cholesterol (127.7 ± 58.2 mg/dL), and Apo-B (101.4 ± 33.4 mg/dL) levels, compared with patients from cluster one. Although the role of vitamin D in the pathogenesis of HF in humans is still uncertain, we applied the molecular mechanisms of in-vitro and animal models to explain our findings. Vitamin D deficiency might contribute to inflammation, remodeling, fibrosis, and atherosclerosis in patients with HF.

Keywords: vitamin D; heart failure; inflammation; seasonal variation; lifestyle; cytokines; lipids; mechanisms; immunoregulatory

---

1. Introduction

It has long been recognized that vitamin D plays a major role in bone and mineral metabolism, but until recent years, it has also been implicated in immunity and cardiovascular health. The first rate-limiting step in the endogenous synthesis of vitamin D is the skin's sun exposure, as ultraviolet B (UVB) radiation is necessary to convert 7-dehydrocholesterol into vitamin D3 (cholecalciferol), with estimates of cutaneous synthesis providing between 80% and 100% of the vitamin D requirements of the body [1]. In the liver, 25-hydroxylase (CYP2R1) converts vitamin D3 into 25-hydroxyvitamin D [25(OH)D], which is then transformed in the kidney by means of 1-alpha-hydroxylase (CYP27B1), into 1,25-dihydroxyvitamin D [1,25(OH)2D3], also known as calcitriol, the hormone's biologically active form [2]. The enzyme 1-alpha-hydroxylase is activated by the parathyroid hormone (PTH) and inhibited by fibroblast growth factor-23 (FGF-23). On the other hand, 25-hydroxyvitamin D3 24-hydroxylase (CYP24A1) is involved in calcitriol's catabolism. This enzyme limits the generation of calcitriol by converting it into hydroxylated derivatives (which will later be excreted), or by converting 25(OH)D3 into 24,25(OH)2D3 or 23,25(OH)2D3, further decreasing its availability for 1-hydroxylation. CYP24A1 is inhibited by PTH and induced by FGF-23 [3]. By feedback mechanisms, both 1-alpha-hydroxylase and 25-hydroxyvitamin D3 24-hydroxylase regulate 1,25(OH)2D3's bioavailability as a means to protect against hypercalcemia [3,4].

Several risk factors have been described to predispose to vitamin D deficiency. Living in higher latitudes (above 35 degrees) is a well-known risk factor [5]; however, vitamin D deficiency has been shown to be highly prevalent even in populations living near the equator [6]. Other risk factors for vitamin D deficiency include skin phototype, sunscreen usage, indoor working environments, minimal outdoor activity, obesity, high body mass index (BMI), and waist circumference (WC), as well as older age, which is accompanied by a 75% decrease in vitamin D synthesis capacity [1,6]. Among these factors, the combination of low UVB availability and/or underexposure, in addition to insufficient dietary intake, have been described as the most important [1].

Notably, nutrition surveillance data from various countries have indicated that vitamin D ingestion is lower than the recommended minimum amount [1,7]. There is also evidence that suggests that the recommended intake established by guidelines (600 IU) is actually insufficient and should be increased to at least 800 IU [5].

Vitamin D also plays a role in immune regulation, as immune cells express 1-alpha-hydroxylase to regulate their own local concentration of calcitriol. This effect has been related to the milieu of cytokines [8], given that adequate levels of serum 25(OH)D have been associated with increased levels of the anti-inflammatory cytokines interleukins (IL) 4 and 10, and to lower levels of the proinflammatory cytokines IL-1 and IL-6 [9]. On the contrary, vitamin D deficiency has been associated with chronic inflammatory states and a proinflammatory cytokine profile. Vitamin D deficiency has also been linked with augmented collagen synthesis, oxidative stress, and fibrosis, which are potential mechanisms underlying cardiovascular diseases, such as heart failure [10].

Heart failure (HF) is one of the most common chronic medical conditions worldwide. It is estimated that as of 2019, more than 6 million Americans are living with this disease [11–13]. HF with reduced ejection fraction (HFrEF) is defined by a left ventricular ejection fraction (LVEF) of < 40% [14]. Most of the risk factors for HFrEF in Western populations have been described in association with ischemic heart disease [15]. It has been proposed that vitamin D might play a role in disease pathogenesis, as serum 25(OH)D levels have been demonstrated to be lower in patients with HF compared with control subjects [16]. Specifically, prospective studies have shown that the risk of developing HF is increased in patients with vitamin D deficiency [17]. One of the mechanistic links regarding this association relies on a proinflammatory cytokine state, including both innate and adaptive immunity [18–20].

Regarding innate immunity, vitamin D deficiency has been shown to increase the expression of nuclear-factor kappa B (NF-κB), leading to a higher secretion and release of the main proinflammatory cytokines, such as IL-6 and monocyte chemoattractant protein-1 (MCP-1) [10]. Cardiomyocytes themselves are activated by hemodynamic stress and are able to secrete several inflammatory cytokines as well [21]. On the other hand, by activation of mitogen-activated protein kinase (MAPK) phosphatase-1 and subsequent inhibition of p38 MAPK, vitamin D has been demonstrated to switch the cytokine profile into an anti-inflammatory state, with inhibition of the production of tumor necrosis factor-alpha (TNF-α) and IL-6 [22]. In the case of adaptive immunity, vitamin D has been found to inhibit the CD4+ T-cell course towards the Th17 lineage [9]. Additionally, vitamin D is able to hinder IL-17 production of those CD4+ T-cells that have been already committed towards the Th17 lineage [23]. Not only does vitamin D exert its effects through immune regulation, but it is also able to control extracellular matrix metabolism. Vitamin D deficiency has been related to increased expression of matrix metalloproteinase (MMP) 2 and 9 [10], as well as to augmented tissue macrophage infiltration [24]. These mechanisms may be associated with some of the structural abnormalities seen in HF, such as ventricular remodeling, tissue fibrosis, and a systemic proinflammatory state. Other mechanisms through which vitamin D deficiency predisposes to HF include: overactivation of the renin-angiotensin-aldosterone system (RAAS); dysfunction of the intracellular calcium handling by the cardiomyocyte; overexpression of procollagen-1, which leads to increased fibrosis; diminished protein kinase A (PKA) levels that result in impaired contractility; and activation of calcineurin signaling, which promotes cardiac hypertrophy [25–28].

Given the evidence provided relating the mechanisms through which vitamin D deficiency is associated with HF, it is important to study the seasonal variation of vitamin D deficiency and the cytokine profile, as well as the lifestyle factors that exert an influence in patients with HF. Thus, the aim of this study is to describe the seasonal variation of vitamin D deficiency and its association with 13 inflammatory cytokines, biochemical, and lifestyle factors during a 12-month follow-up in a cohort of patients with HFrEF, as well as to describe the molecular inflammatory and atherosclerotic mechanisms related to vitamin D deficiency. An original figure summarizing these mechanisms is also shown.

2. Results

2.1. Demographic, Anthropometric, and Lifestyle Parameters

The mean and standard deviation of serum 25(OH)D concentrations, demographic data, lifestyle, and anthropometric characteristics are presented in Table 1. The mean age of the cohort (n = 17) was 64.2 years. Most of the patients in the study were males (82.4%). In order to assess the level of skin pigmentation in our patients, the Fitzpatrick's classification of phototypes was clinically determined. Most of the patients belonged to phototype IV (58.8%), followed by V (29.4%), and lastly by phototype III (11.8%). All of the patients were of Hispanic ethnicity. Heart failure severity was clinically determined by the New York Heart Association (NYHA) classification of functional capacity [29]. All of the patients in our cohort had an NYHA class III status, which describes subjects that are asymptomatic at rest but develop fatigue, dyspnea, or palpitations when performing less than ordinary physical activity. Mean BMI was 28.5 kg/m^2, body fat percentage (BF%) was 30.5%, WC was 99.1 cm, and fat mass was 23.4 kg.

Table 1. Serum 25(OH)D levels, demographic, lifestyle, and anthropometric parameters in patients with heart failure.

Parameter	Mean (Standard Deviation)
Age (years)	64.2 (± 8.9)
Gender	Male 82.4%/Female 17.6%
Phototype	III 11.8%/IV 58.8%/V 29.4%
Smoking	Yes 11.8%/No 88.2%
Height (m)	1.6 (± 0.1)
Weight (kg)	76.8 (± 11.7)
Body fat (%)	30.5 (± 6.3)
Fat mass (kg)	23.4 (± 5.6)
Waist circumference (cm)	99.1 (± 9)
BMI (kg/m^2)	28.5 (± 2.8)
Vitamin D intake (IU/day)	224 (± 113.1)
Sun exposure (min/week)	307.3 (± 444.2)
25(OH)D (ng/mL)	24.3 (± 7.7)

Data are expressed as mean (± standard deviation) unless specified otherwise as a percentage (%). BMI = body mass index; 25(OH)D = 25-hydroxyvitamin D.

Mean vitamin D intake per day was calculated to be 224 ± 113.1 IU; all of the patients were found to have an overall consumption throughout the year of less than 400 IU/day. Sun exposure had a large variability among subjects; therefore, this data was further analyzed by grouping patients into those who reported a null amount of sun exposure (negative) versus those who had any time of sun exposure (positive) per day (Figure 1). Since individual patients reported different amounts of sun exposure throughout the seasons, the data was analyzed considering four observations per patient, each corresponding to a season of the year, with a total of 68 observations. From these, 51 of the observations were categorized as positive and 17 as negative. A vitamin D sufficient status was statistically more prevalent in patients with sun exposure (31.4%) compared to those with no exposure (5.9%) ($p < 0.044$).

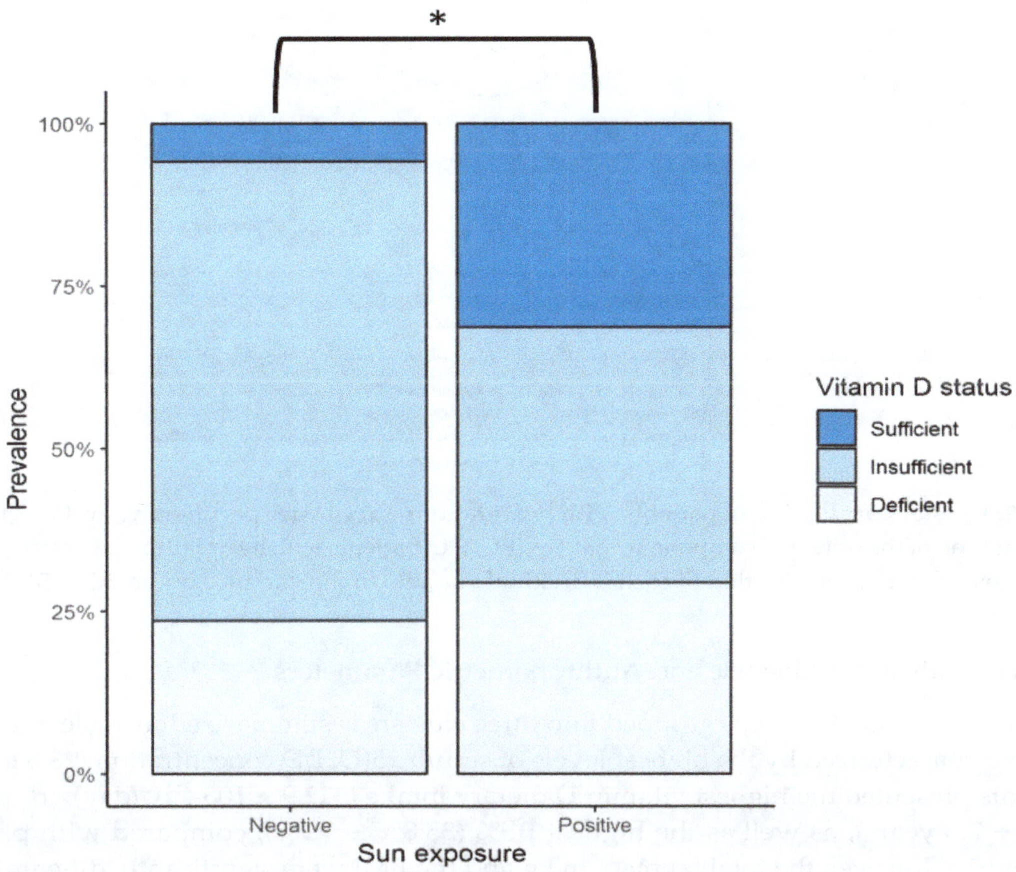

Figure 1. Sun exposure and vitamin D status in patients with heart failure during the 12-month follow up. Negative = observations with null sun exposure; positive = observations with any amount of sun exposure; * represents a statistically significant difference in the prevalence of vitamin D sufficiency in patients with some amount of sun exposure (positive), 31.4%, versus those with null exposure (negative), 5.9% ($p < 0.044$). Sufficient vitamin D status is defined as serum 25(OH)D levels > 30 ng/mL, insufficient as serum 25(OH)D levels > 20 and < 30 ng/mL, and deficient status as serum 25(OH)D levels < 20 ng/mL. [30]. 25(OH)D = 25-hydroxyvitamin D.

2.2. Cluster Analysis

Principal component analysis (PCA) was performed with numeric demographic, anthropometric, and lifestyle variables, as well as with serum 25(OH)D concentration, in order to better understand the nature of the observations in our cohort. The 68 observations (four observations per patient, each one according to the corresponding season) were classified into three clusters by partitioning around medoids (PAM). Graphical representation of the grouping of each observation is shown in Figure 2a, while the contribution of each variable to the total variance of PCA is seen in Figure 2b.

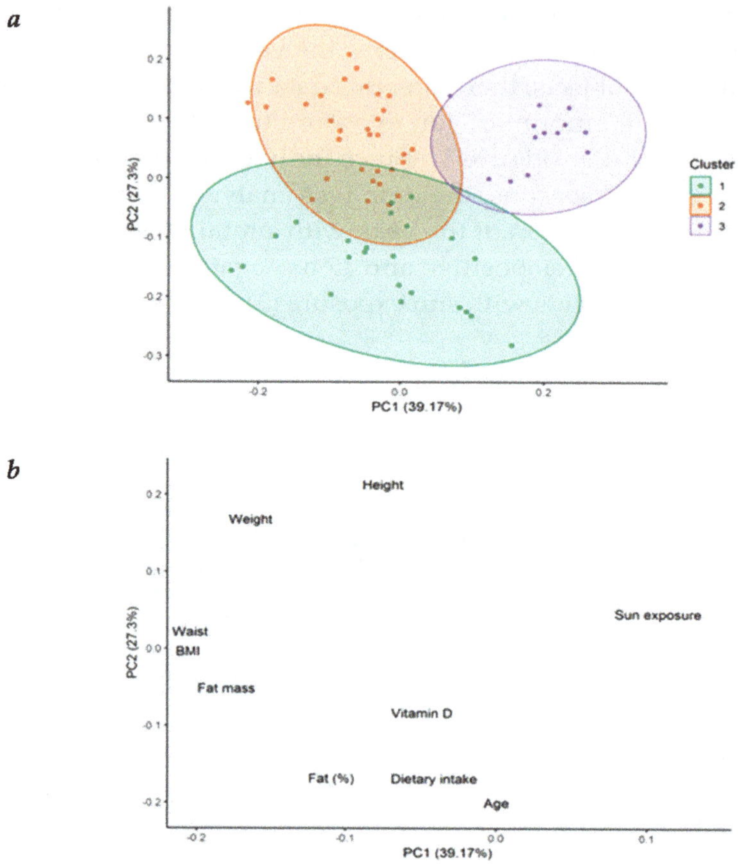

Figure 2. Cluster partitioning in patients with heart failure. (**a**) Cluster partitioning and its graphical representation of the principal component analysis (PCA) in patients with heart failure (HF); (**b**) graphical representation of the contribution of each individual variable to the variance of the PCA. BMI = body mass index.

2.2.1. Cluster Analysis for Lifestyle and Anthropometric Parameters

Differences in data of patients grouped into three clusters is summarized in Table 2. Patients from cluster 1 were characterized by the highest levels of serum 25(OH)D concentration (28.3 ± 8.0 ng/mL). These patients presented the highest vitamin D dietary intake (322.9 ± 103.4 IU/day), in spite of being older (72.2 ± 7.5 years), as well as the highest BF% (35.8% ± 4.9%), compared with patients from clusters 3 and 2. However, the total fat mass in kg and the BMI were significantly different from those shown by patients from cluster 3, but not from those of cluster 2. In contrast, patients from cluster 3 presented the lowest serum 25(OH)D levels (19 ± 4.5 ng/mL). These patients showed the highest amount of sun exposure (1178.5 ± 925.6 min/week) compared with patients from the other two clusters, but lower vitamin D ingestion (174 ± 72.9 IU/day) compared with patients from cluster 1. They also displayed lower BMI (24.6 ± 1.2 kg/m^2), BF% (22.7% ± 3.3%), and fat mass in kg (15.0 ± 2.6 kg) than patients from cluster 1. Finally, patients from cluster 2 showed the highest body weight (85.4 ± 8.0 kg) and WC (103.9 ± 7.1 cm); lower vitamin D intake (173.1 ± 83.9 IU/day), but no difference in sun exposure compared with patients from cluster 1. No significant difference among the clusters was demonstrated for LVEF (%): cluster 1 (28.8% ± 7.1%), cluster 2 (30.5% ± 13.0%), cluster 3 (27.3% ± 4.3%) (Figure A1-Appendix A).

2.2.2. Biochemical and Metabolic Parameters among the Clusters of Patients with HF

Using the same cluster classification, Table 3 shows the differences among clusters for biochemical and metabolic parameters. Patients from cluster 3 were found to present with the highest levels of total cholesterol (TC) (193.9 ± 61.4 mg/dL), low-density lipoprotein (LDL) cholesterol (127.7 ± 58.2 mg/dL), non-high-density lipoprotein (non-HDL) cholesterol (152.3 ± 58.2 mg/dL), Apo-B (101.4 ± 33.4 mg/dL), Apo-B/Apo-A ratio (0.7 ± 0.2), and TC/HDL ratio (4.7 ± 1.4). All of these metabolic parameters were significantly different compared with patients from cluster 1. These patients also presented the lowest insulin levels (8.6 ± 4.5 μU/mL) and Homeostatic Model Assessment (HOMA) index (2.7 ± 1.6), both of which were significantly different regarding cluster 2. Figure 3 shows the PCA, including the biochemical and metabolic variables shown in Table 3.

Table 2. 25(OH)D levels, lifestyle, anthropometrical, and clinical data for patients with heart failure grouped into three clusters according to the PCA analysis.

Parameter	Cluster 1	Cluster 2	Cluster 3
Age (years)	72.2 (± 7.5) $^{b, c}$	60.4 (± 6.6) ^{a}	59.6 (± 6.6) ^{a}
Height (m)	1.56 (± 0.06) $^{b, c}$	1.69 (± 0.06) $^{a, c}$	1.64 (± 0.06) $^{a, b}$
Weight (kg)	70.7 (± 9.8) ^{b}	85.4 (± 8.0) $^{a, c}$	66.3 (± 5.4) ^{b}
Body fat (%)	35.8 (± 4.9) $^{b, c}$	29.8 (± 4.3) $^{a, c}$	22.7 (± 3.3) $^{a, b}$
Fat mass (kg)	25.4 (± 5.6) ^{c}	25.3 (± 2.7) ^{c}	15 (± 2.6) $^{a, b}$
Waist circumference (cm)	98.9 (± 7.7) $^{b, c}$	103.9 (± 7.1) $^{a, c}$	87.7 (± 4.2) $^{a, b}$
BMI (kg/m^2)	28.9 (± 2.8) ^{c}	29.7 (± 1.7) ^{c}	24.6 (± 1.2) $^{a, b}$
Vitamin D intake (IU/day)	322.9 (± 103.4) $^{b, c}$	173.1 (± 83.9) ^{a}	174 (± 72.9) ^{a}
Sun exposure (min/week)	202.2 (± 218.9) ^{c}	171.7 (± 234.2) ^{c}	1178.5 (± 925.6) $^{a, b}$
Vitamin D (ng/mL)	28.3 (± 8.0) $^{b, c}$	23.6 (± 7.2) ^{a}	19 (± 4.5) ^{a}
LVEF (%)	28.8 (± 7.1)	30.5 (± 13.0)	27.3 (± 4.3)

Tukey honest significant difference (HSD); data are expressed as mean (± standard deviation). BMI = body mass index; LVEF = left ventricular ejection fraction. ^{a} = statistical difference when compared vs. cluster 1 ($p < 0.05$); ^{b} = statistical difference when compared vs. cluster 2 ($p < 0.05$); ^{c} = statistical difference when compared vs. cluster 3 ($p < 0.05$). Cluster 1 includes 23 observations from 7 different patients, cluster 2 includes 32 observations from 10 different patients, and cluster 3 includes 13 observations from 4 different patients.

Table 3. Biochemical and metabolic parameters in the three clusters of patients with heart failure.

Analyte (Units)	Cluster 1	Cluster 2	Cluster 3
BNP (pg/mL)	125.5 (± 104.1)	138.5 (± 158.9)	183.1 (± 142.3)
hsCRP (mg/dL)	0.5 (± 1.1)	0.5 (± 0.6)	0.1 (± 0.1)
Calcium (mg/dL)	9.4 (± 0.3) $^{b, c}$	9.2 (± 0.2) ^{a}	9 (± 0.3) ^{a}
PTH (pg/mL)	80.6 (± 54.0)	61.8 (± 23.4)	58.1 (± 15.2)
Total cholesterol (mg/dL)	138.1 (± 50.2) ^{c}	171.5 (± 38.3)	193.9 (± 61.4) ^{a}
LDL (mg/dL)	63.5 (± 35.9) ^{c}	93 (± 32.5)	127.7 (± 58.2) ^{a}
HDL (mg/dL)	38.3 (± 10.8)	42.1 (± 8.5)	41.6 (± 6.8)
non-HDL (mg/dL)	99.8 (± 44.8) ^{c}	128.1 (± 31.0)	152.3 (± 58.2) ^{a}
VLDL (mg/dL)	30 (± 15.3)	36.4 (± 16.1)	39.8 (± 42.6)
Triglycerides (mg/dL)	149.8 (± 76.7)	181.9 (± 80.7)	199 (± 212.8)
Ratio cholesterol/HDL	3.5 (± 0.6) ^{c}	4.1 (± 0.7)	4.7 (± 1.4) ^{a}
Apo A (mg/dL)	139.1 (± 16.6)	141.9 (± 20.2)	134.4 (± 11.6)
Apo B (mg/dL)	70.8 (± 26.1) $^{b, c}$	97.7 (± 18.4) ^{a}	101.4 (± 33.4) ^{a}
Ratio Apo B/Apo A	0.5 (± 0.2) $^{b, c}$	0.7 (± 0.1) ^{a}	0.7 (± 0.2) ^{a}
Glucose (mg/dL)	132.4 (± 50.2)	137.5 (± 54.9)	134 (± 56.4)
Insulin (μU/mL)	16.3 (± 11.3)	20.8 (± 14.7) ^{c}	8.6 (± 4.5) ^{b}
HOMA index	5.2 (± 4.0)	6.3 (± 3.9) ^{c}	2.7 (± 1.6) ^{b}

Tukey honest significant difference (HSD); data are expressed as mean (± standard deviation). BNP = brain natriuretic peptide; hsCRP = high sensitivity C-reactive protein; PTH = parathyroid hormone; LDL = low-density lipoprotein; HDL = high-density lipoprotein; non-HDL = non-high-density lipoprotein; VLDL = very low-density lipoprotein; Apo = apolipoprotein; HOMA = Homeostatic Model Assessment. ^{a} = statistical difference when compared vs. cluster 1 ($p < 0.05$); ^{b} = statistical difference when compared vs. cluster 2 ($p < 0.05$); ^{c} = statistical difference when compared vs. cluster 3 ($p < 0.05$).

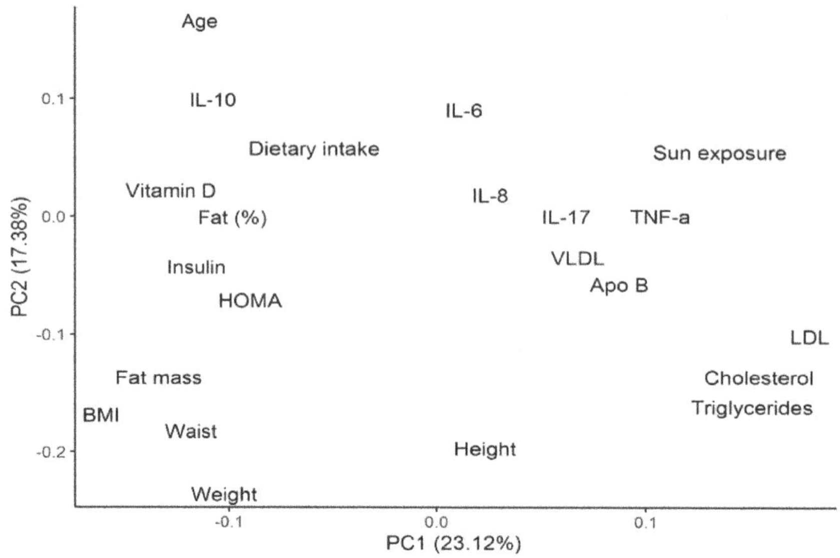

Figure 3. PCA analysis for the metabolic and biochemical variables described in the cluster's analysis. PCA = principal component analysis; IL= interleukin; HOMA = Homeostatic Model Assessment; BMI = body mass index; TNF = tumor necrosis factor; VLDL = very low-density lipoprotein; Apo = apolipoprotein; LDL = low-density lipoprotein.

2.2.3. Cytokine Differences among the Clusters of Patients with Heart Failure

Cytokine profile analysis, according to the patient's cluster grouping, is shown in Table 4. Patients from cluster 1 showed the lowest levels of TNF-α (3.3 ± 4.1 pg/mL) and IL-17A (2.4 ± 2.3 pg/mL), as well as the highest levels of IL-10 (2.7 ± 2.0 pg/mL), IL-6 (6.2 ± 6.9 pg/mL), IL-18 (471.2 ± 400.6 pg/mL), IL-12p70 (4.5 ± 6.0 pg/mL), and interferon (IFN)-α2 (74.5 ± 99.7 pg/mL). Among these cytokines, TNF-α, IL-12p70, IFN-α2, and IL-10 were significantly different from cluster 3. Opposite to these results, patients from cluster 3 showed the highest levels of TNF-α (9.1 ± 3.5 pg/mL), IL-8 (55.6 ± 117.1 pg/mL), and IL-17A (3.5 ± 2.0 pg/mL), as well as the lowest levels of IL-10 (1.0 ± 0.9 pg/mL), IL-12p70 (0.5 ± 0.4 pg/mL), and IFN-α2 (1.1 ± 0.4 pg/mL). From these, TNF-α, IL-12p70, IL-10, and IFN-α2 levels were significantly different regarding cluster 1. Patients from cluster 2 were shown to have significant lower levels of IL-10 (1.1 ± 0.8 pg/mL), IL-12p70 (0.6 ± 0.6 pg/mL), and IFNα-2 (4.3 ± 6.5 pg/mL) compared with those from cluster 1. Figure 3 shows the PCA, including the cytokine variables shown in Table 4.

Table 4. Differences in cytokine concentration for the three clusters of patients with heart failure.

Cytokine (pg/mL)	Cluster 1	Cluster 2	Cluster 3
IFN-α2	74.5 (± 99.7) [b, c]	4.3 (± 6.5) [a]	1.1 (± 0.4) [a]
IFN-Ɣ	65.7 (± 238.1)	48.6 (± 196.2)	8.2 (± 14.7)
TNF-α	3.3 (± 4.1) [c]	5.3 (± 5.8)	9.1 (± 3.5) [a]
MCP-1	543.6 (± 374.9)	490.9 (± 439.4)	252 (± 321.6)
IL-6	6.2 (± 6.9)	3.3 (± 2.1)	4.4 (± 2.6)
IL-8	38.2 (± 82.4)	18.8 (± 34.4)	55.6 (± 117.1)
IL-10	2.7 (± 2.0) [b, c]	1.1 (± 0.8) [a]	1 (± 0.9) [a]
IL-12p70	4.5 (± 6.0) [b, c]	0.6 (± 0.6) [a]	0.5 (± 0.4) [a]
IL-17A	2.4 (± 2.3)	2.8 (± 2.8)	3.5 (± 2.0)
IL-18	471.2 (± 400.6)	284 (± 217.6)	221.9 (± 127.8)
IL-23	36.7 (± 76.8) [b]	3.6 (± 2.8) [a]	3 (± 2.2)
IL-33	0.9 (± 0.6)	1 (± 0.9)	2.1 (± 2.7)

Tukey honest significant difference (HSD); data are expressed as mean (± standard deviation). IFN = interferon; TNF = tumor necrosis factor; MCP = monocyte chemoattractant protein; IL = interleukin. [a] = statistical difference when compared vs. cluster 1 ($p < 0.05$); [b] = statistical difference when compared vs. cluster 2 ($p < 0.05$); [c] = statistical difference when compared vs. cluster 3 ($p < 0.05$).

2.3. *Correlation between 25(OH)D Levels and Ventricular Function, Biochemical, Lifestyle, and Anthropometric Parameters in Patients with Heart Failure*

A significant positive correlation was found between 25(OH)D serum levels and age ($R = 0.386$, $p < 0.01$), BMI ($R = 0.265$, $p < 0.05$), dietary intake of vitamin D-rich foods ($R = 0.276$, $p < 0.05$), and calcium ($R = 0.354$, $p < 0.05$) (Tables 5 and 6). No association was observed between sun exposure and 25(OH)D concentration when the total data was analyzed; however, as was shown in Figure 1, a difference was demonstrated when the observations were subgrouped into null sun exposure or any time of sun exposure. There was no correlation between 25(OH)D levels and ventricular function parameters (LVEF and brain natriuretic peptide [BNP]) (Table 6 and Figure A2-Appendix A).

Table 5. Association of serum 25(OH)D levels with ventricular function, lifestyle, and anthropometric parameters in patients with heart failure for the 12-month follow-up.

Variable	Spearman's Rho
Age (years)	0.386 **
Weight (kg)	0.031
Body fat (%)	0.160
Fat mass (kg)	0.150
Waist circumference (cm)	0.150
BMI (kg/m^2)	0.265 *
Vitamin D intake (IU/day)	0.276 *
Sun exposure (min/week)	−0.075

Spearman's rank correlation test; * = $p < 0.05$; ** = $p < 0.01$. Values represent the four measurements corresponding to each season of the year per patient (only correlations for serum 25(OH)D levels are shown). LVEF = left ventricular ejection fraction; BMI = body mass index.

Table 6. Association of serum 25(OH)D levels with biochemical and metabolic parameters in patients with heart failure for the 12-month follow-up.

Variable	Spearman's Rho
LVEF (%)	0.251
BNP (pg/mL)	0.221
hsCRP (mg/dL)	0.133
Calcium (mg/dL)	0.354 *
PTH (pg/mL)	0.283
Total cholesterol (mg/dL)	−0.479 **
LDL (mg/dL)	−0.507 ***
HDL (mg/dL)	−0.196
non-HDL (mg/dL)	−0.481 **
VLDL (mg/dL)	−0.317 *
Triglycerides (mg/dL)	−0.317 *
Ratio cholesterol/HDL	−0.423 **
Apo A (mg/dL)	−0.299
Apo B (mg/dL)	−0.566 ***
Ratio Apo B/Apo A	−0.496 ***
Glucose (mg/dL)	−0.073
Insulin (μU/mL)	−0.017
HOMA index	−0.077

Spearman's rank correlation test; * = $p < 0.05$; ** = $p < 0.01$; *** = $p < 0.001$. Values represent the four measurements corresponding to each season of the year per patient (only correlations for serum 25(OH)D levels are shown). LVEF = left ventricular ejection fraction; BNP = brain natriuretic peptide; hsCRP = high sensitivity C-reactive protein; PTH = parathyroid hormone; LDL = low-density lipoprotein; HDL = high-density lipoprotein; VLDL = very low-density lipoprotein; Apo = apolipoprotein; HOMA = Homeostatic Model Assessment.

2.4. *Lipid Parameters Are Negatively Correlated with 25(OH)D Levels in Patients with Heart Failure*

A significant inverse correlation was found between serum 25(OH)D concentration and LDL cholesterol ($R = -0.507$, $p < 0.001$), Apo-B ($R = -0.566$, $p < 0.001$), Apo-B/Apo-A ratio ($R = -0.496$,

$p < 0.001$), total cholesterol ($R = -0.479$, $p < 0.01$), non-HDL cholesterol ($R = -0.481$, $p < 0.01$), and triglycerides ($R = -0.317$, $p < 0.05$) (Table 6). No correlation with HDL cholesterol or Apo-A was found. A decision-tree analysis was created in order to identify which variables might have the greatest prediction power to determine 25(OH)D status. Despite multiple variables being associated with serum 25(OH)D levels in the univariate correlation analysis, after multivariate analysis, Apo-B was the only variable that remained with a significant correlation. An Apo-B level > 76 mg/dL was shown to significantly predict a higher risk of being vitamin D insufficient or deficient ($p = 0.025$) (Figure 4). No seasonal variation was found for any of the lipid parameters in the HFrEF patients, nor was there a correlation between serum 25(OH)D levels and glycemic parameters such as fasting glucose, insulin levels, or HOMA index, or any seasonal variation either.

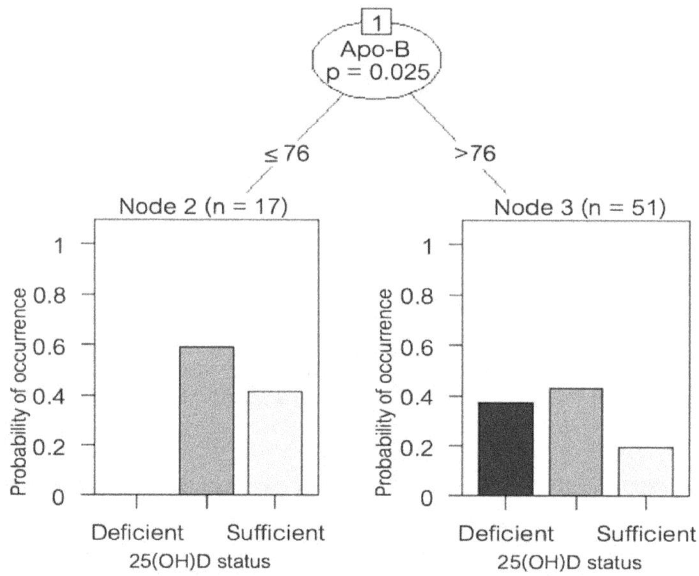

Figure 4. Decision tree predicting vitamin D status in patients with heart failure. Variable name and *p*-value is shown inside the circle; the corresponding lines show cut-off values. Bar graphs at the bottom show 25(OH)D status distribution amongst patients. Apo = apolipoprotein; sufficiency = 25(OH)D ≥ 30 ng/mL, insufficiency = 25(OH)D ≥ 20 and < 30 ng/mL, and deficiency = 25(OH)D < 20 ng/mL [30]. 25(OH)D = 25-hydroxyvitamin D.

2.5. *Inflammatory Cytokines Are Inversely Correlated with 25(OH)D Levels in Patients with Heart Failure*

Table 7 shows a strong inverse correlation between serum 25(OH)D levels and the proinflammatory cytokines IL-1β ($R = -0.779$, $p < 0.001$), TNF-α ($R = -0.530$, $p < 0.001$), IL-6 ($R = -0.418$, $p < 0.01$), and IL-8 ($R = -0.414$, $p < 0.01$), and a weaker negative correlation with IL-17A ($R = -0.309$, $p < 0.05$), IL-18 ($R = -0.349$, $p < 0.05$), and IL-33 ($R = -0.357$, $p < 0.05$) as well. There was no seasonal variation amongst the cytokine milieu. Furthermore, there was no significant correlation between BMI and cytokine levels.

2.6. *Vitamin D Insufficiency/Deficiency Was Highly Prevalent Throughout All Year*

Most of the patients with HF in our cohort were vitamin D insufficient or deficient throughout all of the year (Figure 5a). The highest prevalence of vitamin D insufficiency/deficiency was found to be in winter and spring (82.4%), followed by that in autumn (70.6%), and remaining high during the summer (64.7%). An ANOVA analysis was performed to evaluate whether serum 25(OH)D concentrations varied throughout the year. As observed in Figure 5b and Table 8, 25(OH)D levels were found to be lowest in winter (23.6 ± 7.8 ng/mL), followed by spring (24.0 ± 7.8 ng/mL) and autumn (24.4 ± 8.9 ng/mL), while the highest concentrations were found in summer (25.2 ± 6.8 ng/mL). Although no significant seasonal variation was observed, there was a tendency towards a higher prevalence of vitamin D deficiency during winter.

Table 7. Association of serum 25(OH)D concentration and cytokine levels in patients with heart failure for the 12-month follow-up.

Variable	Spearman's Rho
IL-1β	−0.779 ***
IFN-α	0.464 ***
IFN-ɣ	−0.046
TNF-α	−0.530 ***
MCP-1	0.257
IL-6	−0.418 **
IL-8	−0.414 **
IL-10	0.001
IL-12p70	0.188
IL-17A	−0.309 *
IL-18	−0.349 *
IL-23	0.114
IL-33	−0.357 *

Spearman's rank correlation test; * = $p < 0.05$; ** = $p < 0.01$; *** = $p = 0.001$. Values include the four measurements corresponding to each season of the year. IL = interleukin; IFN = interferon; TNF = tumor necrosis factor; MCP = monocyte chemoattractant protein.

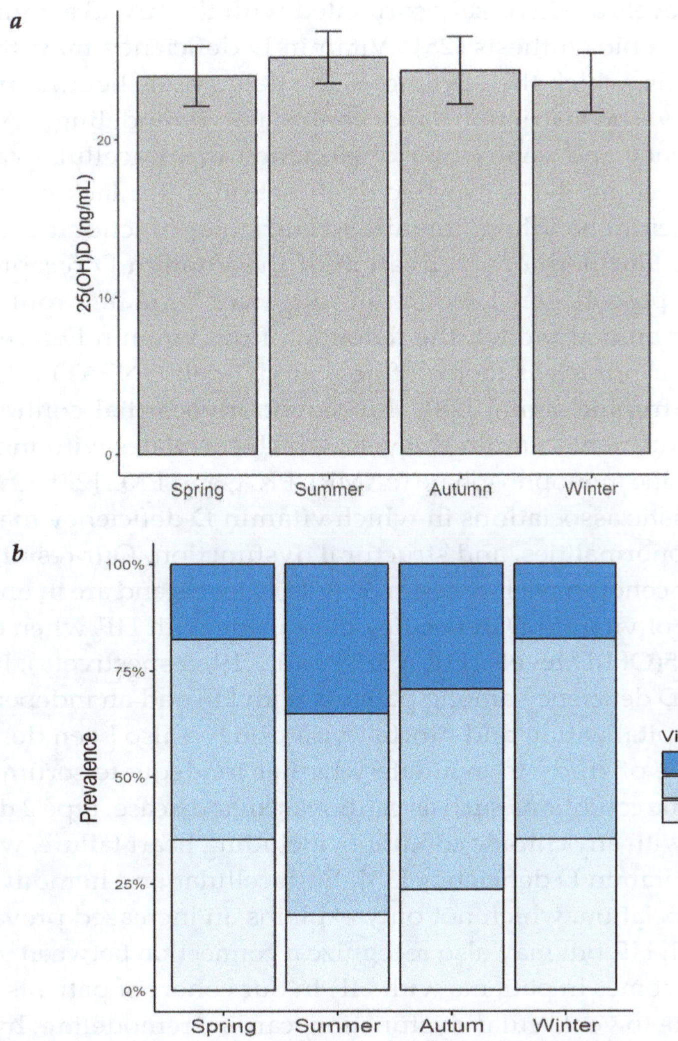

Figure 5. Seasonal variation of serum 25(OH)D concentration and prevalence of vitamin D status in patients with heart failure. (**a**) Seasonal variation of serum 25(OH)D concentration in patients with HF; bar height = mean; error bars = ± standard error; (**b**) prevalence of vitamin D status by season in the same patients. 25(OH)D = 25-hydroxyvitamin D.

Table 8. Seasonal variation of serum 25(OH)D levels and prevalence of deficiency, insufficiency, and sufficiency in patients with heart failure.

Season	25(OH)D (ng/mL)	Vitamin D Deficiency *n* (%)	Vitamin D Insufficiency *n* (%)	Vitamin D Sufficiency *n* (%)
Spring	24 (± 7.8)	6 (35.3)	8 (47.1)	3 (17.6)
Summer	25.2 (± 6.8)	3 (17.6)	8 (47.1)	6 (35.3)
Autumn	24.4 (± 8.9)	4 (23.5)	8 (47.1)	5 (29.4)
Winter	23.6 (± 7.8)	6 (35.3)	8 (47.1)	3 (17.6)

Data are expressed as mean (± standard deviation) for serum 25(OH)D levels, and as absolute value (*n*) and percentage (%) of the population for each season. 25(OH)D = 25-hydroxyvitamin D.

3. Discussion

3.1. Vitamin D Deficiency in the Setting of Patients with HFrEF

One of the core aspects of recent molecular and clinical research into HFrEF has been to better understand the role of vitamin D and the vitamin D receptor in the initiation and progression of HF. There are several mechanisms underlying this association. Studies in animals and humans have shown that serum 25(OH)D levels are inversely correlated with the RAAS activity, possibly because active vitamin D inhibits renin biosynthesis [25]. Vitamin D deficiency may, therefore, contribute to a hyper-activated RAAS axis, which then promotes the deleterious hemodynamic consequences of salt and water retention, vasoconstriction, and ventricular remodeling. Another mechanism associating vitamin D deficiency and ventricular dysfunction is intracellular calcium handling by the cardiomyocyte. In a mouse model of cardiac dysfunction, mice lacking calcitriol have been found to exhibit abnormal calcium handling, impaired ventricular functioning, and adverse cardiac remodeling and fibrosis [26]. Furthermore, activation of the Vitamin D receptor has been shown to regulate the expression of procollagen 1, which in turn may regulate profibrotic activity in the myocardium [27]. In another animal model, the deletion of the vitamin D receptor gene was also found to activate the calcineurin/nuclear factor of activated T-cells (NFAT) intracellular signaling pathway, a potent pro-hypertrophic signal [28]. Moreover, myocardial contractility may also be enhanced in the presence of sufficient vitamin D levels, which correlates with increased intracellular concentrations of cyclic adenosine monophosphate (cAMP), PKA, and PKC [27]. Overall, these findings demonstrate several mechanistic associations in which vitamin D deficiency may participate in HF progression, hemodynamic abnormalities, and structural dysfunction. Our results show that most of the patients with HFrEF in our cohort have low serum 25(OH)D levels and are in line with other studies. A significant high prevalence of vitamin D deficiency in patients with HF, when comparing low and very low vs. normal serum 25(OH)D levels (HR = 1.33 and 2.19, respectively), has been found [31]. A high prevalence of vitamin D deficiency among patients with HF and an independent association of low 25(OH)D levels with hospitalization and mortality rates have also been described [32]. On the other hand, in a different type of study to evaluate whether inadequate serum levels of 25(OH)D predict the prevalence of chronic conditions such as cardiovascular disease, type 2 diabetes, and obesity, among others, no association with any chronic condition, including heart failure, was found; this study did not report prevalence of vitamin D deficiency [33]. Both cellular and hemodynamic mechanisms may be implicated in this association, which not only explains an increased prevalence of vitamin D deficiency among patients with HF, but may also recognize a connection between vitamin D deficiency and higher risk of adverse outcomes in patients with HF. In our cohort of patients with HF, vitamin D deficiency may thus contribute to ventricular dysfunction, cardiac remodeling, hypertrophy, fibrosis, and disease progression by the molecular and cellular signaling mechanisms described above.

3.2. Correlation of Atherosclerotic and Metabolic Parameters with Vitamin D Deficiency in Patients with HFrEF

Diverse types of dyslipidemias have been recognized as risk factors for the development of HF [34], and in conjunction with vitamin D deficiency, they may explain some of the mechanisms for disease progression. Atherosclerosis plays a predominant role in the pathophysiology of ischemic heart disease, which by itself, is the leading cause of HF. LDL-cholesterol particles turn into oxidized LDL cholesterol (oxLDL) by reactive oxygen species. Macrophages, which express high-capacity scavenger receptors that are not down-regulated in the presence of high oxLDL concentration, are modified into foam cells [35]. Clusters of foam cells accumulated in the sub-endothelium, up-regulate the expression of NF-κB, which in turn triggers the membrane expression of vascular cell adhesion protein 1 (VCAM-1) and the endothelial adhesion molecule E-selectin. Another mechanism that increases NF-κB transcription in the endothelial cells is the increased proinflammatory cytokines IL-1, IL-8, and MCP-1 that characterize the inflammatory state in HF [36]. Adhesion molecules VCAM-1 and E-selectin contribute to increased cellular inflammation in the endothelial surface, as macrophages and T-cells are attracted to these proteins [35,36]. This propagates the inflammatory cycle, eventually leading to disturbed blood flow in the vessel's lumen and progression of atherosclerosis.

Regarding these mechanisms, vitamin D may have lipid-regulating effects. Therefore, adequate levels of 25(OH)D might act as a protective factor in coronary disease and HF, but in the case of vitamin D deficiency, there may be deleterious consequences. Figure 6 shows the possible immunomodulatory role of vitamin D regarding inflammation in the context of HF progression. In an animal model of hypercholesterolemia, vitamin D was shown to promote cholesterol efflux from macrophage-derived foam cells by augmenting the expression of ATP-binding membrane cassette transporter types A1 and G1 (ABCA1/G1) [37]. Hepatocyte uptake of cholesterol was also shown to be increased in the presence of higher levels of 25(OH)D concentrations. In addition, vitamin D has also been described to downregulate the c-Jun N-terminal protein kinase 2 (JNK2) cellular pathway in macrophages, which decreases oxLDL uptake and subsequently inhibits transformation into a foam cell phenotype [38]. Given the high prevalence of vitamin D deficiency throughout the four seasons of the year in our cohort of patients with HF, these protective effects of vitamin D may likely be absent. Furthermore, our results show an inverse correlation between 25(OH)D levels and total cholesterol, LDL cholesterol, non-HDL cholesterol, triglycerides, Apo-B, and Apo-B/Apo-A ratio. These correlations may also reflect the mechanisms described above, pointing towards the lack of the possible protective role of vitamin D in the setting of dyslipidemias. Our results are consistent with the prospective study, *The Atherosclerosis Risk in Communities*, in which lower 25(OH)D concentrations were shown to be associated with higher LDL cholesterol and total cholesterol, as well as an overall greater risk of dyslipidemias [39]. Similarly, Forrest et al. found that vitamin D deficiency was significantly more common in individuals with high LDL cholesterol [40].

Dysregulation of glucose metabolism has been linked to vitamin D deficiency and the development, as well as progression, of HF. In patients with established HF, the presence of diabetes mellitus has been associated with increased hospitalization rates and overall increased mortality [34]. Several mechanisms have been described regarding the role of vitamin D in glucose metabolism. In an animal model of vitamin D deficiency, decreased protein kinase B/Akt phosphorylation and reduced expression of glucose transporter 4 (GLUT4) in cardiomyocytes was shown. This, in turn, resulted in insulin resistance by the myocardium, a significant downregulation of the endogenous antioxidant enzymes SOD2 and catalase, and diminished LVEF [41]. The high prevalence of vitamin D deficiency throughout the 12-month follow-up shown in our cohort of patients with HF may thus worsen or predispose them to alterations in glucose metabolism. Moreover, a significant correlation between 25(OH)D levels < 43 ng/mL and impaired fasting glucose (OR = 3.40) and low insulin sensitivity (defined as HOMA index for insulin sensitivity < 90%) (OR = 2.65) has been reported in healthy adults with a median age of 39.4 years old [42]. Specifically, in patients with HF, vitamin D deficiency was shown to be correlated with increased rates of diabetes mellitus when compared with a non-vitamin D deficient group (31.4% vs. 22.8%) [43]. Despite these observations, our results show no correlation between 25(OH)D concentrations and fasting glucose level, insulin concentration, or HOMA index. These findings may be attributed to the low LVEF (below 40%) of all our patients, or to the medications they were taking.

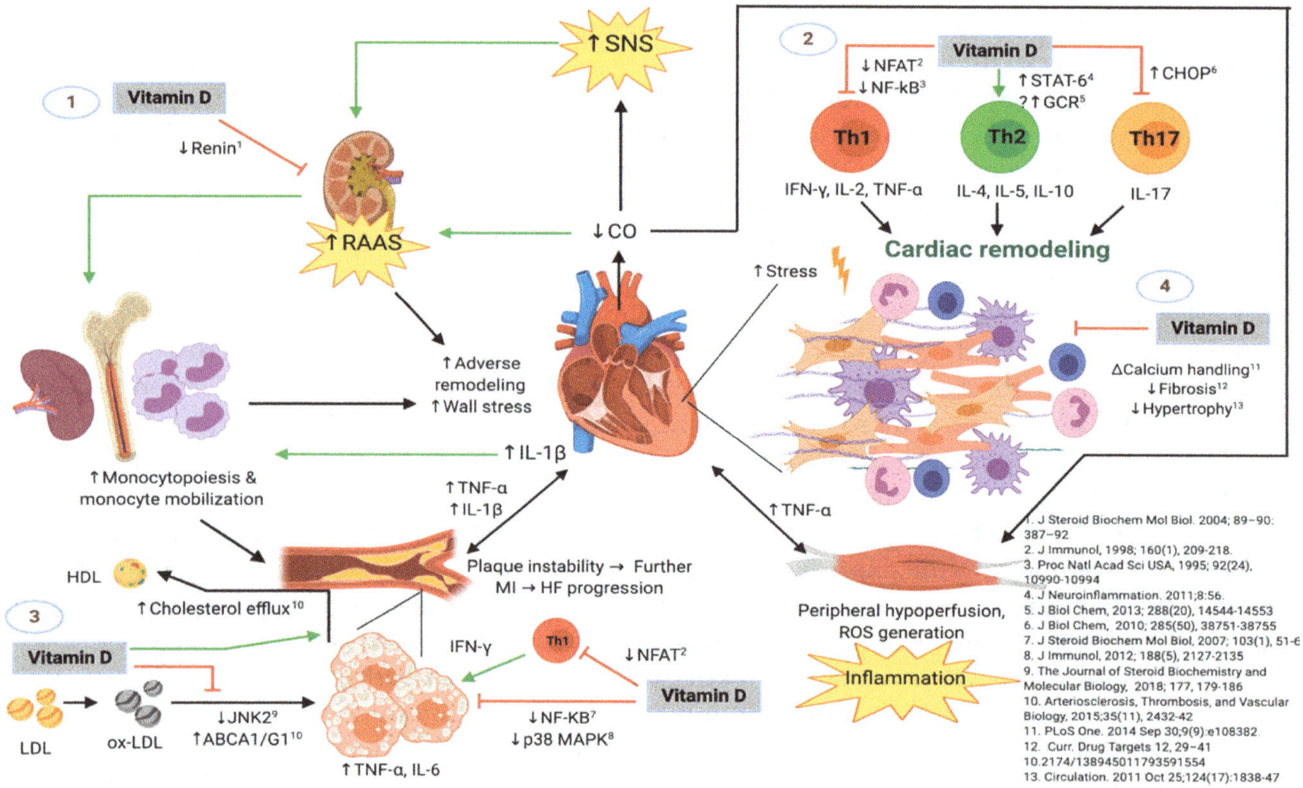

Figure 6. The Possible Immunomodulatory Role of Vitamin D in the Context of Heart Failure (HF) Progression. Green and black lines with arrowheads represent a direct stimulation and a positive correlation, respectively. Red lines ending in perpendicular bars indicate inhibition. (↑) represent an increase in expression, concentration, or activity of the parameter or mechanism. (↓) indicate a decrease in expression, concentration, or activity of the parameter of mechanism. HF is initiated and maintained by chronic maladaptive activation of neurohumoral networks that result from decreased cardiac output (e.g., the sympathetic nervous system [SNS] and the renin-angiotensin-aldosterone system [RAAS]), innate and adaptive immune mechanisms triggered by myocardial damage and stress, and systemic inflammation that results from hypoperfusion of peripheral organs [20,21]. Vitamin D may play a protective role in the progression of HF by interfering with several deleterious pathways [25], which include but are not limited to: (1) inhibiting the release of renin [44], which leads to attenuated RAAS-mediated adverse cardiac remodeling and release of monocytes from bone marrow and lymphoid tissue (an event that is also favored by IL-1β and perhaps other inflammatory cytokines from damaged myocardium) [21]. Monocytes are known to infiltrate damaged myocardium [45] and atheromatous plaques [35], where they exacerbate the local inflammatory response and promote further adverse ventricular remodeling as well as growth and instability of atherosclerotic plaques, respectively. Hence, vitamin D may indirectly attenuate monocyte/macrophage-mediated myocardial damage. (2) Vitamin D may also favor an anti-inflammatory T-helper lymphocyte phenotype by decreasing Th1 [46–48] and Th17 [9,23] cytokine production and favoring the Th2 phenotype [49], which would theoretically promote adequate remodeling and decreased fibrosis, and reduce cardiomyocyte hypertrophy and dysfunction. (3) Vitamin D could also slow the progression of atherosclerotic plaques by inhibiting the

proinflammatory activation of foam cells (macrophages that have phagocytosed ox-LDL particles) through diminished ox-LDL capture [38], increased cholesterol efflux [37], and decreased activation of transcription factors involved in the expression of proinflammatory cytokines such as TNF-α and IL-6 [22,50]. Like the mechanism described above, vitamin D may also act on T-lymphocytes present in atherosclerotic plaques, decreasing IFN-γ production and hence proinflammatory polarization of macrophages/foam cells. This is of relevance, as growth of atherosclerotic plaques results in plaque instability and further myocardial infarction, with consequent exacerbation of the pathogenic loop that characterizes HF. (4) Vitamin D has also been demonstrated to exert direct effects on the cardiomyocyte and interstitium, including modulation of intracellular calcium handling [26], expression of procollagen-1 [27], and hypertrophic calcineurin/NFAT signaling [28]. Abbreviations: HF = heart failure; MI = myocardial infarction; ABCA1/G1 = ATP-binding cassette transporter types A1 and G1; CHOP = C/EBP homologous protein; CO = cardiac output; GCR = glucocorticoid receptor; IFN = interferon; IL = interleukin; JNK2 = c-Jun N-terminal kinase 2; LDL = low-density lipoprotein; HDL = high-density lipoprotein; NFAT = nuclear factor of activated T-cells; NF-κB = nuclear factor kappa-B; ox-LDL = oxidized low-density lipoprotein; p38 MAPK = p38 mitogen-activated protein kinases; RAAS = renin-angiotensin-aldosterone system; SNS = sympathetic nervous system; STAT6 = signal transducer and activator of transcription 6; Th = T-helper; TNF = tumor necrosis factor-alpha. Original image created with BioRender® (BioRender, Toronto, ON, Canada; website URL: https://biorender.com/; accessed on 9 October 2019).

Contrary to what was expected, no correlation was seen between serum 25(OH)D concentrations and LVEF in our cohort. This could be explained by the fact that all of our patients presented abnormally low values of LVEF. Therefore, we could not analyze the whole spectrum of the relationship between vitamin D levels and LVEF.

3.3. Inflammation Pathways Associating Vitamin D Deficiency with HFrEF

Figure 6 shows the possible immunomodulatory role of Vitamin D regarding inflammation in the context of HF progression. HFrEF has long been recognized as a systemic proinflammatory state, with pathways involving activation of both innate and adaptive immunity mechanisms [19,20]. Most likely, a crosstalk between the heart and the peripheral organs in which HF promotes inflammation and vice versa might be present [21]. Hemodynamic stress and volume overload have been described to increment wall stress and cell mechanical damage, which stimulates cardiomyocyte release of proinflammatory cytokines, such as TNF-α, IL-1, MCP-1, and IL-6. On the other hand, peripheral organs respond to these inflammatory signals inducing more deleterious effects, such as: skeletal muscle inflammation (which may itself be secondary to chronic vasoconstriction and hypoperfusion due to decreased cardiac output), adipose tissue inflammation, increased atherogenic progression in the endothelium, augmented monocyte production by the bone marrow, and increased bacterial translocation from the gut [21]. This chronic proinflammatory cycle has been shown to contribute to the deterioration of ventricular function by inducing myocardial contractile dysfunction, hypertrophy, apoptosis, and fibrosis, with subsequent progression of HF [51]. Although systemic inflammation is a central pathogenic hallmark of HF [20], it is currently unclear whether vitamin D deficiency plays a specific role in the pathogenesis of HF through the attributed immunomodulatory functions [52]. However, it has been shown that vitamin D deficiency is indeed associated with HFrEF and increased markers of ongoing inflammation [17,53].

In the context of inflammation, the relationship between vitamin D and the cytokine milieu has been shown to represent a core aspect that leads to a proinflammatory state through several mechanisms. Our results in this cohort of patients with HF show serum 25(OH)D levels to be inversely correlated with the proinflammatory cytokines IL-1β, TNF-α, IL-6, and IL-8, although no correlation with the anti-inflammatory cytokine IL-10 was noted. Vitamin D has been found to inhibit the secretion of proinflammatory cytokines TNF-α and IL-6 by monocytes and macrophages through inhibiting p38 MAPK via induction of MKP1, which results in dephosphorylation of p38 [22]. The MAPK pathway is stimulated by diverse stressors to induce expression of proinflammatory cytokines, not only in immune cells but also in the myocardium itself [54]. Since a high prevalence of vitamin D deficiency was found in our study population, induction of this metabolic pathway is highly probable, which might aggravate the inflammatory status that these patients with HFrEF are already in.

Other mechanisms by means of which vitamin D has been associated with inflammation are related to the vitamin D-activated vitamin D receptor/retinoid X receptor (VDR/RXR) heterodimer. VDR/RXR has been reported to interact with transcription factors such as NF-κB, NFAT, and the glucocorticoid receptor (GCR), all of which participate in the transcription of genes involved in inflammatory processes [52]. NF-κB is involved in the transcription of many proinflammatory cytokines, including TNF-α, IL-1β, and IL-6, among others [55], which are direct mediators of cardiac dysfunction [56]. NF-κB expression and activation has been shown to be downregulated by vitamin D [48,50], which may function as a protective mechanism that would not be present in the setting of vitamin D deficiency. In its own way, NFAT upregulates the expression of IL-2, a crucial cytokine for T-cell replication, activation, and induction of Th1-mediated inflammatory responses [47], which appear to be relevant in HF, as evidenced by the higher number of circulating Th1 cells seen in this condition [57]. NFAT signaling has been shown to be inhibited by vitamin D, preventing this transcription factor from binding to its response elements [46], which further indicates another immunological pathway by which vitamin D deficiency may be deleterious in HF. On the other hand, GCR upregulates the expression of anti-inflammatory cytokines, while downregulating proinflammatory ones [58]. Vitamin D has been found to enhance these GCR-mediated anti-inflammatory activities [59], which may represent an anti-inflammatory mechanism that would be absent in circumstances of vitamin D deficiency. Considering the lines of evidence of the mechanisms and pathways provided, low 25(OH)D levels are expected to be accompanied by increased circulating proinflammatory cytokines, as observed in our cohort, which may possibly contribute to clinical deterioration in these patients.

Regarding one of the main pathways of adaptive immunity, our results show serum 25(OH)D concentrations to be negatively correlated with IL-17A as well. Interestingly, vitamin D has also been shown to inhibit the secretion of the proinflammatory cytokine IL-17 by Th17 cells through a post-transcriptional mechanism [23]. Others have shown that vitamin D suppresses autoimmunity, not only by decreasing the production of IL-17, but also by inhibiting the ability of naïve CD4+ T-cells to commit to the Th17 lineage [9]. The anti-Th17 effects of vitamin D could be of pathophysiological relevance in HFrEF, as IL-17 appears to have a role in adverse cardiac remodeling and myocardial fibrosis [60]. Vitamin D seems to induce a shift from a Th1 towards a Th2 phenotype, as well as to suppress Th17 responses [52]. Hence, it is reasonable to assume that vitamin D deficiency exacerbates the deleterious generalized proinflammatory state in our patients with HFrEF. In opposition to a previous study in our group with healthy adults [6], no significant seasonal variation of any cytokine was observed, which is consistent with the permanent state of inflammation that occurs in the context of HF [19,20].

3.4. Cluster Analysis

In order to characterize the cytokine profile and the 25(OH)D levels in our patients, we performed a cluster analysis, identifying three clusters. Patients from cluster 1 presented the highest circulating levels of 25(OH)D and the highest dietary intake of vitamin D. They showed the lowest significant levels of the proinflammatory cytokines TNF-α and IL-12p70, and the highest levels of the anti-inflammatory cytokine IL-10, compared with patients from the other two clusters, further reflecting the protective role that vitamin D plays in the cytokine milieu. These patients also showed the lowest concentration of total cholesterol, triglycerides, and Apo-B, representing the possible defensive role of vitamin D in atherosclerosis. Patients from cluster 2 had relatively intermediate levels of vitamin D concentration and vitamin D intake, along with intermediate levels of TNF-α, IL-17A, and IL-10 compared with patients from clusters 1 and 3. Finally, and in opposition, patients from cluster 3 presented the lowest serum 25(OH)D levels. These patients showed the highest concentrations of TNF-α, IL-8, and IL-17A, (significant for TNF-α), and the lowest significant levels of IL-10. They also had the highest levels of total cholesterol, LDL cholesterol, Apo-B, and triglycerides, indicating the proinflammatory and atherosclerotic mechanistic roles of vitamin D deficiency described previously. The role of dietary intake as the main lifestyle factor associated with vitamin D deficiency in this setting of patients may also be considered.

3.5. Correlation of Vitamin D Deficiency with Anthropometric and Lifestyle Parameters in Patients with HFrEF

The relationship between vitamin D and anthropometric parameters in the setting of HF has not been thoroughly explored. In the general population, there seems to be a consensus of a negative correlation between serum 25(OH)D concentrations and BMI, WC, and BF% [33,61–64], mainly attributed to sequestration of vitamin D by adipocytes. However, controversy has been found in patients with HF, as no correlation has been reported in this context between serum 25(OH)D levels and body weight, BMI, mid-arm muscle circumference [65], arm lean mass, leg lean mass, and grip strength (rather related to muscle mass and strength) [66]. Similarly, we found no correlation between 25(OH)D levels and BMI, BF%, and fat mass in kg. On the other hand, in a study with 14 HF patients vs. 14 controls, an inverse relationship was found between 25(OH)D levels and BMI [67]. Our results could be explained by the fact that most of our patients belonged to the overweight BMI and BF% category, and WC was within normal limits. Our sample of patients, like most with HF, are rather not obese because of a higher metabolic waste status due to the disease, and hence do not fully represent each of the BMI or BF% categories.

Likewise, lifestyle factors related to vitamin D status in patients with HF have been understudied. In a questionnaire-based study, patients with HF were less exposed to summer outdoor activity at least once a year compared with controls, but no difference was found in fish consumption (the only food source investigated) or vitamin D supplementation. However, serum 25(OH)D levels were not measured [67]. In the previously mentioned cross-sectional case-control study, that included 14 patients with HF vs. 14 controls, no significant differences in 25(OH)D concentration was reported. HF patients were shown to present less weekly sun exposure, but no differences in daily dietary vitamin D intake between the groups was found [67]. In addition, using data from a large population study, no differences were seen among various amounts of vitamin D intake and the incidence (new cases) of HF, but measurement of 25(OH)D levels was not performed either [68]. Our results during the 12-month follow up showed a significant positive correlation between dietary intake of vitamin D-rich foods and serum 25(OH)D concentrations. Regarding sun exposure, when the total population was considered, no correlation was found between serum 25(OH)D levels and sun exposure. Nevertheless, in a sub-analysis in which patients were separated into two groups, those with any amount of sun exposure versus those with no exposure at all, the prevalence of vitamin D sufficiency was significantly greater in patients exposed to the sun compared with those that had no exposure. Our group previously studied the seasonal variation of serum 25(OH)D concentration in a cohort of 23 healthy subjects with a follow-up of 12 months, in which seasonal variation was observed [6]. However, no seasonal variation of 25(OH)D levels was found in our present study, suggesting that sun exposure may not play a dominant role in vitamin D status (as opposed to healthy controls), but rather vitamin D intake seems to play a greater role. Consideration has to be given to our patients' skin phototype. Skin pigmentation represents a significant independent risk factor for vitamin D deficiency because UVB is needed in the initial conversion of 7-dehydrocholesterol into cholecalciferol, which is less available for this reaction in darker skin phototypes, as melanin acts as a light-absorbent protein. Thus, our cohort might be prone to vitamin D deficiency, given that the majority of the subjects belonged to phototypes IV and V.

The recommended daily allowance (RDA) of vitamin D for adults 51–70 years old is 600 IU/day, while that of adults >70 years old is 800 IU/day [69]. Therefore, none of the patients in our cohort met the nutritional requirements for vitamin D intake, as all of them had an average intake throughout the year of less than 400 IU/day. Although the time of sun exposure required for vitamin D synthesis varies considerably depending on the living latitude and the season of the year, it has been estimated that 5 to 30 min of sun exposure between 10 a.m. and 3 p.m. at least two times per week may be a reasonable amount [70]. Most of the patients in our cohort (82.3% during summer, autumn, and spring, and 52.9% during winter) obtained at least this level of sun exposure while living at an adequate latitude. Therefore, vitamin D ingestion might be a lifestyle factor as important or even more significant than sun exposure in determining 25(OH)D levels in the setting of our cohort of patients with HF.

The study has some limitations. The sample size is both small and from a Hispanic ethnicity; thus, our results might not be extrapolated to other populations. Hence, results should be cautiously interpreted. Even though data regarding vitamin D-rich foods intake and sun exposure was obtained through a personal interview, the information given by the patients might still be subjective. However, our study has several strengths. This is a 12-month follow up to approach seasonal variation of vitamin D and cytokines. In-vitro and animal model studies concerning the molecular mechanisms were identified to describe and apply these mechanisms to explain our results, given that studies in humans hardly explain them in such detail. We also emphasize these molecular mechanisms in an original figure presented in this article, which could offer insight for further research.

4. Materials and Methods

4.1. Study Population

We conducted a longitudinal study in a sample of HFrEF patients (49 to 82 years old) following standard treatment. Patients (n = 17) were followed during 12 months. Every three months, corresponding to each of the four seasons of the year, every patient was personally interviewed and evaluated for lifestyle, anthropometric, and laboratory parameters. All of the patients live in northeastern Mexico (city of Monterrey, latitude 25°40′0′′N) and are of Hispanic origin. The Fitzpatrick classification of phototypes, the standardized clinical method to evaluate a person's level of melanin pigmentation, was used to determine the level of skin pigmentation of the patients. Phototype I individuals have fair skin, which burns and peels easily with sun exposure, but does not tan; they usually have light eye and hair color. Phototype VI individuals are dark-skinned; when exposed to the sun, they always tan and never burn [71]. The inclusion criteria were a proved diagnosis of HFrEF (LVEF < 40%) and a New York Heart Association (NYHA) functional class of III or IV [29]. The exclusion criteria were chronic kidney disease, liver disease, LVEF ≥ 40%, chronic use of corticosteroids, ingestion of vitamin D supplements, and being institutionalized. Written informed consent was explained, accepted, and signed by all of the patients. The study was approved on May 14, 2013, by the Ethics and Research Commissions of the School of Medicine of Tecnologico de Monterrey and the Santos y de la Garza Evia Foundation, as well as by the Mexican Secretariat of Health with the project identification code "ESVDIC".

4.2. Vitamin D Intake

Every 3 months, each of the patients were interviewed about regular ingestion of vitamin D-rich foods. Standardized portions of these foods were shown to the patients in order to quantify in a more accurate way the amount of vitamin D ingested per source. The patients were asked about consumption of milk (124 IU/portion), yogurt (120 IU/portion), cheese (20 IU/portion), egg (20 IU/portion), fish (150 IU/portion), and cereal (50 IU/portion). Estimated vitamin D content per food source and portions were determined according to the USDA National Nutrient Database for Standard Reference Release [72].

4.3. Sun Exposure

During each visit, patients were asked for the total amount of time being exposed to the sun (minutes per day [mpd] and days per week [dpw]). Activities involving and not involving physical exercise were both taken into account. Skin characteristics according to the Fitzpatrick classification of phototypes were registered [71].

4.4. Anthropometric Parameters

For each of the seasons, the following anthropometric parameters were measured: height (m), weight (kg), BMI (kg/m^2), WC (cm), BF% (%), and fat mass (kg) according to standardized protocols [73]. The body fat percentage was measured by bioimpedance using a TANITA's BF-350 (Tanita Corporation of America, Inc., Arlington Heights, IL, USA).

4.5. Vitamin D, Biochemical Parameters, and Cytokines

The patients had a blood sample withdrawn by venipuncture for each of the seasons. Calcium concentration was obtained by spectrophotometry with the Calcium 3L79-21 kit (06753/R05) (Abbott Laboratories Diagnostics Division, Chicago, IL, USA), while serum 25(OH)D and PTH levels were measured by chemiluminescence with the Vit D25OH 5P02-25 kit (G5-9160/R01) and the iPTH 8K25-25 kit (G6-5257/-R05), respectively, on the Architect iSystem (Abbott Laboratories Diagnostics Division, Chicago, IL, USA). Serum and plasma were also obtained from these samples, centrifuged, and frozen at −80 °C afterward. Vitamin D status was determined according to the Endocrine Clinical Society Guidelines: sufficiency as serum 25(OH)D ≥ 30 ng/mL, insufficiency as serum 25(OH)D ≥ 20 and < 30 ng/mL, and deficiency as serum 25(OH)D < 20 ng/mL [30]. High-sensitivity C-reactive protein levels were measured by quantitative immunoturbidimetric assay with a CRP Vario 6K26-30 and 6K26-41 kits (Abbott Laboratories Diagnostic Division, Chicago, IL, USA). Fasting glucose levels were determined by the hexokinase (HK)/glucose-6-phosphate dehydrogenase (G-6-PD) method with the Glucose 3L82 reagent (DENKA SEIKEN Co. Ltd., Tokyo, Japan). Insulin concentrations were measured by chemiluminescence, using the ARCHITECT Insulin Reagent 8K41-27 kit (Abbot Laboratories Diagnostic Division, IL, USA). Total cholesterol was determined with the Cholesterol 7D62-21 reagent kit (307166/R04) (Abbot Laboratories Diagnostic Division, Chicago, IL, USA) on the Architect cSystem. HDL cholesterol was measured by the accelerator selective detergent method with the Ultra HDL 3K33-21 (307177-R04) assay (Abbot Laboratories Diagnostic Division, Chicago, IL, USA) on the Architect cSystem. Triglycerides were measured via the glycerol-phosphate-oxidase reaction with the Triglyceride 7D74-21 kit (307170/R03) (Abbot Laboratories Diagnostic Division, Chicago, IL, USA) on the Architect cSystem. LDL cholesterol was calculated using the total cholesterol, HDL cholesterol, and triglyceride determinations previously mentioned [74]. Apo-A and Apo-B were obtained via immunoturbidimetric assays with the Apolipoprotein A1 9D92-21 kit (306769/R03) and the Apolipoprotein B 9D93-21 kit (306770/R03), respectively, using the Architect cSystem (Abbot Laboratories Diagnostic Division, Chicago, IL, USA). BNP was measured by chemiluminescence with the BNP 8K28-28 kit (616-010-R01) (Abbott Laboratories Diagnostics Division, Chicago, IL, USA) on the Architect iSystem. Serum was used to obtain a cytokine profile using the Legendplex Human Inflammation Panel through a multianalyte flow cytometry assay (BioLegend, San Diego, CA, USA). This panel allows determination of 13 cytokines: IL-1β, IFN-α, IFN-γ, TNF-α, MCP-1, IL-6, IL-8, IL-10, IL-12p70, IL-17A, IL-18, IL-23, and IL-33. As recommended by Biolegend's instructions, each experiment was performed in triplicate. The flow cytometer used was FACS-Canto II (Becton Dickinson, Franklin Lakes, NJ, USA). Using the standard curves and the Legendplex Data Analysis software version 7.1 provided by BioLegend (BioLegend, San Diego, CA, USA), the analyte concentration and the serum concentrations were calculated for each of the cytokines.

4.6. Subgrouping Analysis by Cluster

In order to better identify which variables may represent a given profile regarding vitamin D deficiency in patients with HFrEF, a cluster analysis by partitioning around medoids (PAM) was performed. A total of 4 observations per patient were included in this analysis (corresponding to each of the seasons). The 25(OH)D levels, inflammatory cytokines, lifestyle factors, biochemical, and anthropometric parameters were included. Differences among clusters were assessed by ANOVA with Tukey's post-hoc test.

4.7. Statistical Analysis

Principal component analysis (PCA) was performed to explore continuous demographic, anthropometric, and lifestyle variables. Seasonal variation was tested with repeated-measures ANOVA. Categorical variables were evaluated with Fisher's exact test. Univariate association with 25(OH)D concentration was calculated with Spearman's rank correlation test. A conditional inference tree was constructed for vitamin D status prediction according to parameters with statistically significant association in univariate analysis. The R platform (R package version 2.0.7-1; The R Foundation, Vienna, Austria), along with the cluster [75] and party [76] packages, were used.

5. Conclusions

Several lines of evidence establish the mechanistic and metabolic roles of vitamin D deficiency contributing to the inflammatory, immunomodulatory, and atherosclerotic status of patients with HF. Our results in this 12-month follow-up of patients with HFrEF are consistent with previous observations of a high prevalence of vitamin D deficiency in these type of patients. We found no seasonal variation of 25(OH)D levels, nor of the proinflammatory cytokine profile. Serum 25(OH)D concentrations correlated with dietary intake of vitamin D-rich foods. When analyzing our total population, no correlation was seen between 25(OH)D levels and sun exposure; nonetheless, when subgrouping the patients into positive (any amount of sun exposure) and negative (no sun exposure), there was a higher prevalence of vitamin D sufficiency in those belonging to the positive group. Considering the inflammatory state observed in the setting of HF, 25(OH)D levels were inversely correlated with the proinflammatory cytokines IL-1β, TNF-α, IL-6, IL-8, IL-17A, IL-18, and IL-33. Total cholesterol, LDL cholesterol, and triglycerides were also negatively correlated with 25(OH)D concentrations. Cluster analysis to better identify different patient profiles related to vitamin D status revealed that patients with the highest levels of 25(OH)D showed the highest dietary intake of vitamin D-rich foods, along with the lowest concentration of TNF-α, IL-17A, total cholesterol, triglycerides, and Apo-B. Overall, these results point towards the lifestyle factors and lipid parameters related to adequate levels of 25(OH)D. In addition, the protective anti-inflammatory role that vitamin D has in the setting of HFrEF was shown in this group of patients. Some of the pathways underlying these mechanisms have been described mostly in in-vitro and animal models: inhibition of renin biosynthesis; less detrimental ventricular remodeling by inhibition of procollagen-1 expression; increased myocardial contractility; and downregulation of JNK2, calcineurin/NFAT, and NF-κB cellular pathways. Induction of cholesterol efflux from foam cells; increased cholesterol uptake by hepatocytes; adequate regulation of GLUT4 expression in cardiomyocytes; and inhibition of the secretion of proinflammatory cytokines by downregulation of the MAPK pathway, have been attributed to vitamin D. Future studies are necessary in patients with HF to establish the molecular mechanisms involved in the pathogenesis of this disease.

Author Contributions: Conceptualization, L.E.-M. and G.G.-R.; methodology, L.E.-M., G.G.-R., C.E.; software, J.R.V.-C.; validation, L.E.-M., G.G.-R., C.E., A.M.G.-G., J.R.V.-C., E.C.C., A.S.H.-D., D.N.R.-V.; formal analysis, J.R.V.-C.; investigation, A.M.G.-G., E.C.C., A.S.H.-D., D.N.R.-V.; resources, L.E.-M., G.G.-R., C.E., A.M.G.-G.; data curation, A.S.H.-D., D.N.R.-V., A.M.G.-G., E.C.C.; writing—original draft preparation, D.N.R.-V., A.S.H.-D., A.M.G.-G.; writing—review and editing, L.E.-M., D.N.R.-V., A.S.H.-D., A.M.G.-G., J.R.V.-C.; visualization, L.E.-M., D.N.R.-V., A.S.H.-D.; supervision, L.E.-M., G.G.-R., E.C.C.; project administration, L.E.-M., G.G.-R.; funding acquisition, L.E.-M., G.G.-R.

Acknowledgments: The authors would like to acknowledge the invaluable fieldwork of Mariana Peschard-Franco [1], Gustavo Gutierrez-DelBosque [1], Gerardo Mendoza-Lara [1], Bianca Nieblas [1], and Sofia Tenorio-Martínez [1]. [1] Tecnologico de Monterrey, Center for Research in Clinical Nutrition, Escuela de Medicina, 64710 Monterrey, N.L., Mexico.

Abbreviations

HF	Heart failure
LDL	Low density lipoprotein
Apo	Apolipoprotein
IL	Interleukin
TNF	Tumor necrosis factor
BMI	Body mass index
UVB	Ultraviolet B-type
25(OH)D	25-hydroxyvitamin D
1,25(OH)2D3	1,25-dihydroxyvitamin D (calcitriol)
PTH	Parathyroid hormone
FGF-23	Fibroblast growth factor 23
WC	Waist circumference
IU	International units
LVEF	Left ventricular ejection fraction
HFrEF	Heart failure with reduced ejection fraction
HFpEF	Heart failure with preserved ejection fraction
HFmrEF	Heart failure with mid-range ejection fraction
RAAS	Renin angiotensin aldosterone system
PK	Protein kinase
NF-κB	Nuclear-factor kappa B
MCP-1	Monocyte chemoattractant protein-1
MAPK	Mitogen-activated protein kinase
MMP	Matrix metalloproteinase
NYHA	New York Heart Association
USDA	United States Department of Agriculture
IFN	Interferon
PCA	Principal component analysis
HSD	Honest significance difference
PMA	Partitioning around medoids
HDL	High density lipoprotein
HOMA	Homeostatic model assessment
BNP	Brain natriuretic peptide
ANOVA	Analysis of variance
cAMP	Cyclic adenosine monophosphate
NFAT	Nuclear factor of activated T-cells
oxLDL	Oxidized low-density lipoprotein
APC	Antigen-presenting cells
JNK2	c-Jun N-terminal protein kinase 2
GLUT4	Glucose transporter 4
VDR/RXR	Vitamin D receptor/Retinoid X receptor
GCR	Glucocorticoid receptor

Appendix A

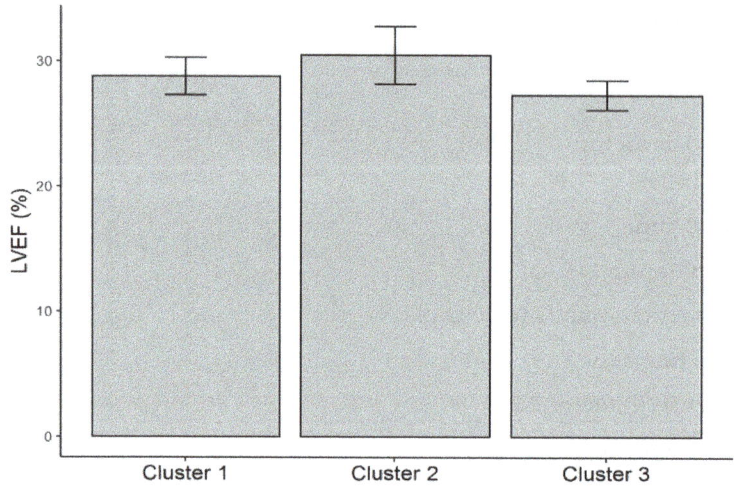

Figure A1. LVEF (%) values for each of the clusters. Mean and standard error (vertical bars) are shown. There was no significant difference of this parameter among clusters. LVEF = left ventricular ejection fraction.

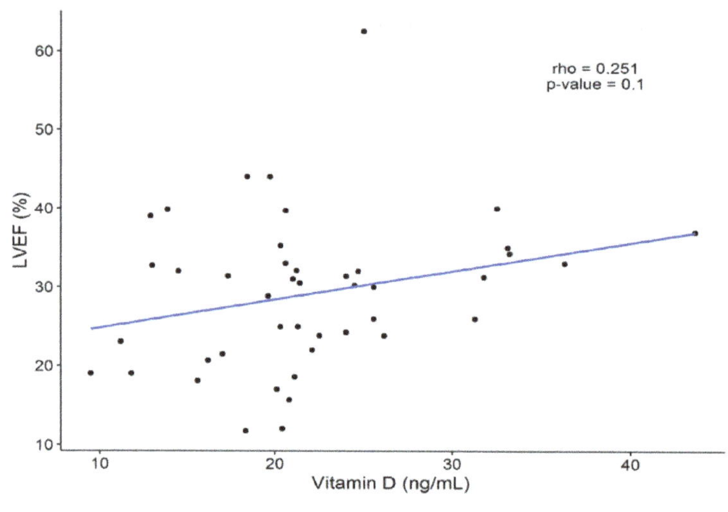

Figure A2. Linear correlation between LVEF (%) and 25(OH)D concentration. A weak positive correlation was found ($R = 0.251$), but no statistical significance was seen. LVEF = left ventricular ejection fraction; 25(OH)D = 25-hydroxivitamin D.

References

1. Cashman, K.D. Vitamin D Deficiency: Defining, Prevalence, Causes, and Strategies of Addressing. *Calcif. Tissue Int.* **2019**, 1–16. [CrossRef] [PubMed]
2. Jeon, S.M.; Shin, E.A. Exploring vitamin D metabolism and function in cancer. *Exp. Mol. Med.* **2018**, *50*, 20. [CrossRef] [PubMed]
3. Veldurthy, V.; Wei, R.; Campbell, M.; Lupicki, K.; Dhawan, P.; Christakos, S. 25-Hydroxyvitamin D_3 24-Hydroxylase: A Key Regulator of $1,25(OH)_2D_3$ Catabolism and Calcium Homeostasis. *Vitam. Horm.* **2016**, *100*, 137–150. [CrossRef] [PubMed]
4. Dhawan, P.; Peng, X.; Sutton, A.L.; MacDonald, P.N.; Croniger, C.M.; Trautwein, C.; Centrella, M.; McCarthy, T.L.; Christakos, S. Functional cooperation between CCAAT/enhancer-binding proteins and the vitamin D receptor in regulation of 25-hydroxyvitamin D3 24-hydroxylase. *Mol. Cell. Biol.* **2005**, *25*, 472–487. [CrossRef] [PubMed]
5. Holick, M.F. Vitamin D deficiency. *N. Engl. J. Med.* **2007**, *357*, 266–281. [CrossRef]

6. Elizondo-Montemayor, L.; Castillo, E.C.; Rodríguez-López, C.; Villarreal-Calderón, J.R.; Gómez-Carmona, M.; Tenorio-Martínez, S.; Nieblas, B.; García-Rivas, G. Seasonal Variation in Vitamin D in Association with Age, Inflammatory Cytokines, Anthropometric Parameters, and Lifestyle Factors in Older Adults. *Mediat. Inflamm.* **2017**, *2017*, 5719461. [CrossRef]
7. Herrick, K.A.; Storandt, R.J.; Afful, J.; Pfeiffer, C.M.; Schleicher, R.L.; Gahche, J.J.; Potischman, N. Vitamin D status in the United States, 2011–2014. *Am. J. Clin. Nutr.* 2019. [CrossRef]
8. Peterson, C.A.; Heffernan, M.E. Serum tumor necrosis factor-alpha concentrations are negatively correlated with serum 25(OH)D concentrations in healthy women. *J. Inflamm. (Lond.)* **2008**, *5*, 10. [CrossRef]
9. Tang, J.; Zhou, R.; Luger, D.; Zhu, W.; Silver, P.B.; Grajewski, R.S.; Su, S.B.; Chan, C.C.; Adorini, L.; Caspi, R.R. Calcitriol suppresses antiretinal autoimmunity through inhibitory effects on the Th17 effector response. *J. Immunol.* **2009**, *182*, 4624–4632. [CrossRef]
10. Rai, V.; Agrawal, D.K. Role of Vitamin D in Cardiovascular Diseases. *Endocrinol. Metab. Clin. N. Am.* **2017**, *46*, 1039–1059. [CrossRef]
11. Benjamin, E.J.; Muntner, P.; Alonso, A.; Bittencourt, M.S.; Callaway, C.W.; Carson, A.P.; Chamberlain, A.M.; Chang, A.R.; Cheng, S.; Das, S.R.; et al. Heart Disease and Stroke Statistics-2019 Update: A Report From the American Heart Association. *Circulation* **2019**, *139*, e56–e528. [CrossRef] [PubMed]
12. Savarese, G.; Lund, L.H. Global Public Health Burden of Heart Failure. *Card. Fail. Rev.* **2017**, *3*, 7–11. [CrossRef]
13. Ciapponi, A.; Alcaraz, A.; Calderón, M.; Matta, M.G.; Chaparro, M.; Soto, N.; Bardach, A. Burden of Heart Failure in Latin America: A Systematic Review and Meta-analysis. *Rev. Esp. Cardiol. (Engl. Ed.)* **2016**, *69*, 1051–1060. [CrossRef] [PubMed]
14. Ponikowski, P.; Voors, A.A.; Anker, S.D.; Bueno, H.; Cleland, J.G.; Coats, A.J.; Falk, V.; González-Juanatey, J.R.; Harjola, V.P.; Jankowska, E.A.; et al. 2016 ESC Guidelines for the diagnosis and treatment of acute and chronic heart failure: The Task Force for the diagnosis and treatment of acute and chronic heart failure of the European Society of Cardiology (ESC). Developed with the special contribution of the Heart Failure Association (HFA) of the ESC. *Eur. J. Heart Fail.* **2016**, *18*, 891–975. [CrossRef] [PubMed]
15. Ziaeian, B.; Fonarow, G.C. Epidemiology and aetiology of heart failure. *Nat. Rev. Cardiol.* **2016**, *13*, 368–378. [CrossRef] [PubMed]
16. Saponaro, F.; Saba, A.; Frascarelli, S.; Frontera, C.; Clerico, A.; Scalese, M.; Sessa, M.R.; Cetani, F.; Borsari, S.; Pardi, E.; et al. Vitamin D measurement and effect on outcome in a cohort of patients with heart failure. *Endocr. Connect.* **2018**, *7*, 957–964. [CrossRef] [PubMed]
17. D'Amore, C.; Marsico, F.; Parente, A.; Paolillo, S.; De Martino, F.; Gargiulo, P.; Ferrazzano, F.; De Roberto, A.M.; La Mura, L.; Marciano, C.; et al. Vitamin D deficiency and clinical outcome in patients with chronic heart failure: A review. *Nutr. Metab. Cardiovasc. Dis.* **2017**, *27*, 837–849. [CrossRef]
18. Shirazi, L.F.; Bissett, J.; Romeo, F.; Mehta, J.L. Role of Inflammation in Heart Failure. *Curr. Atheroscler. Rep.* **2017**, *19*, 27. [CrossRef]
19. Mann, D.L. Innate immunity and the failing heart: The cytokine hypothesis revisited. *Circ. Res.* **2015**, *116*, 1254–1268. [CrossRef]
20. Sánchez-Trujillo, L.; Vázquez-Garza, E.; Castillo, E.C.; García-Rivas, G.; Torre-Amione, G. Role of Adaptive Immunity in the Development and Progression of Heart Failure: New Evidence. *Arch. Med. Res.* **2017**, *48*, 1–11. [CrossRef]
21. Van Linthout, S.; Tschöpe, C. Inflammation—Cause or Consequence of Heart Failure or Both? *Curr. Heart Fail. Rep.* **2017**, *14*, 251–265. [CrossRef] [PubMed]
22. Zhang, Y.; Leung, D.Y.; Richers, B.N.; Liu, Y.; Remigio, L.K.; Riches, D.W.; Goleva, E. Vitamin D inhibits monocyte/macrophage proinflammatory cytokine production by targeting MAPK phosphatase-1. *J. Immunol.* **2012**, *188*, 2127–2135. [CrossRef] [PubMed]
23. Chang, S.H.; Chung, Y.; Dong, C. Vitamin D suppresses Th17 cytokine production by inducing C/EBP homologous protein (CHOP) expression. *J. Biol. Chem.* **2010**, *285*, 38751–38755. [CrossRef] [PubMed]
24. Riek, A.E.; Oh, J.; Bernal-Mizrachi, C. 1,25(OH)2 vitamin D suppresses macrophage migration and reverses atherogenic cholesterol metabolism in type 2 diabetic patients. *J. Steroid Biochem. Mol. Biol.* **2013**, *136*, 309–312. [CrossRef]
25. Wu, M.; Xu, K.; Wu, Y.; Lin, L. Role of Vitamin D in Patients with Heart Failure with Reduced Ejection Fraction. *Am. J. Cardiovasc. Drugs.* **2019**, 1–12. [CrossRef]

26. Choudhury, S.; Bae, S.; Ke, Q.; Lee, J.Y.; Singh, S.S.; St-Arnaud, R.; Monte, F.D.; Kang, P.M. Abnormal calcium handling and exaggerated cardiac dysfunction in mice with defective vitamin d signaling. *PLoS ONE* **2014**, *9*, e108382. [CrossRef]
27. Meems, L.M.; van der Harst, P.; van Gilst, W.H.; de Boer, R.A. Vitamin D biology in heart failure: Molecular mechanisms and systematic review. *Curr. Drug Targets* **2011**, *12*, 29–41. [CrossRef]
28. Chen, S.; Law, C.S.; Grigsby, C.L.; Olsen, K.; Hong, T.T.; Zhang, Y.; Yeghiazarians, Y.; Gardner, D.G. Cardiomyocyte-specific deletion of the vitamin D receptor gene results in cardiac hypertrophy. *Circulation* **2011**, *124*, 1838–1847. [CrossRef]
29. The Joint Commission. *New York Heart Association (NYHA) Classification*; Measures, J.C.N.Q., Ed.; The Joint Commission: Washington, DC, USA, 2016.
30. Holick, M.F.; Binkley, N.C.; Bischoff-Ferrari, H.A.; Gordon, C.M.; Hanley, D.A.; Heaney, R.P.; Murad, M.H.; Weaver, C.M.; Society, E. Evaluation, treatment, and prevention of vitamin D deficiency: An Endocrine Society clinical practice guideline. *J. Clin. Endocrinol. Metab.* **2011**, *96*, 1911–1930. [CrossRef]
31. Anderson, J.L.; May, H.T.; Horne, B.D.; Bair, T.L.; Hall, N.L.; Carlquist, J.F.; Lappé, D.L.; Muhlestein, J.B.; Group, I.H.C.I.S. Relation of vitamin D deficiency to cardiovascular risk factors, disease status, and incident events in a general healthcare population. *Am. J. Cardiol.* **2010**, *106*, 963–968. [CrossRef]
32. Belen, E.; Sungur, A.; Sungur, M.A. Vitamin D levels predict hospitalization and mortality in patients with heart failure. *Scand. Cardiovasc. J.* **2016**, *50*, 17–22. [CrossRef] [PubMed]
33. Cartier, J.L.; Kukreja, S.C.; Barengolts, E. Lower Serum 25-Hydroxyvitamin D Is Associated with Obesity but Not Common Chronic Conditions: An Observational Study of African American and Caucasian Male Veterans. *Endocr. Pract.* **2017**, *23*, 271–278. [CrossRef] [PubMed]
34. Bozkurt, B.; Aguilar, D.; Deswal, A.; Dunbar, S.B.; Francis, G.S.; Horwich, T.; Jessup, M.; Kosiborod, M.; Pritchett, A.M.; Ramasubbu, K.; et al. Contributory Risk and Management of Comorbidities of Hypertension, Obesity, Diabetes Mellitus, Hyperlipidemia, and Metabolic Syndrome in Chronic Heart Failure: A Scientific Statement From the American Heart Association. *Circulation* **2016**, *134*, e535–e578. [CrossRef] [PubMed]
35. Libby, P.; Buring, J.E.; Badimon, L.; Hansson, G.K.; Deanfield, J.; Bittencourt, M.S.; Tokgözoğlu, L.; Lewis, E.F. Atherosclerosis. *Nat. Rev. Dis. Primers.* **2019**, *5*, 56. [CrossRef]
36. Gimbrone, M.A.; García-Cardeña, G. Endothelial Cell Dysfunction and the Pathobiology of Atherosclerosis. *Circ. Res.* **2016**, *118*, 620–636. [CrossRef]
37. Yin, K.; You, Y.; Swier, V.; Tang, L.; Radwan, M.M.; Pandya, A.N.; Agrawal, D.K. Vitamin D Protects Against Atherosclerosis via Regulation of Cholesterol Efflux and Macrophage Polarization in Hypercholesterolemic Swine. *Arterioscler. Thromb. Vasc. Biol.* **2015**, *35*, 2432–2442. [CrossRef]
38. Oh, J.; Riek, A.E.; Zhang, R.M.; Williams, S.A.S.; Darwech, I.; Bernal-Mizrachi, C. Deletion of JNK2 prevents vitamin-D-deficiency-induced hypertension and atherosclerosis in mice. *J. Steroid Biochem. Mol. Biol.* **2018**, *177*, 179–186. [CrossRef]
39. Faridi, K.F.; Zhao, D.; Martin, S.S.; Lupton, J.R.; Jones, S.R.; Guallar, E.; Ballantyne, C.M.; Lutsey, P.L.; Michos, E.D. Serum vitamin D and change in lipid levels over 5 y: The Atherosclerosis Risk in Communities study. *Nutrition* **2017**, *38*, 85–93. [CrossRef]
40. Forrest, K.Y.; Stuhldreher, W.L. Prevalence and correlates of vitamin D deficiency in US adults. *Nutr. Res.* **2011**, *31*, 48–54. [CrossRef]
41. Nizami, H.L.; Katare, P.; Prabhakar, P.; Kumar, Y.; Arava, S.K.; Chakraborty, P.; Maulik, S.K.; Banerjee, S.K. Vitamin D Deficiency in Rats Causes Cardiac Dysfunction by Inducing Myocardial Insulin Resistance. *Mol. Nutr. Food Res.* **2019**, *63*, e1900109. [CrossRef]
42. Mayer, O.; Seidlerová, J.; Černá, V.; Kučerová, A.; Karnosová, P.; Hronová, M.; Wohlfahrt, P.; Fuchsová, R.; Filipovský, J.; Cífková, R.; et al. Serum Vitamin D Status, Vitamin D Receptor Polymorphism, and Glucose Homeostasis in Healthy Subjects. *Horm. Metab. Res.* **2018**, *50*, 56–64. [CrossRef] [PubMed]
43. Cubbon, R.M.; Lowry, J.E.; Drozd, M.; Hall, M.; Gierula, J.; Paton, M.F.; Byrom, R.; Kearney, L.C.; Barth, J.H.; Kearney, M.T.; et al. Vitamin D deficiency is an independent predictor of mortality in patients with chronic heart failure. *Eur. J. Nutr.* **2019**, *58*, 2535–2543. [CrossRef] [PubMed]
44. Li, Y.C.; Qiao, G.; Uskokovic, M.; Xiang, W.; Zheng, W.; Kong, J. Vitamin D: A negative endocrine regulator of the renin-angiotensin system and blood pressure. *J. Steroid Biochem. Mol. Biol.* **2004**, *89*, 387–392. [CrossRef] [PubMed]

45. Epelman, S.; Liu, P.P.; Mann, D.L. Role of innate and adaptive immune mechanisms in cardiac injury and repair. *Nat. Rev. Immunol.* **2015**, *15*, 117–129. [CrossRef] [PubMed]
46. Takeuchi, A.; Reddy, G.S.; Kobayashi, T.; Okano, T.; Park, J.; Sharma, S. Nuclear factor of activated T cells (NFAT) as a molecular target for 1alpha,25-dihydroxyvitamin D3-mediated effects. *J. Immunol.* **1998**, *160*, 209–218.
47. Hermann-Kleiter, N.; Baier, G. NFAT pulls the strings during CD4± T helper cell effector functions. *Blood* **2010**, *115*, 2989–2997. [CrossRef]
48. Yu, X.P.; Bellido, T.; Manolagas, S.C. Down-regulation of NF-kappa B protein levels in activated human lymphocytes by 1,25-dihydroxyvitamin D3. *Proc. Natl. Acad. Sci. USA* **1995**, *92*, 10990–10994. [CrossRef]
49. Sloka, S.; Silva, C.; Wang, J.; Yong, V.W. Predominance of Th2 polarization by vitamin D through a STAT6-dependent mechanism. *J. Neuroinflamm.* **2011**, *8*, 56. [CrossRef]
50. Stio, M.; Martinesi, M.; Bruni, S.; Treves, C.; Mathieu, C.; Verstuyf, A.; d'Albasio, G.; Bagnoli, S.; Bonanomi, A.G. The Vitamin D analogue TX 527 blocks NF-kappaB activation in peripheral blood mononuclear cells of patients with Crohn's disease. *J. Steroid Biochem. Mol. Biol.* **2007**, *103*, 51–60. [CrossRef]
51. Zhang, Y.; Bauersachs, J.; Langer, H.F. Immune mechanisms in heart failure. *Eur. J. Heart Fail.* **2017**, *19*, 1379–1389. [CrossRef]
52. Wöbke, T.K.; Sorg, B.L.; Steinhilber, D. Vitamin D in inflammatory diseases. *Front. Physiol.* **2014**, *5*, 244. [CrossRef] [PubMed]
53. Liu, L.C.; Voors, A.A.; van Veldhuisen, D.J.; van der Veer, E.; Belonje, A.M.; Szymanski, M.K.; Silljé, H.H.; van Gilst, W.H.; Jaarsma, T.; de Boer, R.A. Vitamin D status and outcomes in heart failure patients. *Eur. J. Heart Fail.* **2011**, *13*, 619–625. [CrossRef] [PubMed]
54. Li, M.; Georgakopoulos, D.; Lu, G.; Hester, L.; Kass, D.A.; Hasday, J.; Wang, Y. p38 MAP kinase mediates inflammatory cytokine induction in cardiomyocytes and extracellular matrix remodeling in heart. *Circulation* **2005**, *111*, 2494–2502. [CrossRef] [PubMed]
55. Liu, T.; Zhang, L.; Joo, D.; Sun, S.C. NF-κB signaling in inflammation. *Signal Transduct. Target Ther.* **2017**, *2*. [CrossRef] [PubMed]
56. Gullestad, L.; Ueland, T.; Vinge, L.E.; Finsen, A.; Yndestad, A.; Aukrust, P. Inflammatory cytokines in heart failure: Mediators and markers. *Cardiology* **2012**, *122*, 23–35. [CrossRef] [PubMed]
57. Fukunaga, T.; Soejima, H.; Irie, A.; Sugamura, K.; Oe, Y.; Tanaka, T.; Kojima, S.; Sakamoto, T.; Yoshimura, M.; Nishimura, Y.; et al. Expression of interferon-gamma and interleukin-4 production in CD4± T cells in patients with chronic heart failure. *Heart Vessels* **2007**, *22*, 178–183. [CrossRef]
58. Baschant, U.; Tuckermann, J. The role of the glucocorticoid receptor in inflammation and immunity. *J. Steroid Biochem. Mol. Biol.* **2010**, *120*, 69–75. [CrossRef]
59. Zhang, Y.; Leung, D.Y.; Goleva, E. Vitamin D enhances glucocorticoid action in human monocytes: Involvement of granulocyte-macrophage colony-stimulating factor and mediator complex subunit 14. *J. Biol. Chem.* **2013**, *288*, 14544–14553. [CrossRef]
60. Feng, W.; Li, W.; Liu, W.; Wang, F.; Li, Y.; Yan, W. IL-17 induces myocardial fibrosis and enhances RANKL/OPG and MMP/TIMP signaling in isoproterenol-induced heart failure. *Exp. Mol. Pathol.* **2009**, *87*, 212–218. [CrossRef]
61. Cheng, S.; Massaro, J.M.; Fox, C.S.; Larson, M.G.; Keyes, M.J.; McCabe, E.L.; Robins, S.J.; O'Donnell, C.J.; Hoffmann, U.; Jacques, P.F.; et al. Adiposity, cardiometabolic risk, and vitamin D status: The Framingham Heart Study. *Diabetes* **2010**, *59*, 242–248. [CrossRef]
62. Pantovic, A.; Zec, M.; Zekovic, M.; Obrenovic, R.; Stankovic, S.; Glibetic, M. Vitamin D Is Inversely Related to Obesity: Cross-Sectional Study in a Small Cohort of Serbian Adults. *J. Am. Coll. Nutr.* **2019**, *38*, 405–414. [CrossRef] [PubMed]
63. Gu, J.K.; Charles, L.E.; Millen, A.E.; Violanti, J.M.; Ma, C.C.; Jenkins, E.; Andrew, M.E. Associations between adiposity measures and 25-hydroxyvitamin D among police officers. *Am. J. Hum Biol.* **2019**, *31*, e23274. [CrossRef] [PubMed]
64. Hannemann, A.; Thuesen, B.H.; Friedrich, N.; Völzke, H.; Steveling, A.; Ittermann, T.; Hegenscheid, K.; Nauck, M.; Linneberg, A.; Wallaschofski, H. Adiposity measures and vitamin D concentrations in Northeast Germany and Denmark. *Nutr. Metab. (Lond.)* **2015**, *12*, 24. [CrossRef] [PubMed]
65. Price, R.J.; Witham, M.D.; McMurdo, M.E. Defining the nutritional status and dietary intake of older heart failure patients. *Eur. J. Cardiovasc. Nurs.* **2007**, *6*, 178–183. [CrossRef] [PubMed]

66. Loncar, G.; Bozic, B.; von Haehling, S.; Düngen, H.D.; Prodanovic, N.; Lainscak, M.; Arandjelovic, A.; Dimkovic, S.; Radojicic, Z.; Popovic, V. Association of adiponectin with peripheral muscle status in elderly patients with heart failure. *Eur. J. Intern. Med.* **2013**, *24*, 818–823. [CrossRef]
67. DiCarlo, C.; Schmotzer, B.; Vest, M.; Boxer, R. Body mass index and 25 hydroxyvitamin D status in patients with and without heart failure. *Congest. Heart Fail.* **2012**, *18*, 133–137. [CrossRef]
68. Robbins, J.; Petrone, A.B.; Gaziano, J.M.; Djoussé, L. Dietary vitamin D and risk of heart failure in the Physicians' Health Study. *Clin. Nutr.* **2016**, *35*, 650–653. [CrossRef]
69. National Academy of Sciences. *Dietary Reference Intakes for Adequacy: Calcium and Vitamin D*; Institute of Medicine of the National Academies: Washington, DC, USA, 2011. Available online: https://www.ncbi.nlm.nih.gov/books/NBK56070/pdf/Bookshelf_NBK56070.pdf (accessed on 12 September 2019).
70. National Institutes of Health; ODS. *Vitamin D: Fact Sheet for Health Professionals*; Office of Dietary Supplements, National Institutes of Health: Bethesda, MD, USA, 2019. Available online: https://ods.od.nih.gov/factsheets/VitaminD-HealthProfessional/ (accessed on 12 September 2019).
71. U.S. Department of Health & Human Services. *USDA National Nutrient Database for Standard Reference Release 28*; National Institutes of Health, Office of Dietary Supplements: Bethesda, MD, USA, 2015. Available online: https://ods.od.nih.gov/pubs/usdandb/VitaminD-Content.pdf (accessed on 13 September 2019).
72. Fitzpatrick, T.B. The validity and practicality of sun-reactive skin types I through VI. *Arch. Dermatol.* **1988**, *124*, 869–871. [CrossRef]
73. Centers for Disease Control and Prevention. *National Health and Nutrition Examination Survey (NHANES): Anthropometry Procedures Manual*; National Center for Health Statistics: Hyattsville, MD, USA, 2017. Available online: https://wwwn.cdc.gov/nchs/data/nhanes/2017-2018/manuals/2017_Anthropometry_Procedures_Manual.pdf (accessed on 12 September 2019).
74. Krishnaveni, P.; Gowda, V.M.N. Assessing the Validity of Friedewald's Formula and Anandraja's Formula For Serum LDL-Cholesterol Calculation. *J. Clin. Diagn. Res.* **2015**, *9*, BC01–BC04. [CrossRef]
75. Maechler, M.; Rousseeuw, P.; Struyf, A.; Hubert, M.; Hornik, K. *Cluster: Cluster Analysis Basics and Extensions*, R package version 2.0.7-1; The R Foundation: Vienna, Austria, 2018.
76. Hothorn, T.; Hornik, K.; Zeileis, A. Unbiased Recursive Partitioning: A Conditional Inference Framework. *J. Comput. Graph. Stat.* **2006**, *15*, 651–674. [CrossRef]

6

Marine Omega-3 (N-3) Fatty Acids for Cardiovascular Health: An Update for 2020

Jacqueline K. Innes [1] and Philip C. Calder [1,2,*]

1. School of Human Development and Health, Faculty of Medicine, University of Southampton, Southampton SO16 6YD, UK; innesjackie@gmail.com
2. National Institute for Health Research Southampton Biomedical Research Centre, University Hospital Southampton NHS Foundation Trust and University of Southampton, Southampton SO16 6YD, UK

* Correspondence: pcc@soton.ac.uk

Abstract: The omega-3 (n-3) fatty acids, eicosapentaenoic acid (EPA) and docosahexaenoic acid (DHA), are found in seafood (especially fatty fish), supplements and concentrated pharmaceutical preparations. Long-term prospective cohort studies consistently demonstrate an association between higher intakes of fish, fatty fish and marine n-3 fatty acids (EPA + DHA) or higher levels of EPA and DHA in the body and lower risk of developing cardiovascular disease (CVD), especially coronary heart disease (CHD) and myocardial infarction (MI), and cardiovascular mortality in the general population. This cardioprotective effect of EPA and DHA is most likely due to the beneficial modulation of a number of known risk factors for CVD, such as blood lipids, blood pressure, heart rate and heart rate variability, platelet aggregation, endothelial function, and inflammation. Evidence for primary prevention of CVD through randomised controlled trials (RCTs) is relatively weak. In high-risk patients, especially in the secondary prevention setting (e.g., post-MI), a number of large RCTs support the use of EPA + DHA (or EPA alone) as confirmed through a recent meta-analysis. This review presents some of the key studies that have investigated EPA and DHA in the primary and secondary prevention of CVD, describes potential mechanisms for their cardioprotective effect, and evaluates the more recently published RCTs in the context of existing scientific literature.

Keywords: eicosapentaenoic acid; docosahexaenoic acid; omega-3 polyunsaturated fatty acids; cardiovascular disease; coronary heart disease

---

1. Marine Omega-3 Fatty Acids: Sources and Intakes

Omega-3 (n-3) fatty acids are a family of polyunsaturated fatty acids. They are characterised by, and named according to, the presence of the closest double bond to the methyl end of the hydrocarbon (acyl) chain being on carbon number three, if the methyl carbon is counted as number one. The most functionally important n-3 fatty acids appear to be eicosapentaenoic acid (EPA; 20:5n-3) and docosahexaenoic acid (DHA; 22:6n-3) [1]; however, roles for docosapentaenoic acid (22:5n-3) have also emerged now [2]. The best dietary source of EPA and DHA (and also docosapentaenoic acid) is seafood, especially fatty fish (also called 'oily fish'). The blubber and tissues of sea mammals, such as whales and seals, also contain EPA and DHA in significant amounts. Various supplements, including fish oils, cod liver oil, krill oil and some algal oils, contain EPA and DHA. Finally, concentrated pharmaceutical-grade preparations of EPA and DHA, or EPA alone, are available. Typical values for the EPA and DHA content of selected fish, n-3 fatty acid supplements and pharmaceutical preparations are shown in Table 1. EPA and DHA are often referred to as marine n-3 fatty acids because of their association with seafood.

Table 1. Content of EPA and DHA in fatty fish, lean fish, supplements and pharmaceuticals.

Fish Type	Typical EPA + DHA per Adult Serving	Comment
Fatty (e.g., salmon, trout, mackerel, sardines and herring)	1–3.5 g	Usually more EPA than DHA; content depends on the type of fish, season, water temperature, diet, stage of life cycle, wild or farmed and method of cooking
Lean (e.g., cod, plaice, haddock and sea bass)	0.1–0.3 g	Usually more EPA than DHA
Supplement Type	**Typical EPA + DHA Content per g of oil**	
Cod liver oil	200 mg	Usually more EPA than DHA
Standard "fish oil"	300 mg	Usually more EPA than DHA
Fish oil concentrate	450–600 mg	Usually more EPA than DHA
Tuna oil	460 mg	More DHA than EPA
Krill oil	205 mg	Usually more EPA than DHA; some in phospholipid form
Algal oil	400 mg	Mainly DHA
Flaxseed oil	0 mg	Contains α-linolenic acid, but not EPA or DHA
Pharmaceuticals	**Typical EPA + DHA Content per g of oil**	
Omacor/Lovaza	460 mg EPA + 380 mg DHA	In ethyl ester form
Omtryg	465 mg EPA + 375 mg DHA	In ethyl ester form
Epanova	550 mg EPA + 200 mg DHA	In free fatty acid form
Vascepa/icosapent ethyl	900 mg EPA	In ethyl ester form

Abbreviations: DHA, docosahexaenoic acid; EPA, eicosapentaenoic acid.

The various n-3 fatty acids are related metabolically to one another, and the pathway of conversion of plant-derived n-3 fatty acids (e.g., α-linolenic acid (ALA; 18:3n-3)) to EPA and then to DHA is shown in Figure 1. Studies in humans have identified that there is a fairly low rate of conversion of ALA along this pathway, especially all the way to DHA [3,4]. It is now recognised that this conversion is influenced by several factors, including the stage of life course, age, sex, various hormones, genetics and diseases [4].

The intake of EPA and DHA from diet is strongly influenced by fish consumption because fish, in general, and fatty fish, in particular, are the richest dietary source of these fatty acids. The intake of fish and fatty fish is high in some countries, such as Japan, but it is low in many Western countries, including the USA and the United Kingdom. As a result, the intake of EPA + DHA among adults varies among different populations and is low in most Western countries; it is generally considered that in non-fatty fish eaters, the intake of EPA + DHA is <0.2 g/day [5,6]. This is lower than the recommended intake for the general population [7–9]. Nevertheless, despite these low intakes, it is evident that the recommendations (typically 0.2–0.5 g/day depending upon the authority making the recommendation) can be met by including fatty fish in the diet on a regular basis or, if that is not possible, by using supplements that contain EPA and DHA (Table 1).

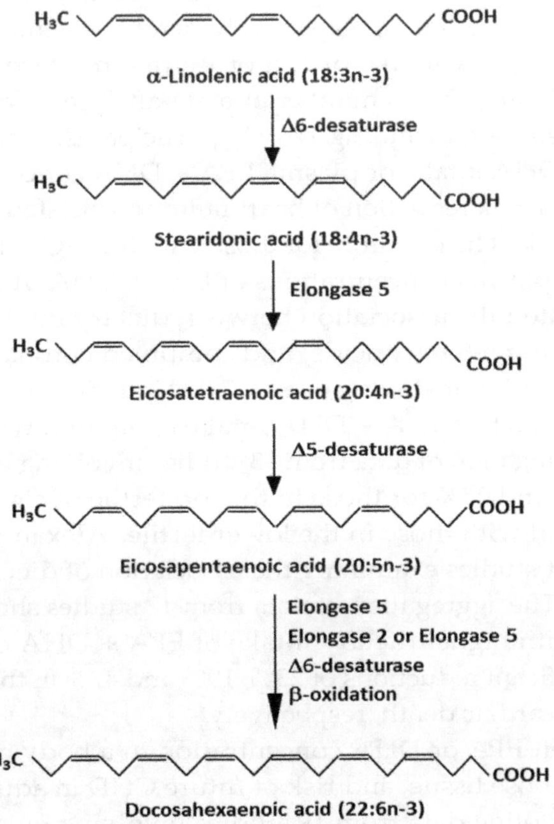

Figure 1. Metabolic pathway of conversion of the plant essential n-3 fatty acid, α-linolenic acid (18:3n-3), to eicosapentaenoic acid (20:5n-3) and docosahexaenoic acid (22:6n-3).

2. Strong Evidence for a Protective Effect of EPA and DHA Towards Cardiovascular Disease Emerges from Ecological, Case Control and Cohort Studies

The potential for EPA and DHA to have a role in reducing the risk of cardiovascular disease (CVD) was first identified by studies in the Greenland Inuit, where the low rate of mortality from myocardial infarction (MI) and ischaemic heart disease [10,11] was linked to the very high dietary intake of EPA and DHA [12]. These observations were replicated in other native Arctic populations [13] and the Japanese population [14]. Subsequently, substantial evidence accumulated from epidemiological and case-control studies in Western populations indicating that consumption of fish, fatty fish, or EPA and

DHA is associated with reduced risk of mortality from CVD, especially coronary heart disease (CHD) (reviewed in [15]). For example, in the Nurse's Health Study, there was an inverse dose-dependent association of risk for developing CHD, having a non-fatal MI or dying from CHD across quintiles of intake of EPA + DHA [16]. The risk for all three outcomes was about 50% in the group with the highest intake compared with the group with the lowest intake of EPA+DHA. The intake of EPA and DHA is highly correlated with their concentrations in blood lipids and red blood cells [17]. A number of studies have associated the concentrations of EPA + DHA (often expressed as a proportion of total fatty acids) in blood plasma or serum, plasma lipid fractions, whole blood, red blood cells and adipose tissue with lower cardiovascular morbidity and mortality (reviewed in [15]). For example, in the Physician's Health Study, there was an inverse dose-dependent association of risk for sudden death across quartiles of whole blood EPA + DHA, with an 80% lower risk in those with the highest whole blood EPA+DHA concentration compared to those with the lowest whole blood EPA + DHA concentration [18]. More recently, the largest prospective cohort study conducted to date included ~420,000 participants from the National Institutes of Health AARP Diet and Health Study with a 16-year follow-up and reported a significant inverse association between fish and EPA + DHA intake and various mortality outcomes [19]. Comparing the highest with lowest quintiles of fish intake, both men and women had 10% lower CVD mortality. EPA + DHA intake was associated with 15% and 18% lower CVD mortality in men and women, respectively, across extreme quintiles.

Cohort studies associating the intake of fish or marine n-3 fatty acids with cardiovascular or coronary outcomes have been subject to a number of meta-analyses. These include a 2012 aggregation of seven prospective cohort studies, including 176,441 participants, which investigated the association between dietary fish, EPA+DHA intake or plasma EPA + DHA concentrations and heart failure [20]. The investigators found a 15% risk reduction of heart failure associated with the highest versus lowest fish intake and a 14% lower risk of heart failure for those with the highest intake compared to those with the lowest dietary intake or plasma concentrations of EPA + DHA. A comprehensive meta-analysis, published in 2014, investigated the association between dietary intakes or blood levels of different classes of fatty acids (including n-3 fatty acids) and combined coronary disease outcomes [21]. The aggregation of data from 16 studies involving over 422,000 individuals showed a risk reduction of 13% for those in the top tertile of dietary EPA + DHA intake compared with those in the lower tertile of intake. Furthermore, the aggregation of data from 13 studies involving over 20,000 individuals showed risk reductions of 22%, 21% and 25% for those in the top tertile of circulating EPA, DHA and EPA + DHA, respectively, compared with those in the lower tertile. Alexander et al. [22] brought together data from prospective cohort studies examining the association of dietary EPA and DHA with risk of various coronary outcomes. The aggregation of data from 17 studies showed an 18% risk reduction for any CHD event for those with higher dietary intake of EPA + DHA compared to those with lower intake. There were also significant reductions of 23%, 19% and 47% in the risk for fatal coronary events, coronary death and sudden cardiac death, respectively.

The association between EPA or DHA concentration in a body compartment, such as plasma, serum, red blood cells or adipose tissue, and risk of future CHD in adults who were healthy at study entry was investigated by pooling data from 19 studies involving over 45,000 individuals [23]. EPA and DHA were each independently associated with a lower risk of fatal CHD, with a 10% lower risk for each one standard deviation increase in content [23]. The omega-3 index is the red blood cell content of EPA+DHA expressed as a proportion of total fatty acids [24]. Omega-3 index is a marker of both long-term dietary intake of these fatty acids and their tissue levels and is suggested to be a marker of CHD risk [24]. Harris et al. [25] used data from 10 cohort studies and identified a 15% reduction in risk of fatal CHD for each one standard deviation increase in omega-3 index.

3. Mechanisms by which EPA and DHA Reduce the Risk of Cardiovascular Disease

Prospective cohort studies have the advantage of a very long follow-up time to observe health outcomes in what starts as a generally healthy study population, something which is typically not possible in randomised control trials (RCTs). There are well-recognised limitations of such cohort studies, including the lack of ability to show causation. Despite this significant limitation, the considerable number of large prospective cohort studies conducted to date that have consistently shown an inverse association between dietary, blood or tissue EPA and DHA and incidence of mortality from CVD provide important evidence for the key role of marine n-3 fatty acids in the prevention of CVD. As such, there has been much interest in the mechanisms by which n-3 fatty acids, specifically EPA and DHA, achieve their cardioprotective action, with much attention being focused on the potential modulation of key cardiovascular risk factors. These risk factors include high blood pressure, high serum triglycerides, low high-density lipoprotein (HDL)-cholesterol, elevated post-prandial lipaemia, endothelial dysfunction, cardiac arrhythmia, heart rate and heart rate variability and a tendency towards thrombosis and inflammation. Large numbers of studies, including many RCTs, in humans have investigated the effect of the combination of EPA and DHA on these risk factors and many of these studies have been included in a number of meta-analyses performed in recent years (Table 2). These meta-analyses demonstrate that EPA and DHA lower triglycerides [26], lower the blood pressure (both systolic and diastolic) [26,27], reduce the heart rate and increase heart rate variability [26,28–30] and reduce platelet aggregation [31], whilst appearing to increase both low density lipoprotein (LDL)- and HDL-cholesterol [26]. Regarding vascular endothelial function, EPA and DHA have been demonstrated to improve flow-mediated dilatation [32,33] and arterial compliance [34]. Concerning the effect of EPA and DHA on inflammation, several meta-analyses have reported that they lower blood concentrations of the acute phase protein, C-reactive protein (CRP), and the pro-inflammatory cytokines, tumour necrosis factor (TNF)-α and interleukin (IL)-6 [26,35], although the effect may be dependent on the health status of the individual. Furthermore, EPA and DHA have been reported to decrease the plasma or serum concentrations of pro-inflammatory eicosanoids like thromboxane B_2 and leukotriene B_4 [36].

Whilst the majority of the scientific evidence base to-date has focused on the administration of EPA and DHA in combination (as occurs naturally in fish and most supplements), there has been much interest in the potential for EPA and DHA to have independent roles in cardiovascular risk reduction. A recent systematic review of the scientific literature concluded that EPA and DHA appear to have differential effects on a number of cardiometabolic outcomes [37]. For example, regarding modulation of blood lipids, whilst both EPA and DHA lowered blood triglycerides, there was evidence for a slightly larger triglyceride-lowering effect for DHA [38,39]. Whilst neither EPA nor DHA affected total cholesterol concentrations to a significant degree, there was an independent effect on other blood lipid parameters, with EPA lowering the HDL3-cholesterol subfraction and DHA increasing the more cardioprotective HDL2-cholesterol [40,41]. DHA also increased LDL-cholesterol more than EPA, an effect observed more in men than in women, and increased LDL particle size, an effect which was not observed with EPA [39–41]. From the more limited trial data, DHA appears to be more effective than EPA at lowering blood pressure and heart rate in normotensive individuals, whilst neither EPA nor DHA had any effect in hypertensive diabetic patients [40–43]. DHA also appeared to increase vasodilatory effects and reduce constrictor effects in the vasculature [44]. Both EPA and DHA were equally effective at increasing systemic arterial compliance [45]. In terms of platelet function, only EPA decreased platelet count and volume [46], whilst only DHA decreased collagen-stimulated platelet aggregation and platelet-derived thromboxane B_2 [47]. Interestingly, neither EPA nor DHA had any effect on fibrinolytic function [47]. Furthermore, from the limited comparative studies available, DHA seemed to be more effective than EPA at lowering a wide range of pro-inflammatory biomarkers in subjects with subclinical inflammation [39,48]. Both EPA and DHA, however, were effective at reducing biomarkers of oxidative stress (F2 isoprostanes) [49–51]. Thus, whilst there are relatively few trials that have been conducted to date that directly compare EPA and DHA, the limited data suggest that EPA and DHA have different effects with regard to cardiovascular risk factors. More research, however, is necessary to be more certain about this.

Table 2. Selected meta-analyses of the effect of marine n-3 fatty acids on cardiovascular risk factors.

Study	Cardiovascular Risk Factors Assessed	Study Design	Form and Dosage of n-3 Fatty Acids	Duration of n-3 Fatty Acid Treatment	Pooled Effects of n-3 Fatty Acids Versus Placebo
AbuMweis et al., 2018 [26]	Blood lipids, heart rate, blood pressure, inflammatory markers, platelet function and flow-mediated dilatation	Meta-analysis of 171 RCTs (up to Feb 2013) in participants in various states of health (note: the number of studies used for the analysis of different outcomes varied from 110 for triglycerides and HDL-cholesterol to 9 for flow-mediated dilatation)	Oral marine n-3 fatty acid supplements providing 0.18–15 g/d EPA+DHA	4–240 weeks	Significant dose-dependent decrease in triglycerides (MD = −0.368 mmol/L; 95% CI: −0.427–−0.309) Significant decrease in systolic blood pressure (MD = −2.195 mmHg; 95% CI: −3.171–−1.217) Significant decrease in diastolic blood pressure (MD = −1.37 mmHg; 95% CI: −2.415–−0.325) Significant decrease in heart rate (MD = −1.37 bpm; 95% CI: −2.41–−0.325) Significant decrease in CRP (MD = −0.343 mg/L; 95% CI: −0.454–−0.232) Significant increase in LDL-cholesterol (MD = 0.150 mmol/L; 95% CI: 0.058–0.243) and HDL-cholesterol (MD = 0.039 mmol/L; 95% CI: 0.024–0.054) No significant effect on total cholesterol, TNF-α, fibrinogen, platelet count, soluble intercellular adhesion molecule 1, soluble vascular cell adhesion molecule 1 or flow-mediated dilatation
Gao et al., 2013 [31]	Platelet aggregation	Meta-analysis of 15 RCTs (up to Jul 2011) including 742 participants in various states of health	Oral marine n-3 fatty acid supplements providing 0.84–6.8 g/d EPA+DHA	2–16 weeks	Significant decrease in adenosine diphosphate-induced platelet aggregation (SMD = −1.23; 95% CI: −2.24–−0.23; p = 0.02) Significant decrease in platelet aggregation units (SMD = −6.78; 95% CI: −12.58–−0.98; p = 0.02) Non-significant trend towards decreased collagen-induced and arachidonic acid-induced platelet aggregation Greater effect observed in non-healthy participants
Hidayat et al., 2017 [30]	Heart rate	Meta-analysis of 51 RCTs (up to May 2017) including ~3000 participants in various states of health	Oral marine n-3 fatty acid supplements providing 0.5–15.0 g/d EPA+DHA	2–52 weeks	Significant decrease in heart rate (WMD = −2.23 bpm; 95% CI: −3.07–−1.40); observed to be due to DHA, not EPA
Jiang et al., 2016 [36]	Pro-inflammatory eicosanoids	Meta-analysis of 18 RCTS (up to November 2015) including 826 subjects in various states of health	Oral marine n-3 fatty acid supplements providing 0.18–4.05 g/d EPA+DHA or EPA alone	4–24 weeks	Significant decrease in serum/plasma thromboxane B_2 in participants with high risk of CVD (SMD = −1.26; 95% CI: −1.65–−0.86) Significant decrease in neutrophil leukotriene B_4 in unhealthy subjects (SMD = −0.59; 95% CI: −1.02–−0.16)
Li et al., 2014 [35]	Pro-inflammatory cytokines	Meta-analysis of 68 RCTs (up to 2013) including 4601 participants in various states of health	Oral marine n-3 fatty acid supplements or dietary intake providing 0.3–6.6 g/d EPA+DHA	4–12 months	Participants with chronic disease: Significant decrease in CRP (WMD = −0.20 mg/L; 95% CI: −0.28–−0.12) and IL-6 (WMD = −0.22 pg/mL; 95%CI: −0.38–−0.06) No significant effect on TNF-α Healthy participants: Significant decrease in CRP (WMD = −0.18 mg/L; 95% CI: −0.28–−0.08) and TNF-α (WMD = −0.12 pg/mL; 95% CI: −0.16–−0.07) No significant effect on IL-6

Table 2. *Cont.*

Study	Cardiovascular Risk Factors Assessed	Study Design	Form and Dosage of n-3 Fatty Acids	Duration of n-3 Fatty Acid Treatment	Pooled Effects of n-3 Fatty Acids Versus Placebo
Miller et al., 2014 [27]	Blood pressure	Meta-analysis of 70 RCTs (up to February 2013) in normotensive and hypertensive subjects	Oral marine n-3 fatty acids from seafood, fortified foods, fish oil, algal oil and purified ethyl esters; mean EPA+DHA dose: 3.8 g/d	>3 weeks (mean study duration: 69 days)	Significant decrease in systolic blood pressure (WMD = −1.52 mmHg; 95% CI: −2.25–−0.79) Significant decrease in diastolic blood pressure (WMD = −0.99 mmHg; 95% CI: −1.54–−0.44) Significant decrease in systolic blood pressure (WMD = −4.51 mmHg; 95% CI: −6.12–−2.83) and diastolic blood pressure (WMD = −3.05 mmHg; 95% CI: −4.35–−1.74) in hypertensive individuals
Mozaffarian et al., 2005 [28]	Heart rate	Meta-analysis of 30 RCTs (up to January 2005) including 1678 healthy participants	Oral marine n-3 fatty acid supplements; median EPA+DHA intake: 3.5 g/d	>2 weeks (median study duration: 8 weeks)	Significant decrease in heart rate (WMD = −1.6 bpm; 95% CI: 0.6–2.5) In those with baseline heart rate ≥ 69 bpm, heart rate decreased by 2.5 bpm (95% CI: 1.4–3.5)
Pase et al., 2011 [34]	Arterial stiffness	Meta-analysis of 10 RCTs (up to September 2010) including 550 participants in various states of health	Oral marine n-3 fatty acid supplements providing 0.64–3 g/d EPA+DHA	6–105 weeks	Significant improvement in pulse wave velocity (SMD = 0.33; 95% CI: 0.12–0.56) Significant improvement in arterial compliance (SMD = 0.48; 95% CI: 0.24–0.72)
Wang et al., 2012 [33]	Vascular endothelial function	Meta-analysis of 16 RCTs (up to August 2011) including 901 participants in various states of health	Oral marine n-3 fatty acid supplements and dietary intake providing 0.45–4.7 g/d EPA+DHA	2 weeks to 12 months (median: 56 days)	Significant increase in flow-mediated dilatation (WMD = 2.3%; 95% CI: 0.89–3.72) No significant change in endothelium-independent vasodilation
Xin et al., 2012 [32]	Vascular endothelial function	Meta-analysis of 16 RCTs (up to February 2012) including 1385 participants in various states of health	Oral marine n-3 fatty acid supplements providing 0.45–4.53 g/d EPA+DHA	2-52 weeks	Significant increase in flow-mediated dilatation (WMD = 1.49%; 95% CI: 0.48–2.5)
Xin et al., 2013 [29]	Heart rate variability	Meta-analysis of 15 RCTS including 692 participants in various states of health	Oral marine n-3 fatty acid supplements providing 0.64–5.9 g/d EPA+DHA	6-24 weeks	Significant increase in high frequency power value of heart rate variability (SMD = 0.30). A sensitivity analysis demonstrated a significant reduction in low frequency power/high frequency power ratio with >1 g/d EPA+DHA

Abbreviations: CI, confidence interval; CVD, cardiovascular disease; CRP, C-reactive protein; DHA, docosahexaenoic acid; EPA, eicosapentaenoic acid; HDL, high-density lipoprotein; IL-6, interleukin-6; LDL, low-density lipoprotein; MD, mean difference; RCT, randomized controlled trial; SMD, standard mean difference; TNF-α, tumour necrosis factor-α; WMD, weighted mean difference.

4. RCTs of Primary Prevention of Cardiovascular Disease with Marine n-3 Fatty Acids

When compared to the large number of observational studies investigating the association between marine n-3 fatty acid exposure and cardiovascular outcomes that have been conducted to date (Section 2), only a few RCTs of sufficient size or duration have investigated the cardioprotective effects of marine n-3 fatty acids in generally healthy populations. The open-label, Japan EPA Lipid Intervention Study (JELIS) directly investigated the use of 1.8 g/d EPA (as an ethyl ester) plus statin versus statin alone in 18,645 hypercholesterolaemic participants [52]. A number of the participants were on existing cardiovascular medication (in addition to statin) and the study included hypercholesterolemic, but otherwise, healthy subjects as well as those with pre-existing CHD, with all patients being followed up for ~5 years. The primary outcome was any major coronary event, including sudden cardiac death, fatal and non-fatal MI and other non-fatal events, including unstable angina pectoris, angioplasty, stenting, and coronary artery bypass grafting. The addition of EPA to statin had no effect over statin alone on the primary outcome in the primary prevention arm of the trial. Two large primary prevention RCTs were published in late 2018 [53,54]. The ASCEND (A Study of Cardiovascular Events iN Diabetes) trial randomised 15,480 people with diabetics and no evidence of CVD to receive either marine n-3 fatty acids (840 mg/d EPA + DHA) or olive oil placebo [53]. The primary outcome was the first serious vascular event and after a mean follow-up of 7.4 years, there was no difference in the primary outcome between the two groups. In exploratory analyses, there were significantly fewer deaths from vascular events in the marine n-3 fatty acid arm (rate ratio: 0.81; 95% CI: 0.67–0.99), as well as a trend towards reduced risk of death from CHD (rate ratio: 0.79; 95% CI: 0.61–1.02). The Vitamin D and Omega-3 Trial (VITAL) trial randomised 25,871 healthy participants aged over 50 years (men) and 55 years (women) to receive marine n-3 fatty acids (840 mg/d EPA+DHA) and/or vitamin D (2000 IU/d) or placebo [54]. After a median follow-up of 5.3 years, there was no difference in the primary outcome of major cardiovascular events (a composite of MI, stroke or death from cardiovascular causes) in those participants supplemented with marine n-3 fatty acids versus placebo. An analysis of the individual components of the composite showed a significant reduction in the n-3 fatty acid arm in MI (hazard ratio: 0.72; 95% CI: 0.59–0.90) and CHD (hazard ratio: 0.83; 95% CI: 0.71–0.97). Correspondingly, there was also a reduced risk of death from these two non-prespecified outcomes (for MI—hazard ratio: 0.50, 95% CI: 0.26–0.97; for CHD—hazard ratio: 0.76, 95% CI: 0.49–1.16). Thus, whilst RCT evidence in primary prevention is less clear than that from the prospective cohort studies, there is now some indication of benefit from marine n-3 fatty acids towards cardiovascular health, especially CHD, from recent large and long RCTs, such as ASCEND and VITAL.

5. RCTs of Secondary Prevention of Cardiovascular Disease with Marine n-3 Fatty Acids

A number of large, randomized, controlled, secondary prevention trials or trials in high-risk patients have been conducted to investigate the effect of EPA and DHA in patients with established CVD. These trials generate a changing picture with time.

5.1. Secondary Prevention Trials and Meta-Analyses Published Prior to 2010

Several large, secondary prevention trials of marine n-3 fatty acids were conducted prior to 2010. The Diet and Reinfarction Trial (DART) included 2,033 recent (mean: 41 days) MI survivors, who were given dietary advice concerning fat, fish and fibre intake and followed up for 2 years [55]. Those patients advised to eat at least two portions of fatty fish per week (or to take fish oil supplements) had a 29% reduction in total mortality as well as a reduced risk of death from ischaemic heart disease at 2 years compared to those patients given other advice. The landmark Gruppo Italiano per lo Studio della Sopravvivenza nell'Infarto miocardico (GISSI)–Prevenzione trial investigated the effect of supplementation with 840 mg/d EPA+DHA in 11,324 recent (≤3 months) MI survivors versus vitamin E supplementation, supplementation with both EPA + DHA and vitamin E, and placebo control [56]. After 3.5 years, patients who received EPA + DHA had a 20% reduction in total mortality, 30% reduction in cardiovascular death and 45% decrease in sudden death compared to those that did not receive EPA + DHA. There was no benefit reported on non-fatal MI or stroke. The beneficial effect of EPA + DHA on total mortality and sudden cardiac death was observed after 3 months and 4 months of supplementation, respectively, and raised interest in the potential anti-arrhythmic action of EPA and DHA [57]. The GISSI investigators undertook a separate RCT in 6,975 patients with chronic heart failure (GISSI-HF) to investigate the effect of 840 mg/d EPA+DHA versus placebo over a period of ~4 years in this patient population [58]. The investigators reported a small (9%), but significant, reduction in all-cause mortality and a small (8%) reduction in combined all-cause mortality or admission to hospital for cardiovascular reasons in this high-risk population following supplementation with marine n-3 fatty acids. In line with the increased prescription of statins to prevent all-cause mortality and cardiovascular events at this time, JELIS directly investigated the use of 1.8 g/d EPA (as an ethyl ester) plus statin versus statin alone in 18,645 hypercholesterolaemic participants who were followed up for ~5 years [52]. As mentioned above, the addition of EPA to statin had no effect over statin alone in the primary prevention arm of JELIS, but in the secondary prevention arm, EPA caused a 19% decrease in non-fatal coronary events compared with the statin alone group [52]. Unlike GISSI, JELIS found no beneficial effect on cardiovascular mortality. A subsequent analysis found an inverse association between plasma EPA levels and risk of major coronary events; participants with the highest levels of plasma EPA (≥150 μg/mL) were 20% less likely to experience a major coronary event [59].

Meta-analyses of RCTs conducted prior to 2010 confirmed the reductions in mortality seen in individual trials of marine n-3 fatty acids ([60–63]; Table 3). For example, a 2002 meta-analysis of 11 RCTs in 15,806 patients with CHD found 20% lower risk of non-fatal MI, 30% lower risk of fatal MI, 30% lower risk for sudden death and 20% lower risk for all-cause mortality in patients who received marine n-3 fatty acids versus control [60]. Another meta-analysis from 2002 of 14 RCTs and 20,260 participants, both with and without CVD, found a 23% reduction in overall mortality and 32% reduction in cardiac mortality for those patients who were given marine n-3 fatty acids versus controls [61]. A further meta-analysis in 2009 focused on 8 RCTs and 20,997 patients with CHD found a 57% reduction in sudden death in patients with prior MI who were taking marine n-3 fatty acids compared with placebo [62]. In 2009, a meta-analysis of 11 RCTs representing 39,044 patients with all stages of CVD, including both low- and high-risk patients, found a 13% reduction in cardiovascular death and in sudden death and an 8% reduction in all-cause mortality in high-risk patients who were taking marine n-3 fatty acids compared to controls [63]. The investigators also found an 8% reduction in non-fatal cardiovascular events in moderate-risk patients.

5.2. RCTs with Marine n-3 Fatty Acids in High-Risk Patients Published in the Period 2010–2013

Three RCTs published in 2010 failed to replicate the findings of earlier trials [64–66]. The OMEGA study investigated the effect of supplementation with 840 mg/d EPA + DHA for 1 year in 3,851 early post-MI patients, with the primary endpoint of sudden cardiac death [64]. Marine n-3 fatty acids did not decrease the rate of sudden cardiac death, total mortality, major adverse cerebrovascular and cardiovascular events or revascularisation compared to control. The Supplémentation en Folates et Omega-3 (SU.FOL.OM3) trial investigated the effect of supplementation of B vitamins and/or marine n-3 fatty acids (600 mg/d EPA + DHA) in 2,501 patients with documented MI, unstable angina or ischaemic stroke for ~5 years [65]; the primary outcomes were cardiovascular death, stroke and non-fatal MI. Marine n-3 fatty acids did not have any effect on these outcomes. The Alpha Omega study included 4,837 post-MI patients who were given margarine fortified with low doses of EPA + DHA (400 mg/d), ALA (2 g/d), EPA + DHA + ALA or placebo, and followed up for 40 months [66]. There was no reduction in cardiovascular events in any group. On further analysis, those patients with diabetes in the EPA + DHA as well as ALA-fortified margarine groups, however, experienced a reduction in fatal CHD and arrhythmia-related events [66].

The Outcome Reduction with an Initial Glargine Intervention (ORIGIN) trial, published in 2012, assessed the effect of supplementation with 840 mg/d EPA + DHA in 12,536 dysglycaemic patients at high risk of cardiovascular events, together with insulin glargine or standard care for a median of 6 years [67]. No effect of marine n-3 fatty acids was reported for total mortality, death from cardiovascular causes or arrhythmia compared to placebo. The Risk and Prevention Study, published in 2013, investigated the effect of supplementation with 840 mg/d marine n-3 fatty acids in 12,513 patients with multiple cardiovascular risk factors or atherosclerotic vascular disease (but no MI) for a median of 5 years, and reported no effect on hospitalisation or death from cardiovascular causes compared to placebo [68]. In a prespecified subgroup analysis, compared with placebo, marine n-3 fatty acids resulted in an 18% lower incidence of the revised primary endpoint among women. Most of the secondary endpoints (e.g., fatal or non-fatal MI or stroke, fatal or non-fatal coronary event, and sudden death) did not differ between groups; however, admissions for heart failure were significantly lower in the marine n-3 fatty acid group.

Whilst these RCTs failed to show any benefit of marine n-3 fatty acids, they did have acknowledged limitations [69,70], which are worthy of mention. OMEGA was underpowered to detect any benefit on its primary outcome, sudden cardiac death, as power calculations were based on earlier RCTs in patients without more recent treatments and hence with higher background rates of sudden cardiac death compared to those seen in OMEGA. Furthermore, reported fish consumption was relatively high among the enrolled patients and increased during the trial, thereby increasing dietary EPA + DHA intake and introducing a confounding factor. The trial also had a relatively short follow-up period of just one year. Regarding SU.FOL.OM3, the length of time between the occurrence of primary cardiovascular event and the commencement of supplementation (median of 101 days) was longer than that of GISSI-Prevenzione (≤3 months) and the dose of EPA + DHA used was lower than that of GISSI-Prevenzione (840 mg/d EPA + DHA) and JELIS (1.8 g/d EPA). There were also fewer than expected background cardiac deaths, perhaps also due to more effective pharmacological management of cardiovascular risk factors. With respect to Alpha Omega, despite the long follow-up time, the dose of EPA+DHA used was modest and enrolment to the trial occurred on average at 4 years post-MI, despite the existence of data suggesting that early intervention with EPA + DHA is required to see a beneficial effect post-MI. ORIGIN included a large number of participants taking effective cardiovascular risk-reducing medications compared to earlier trials, and this may have made the cardioprotective effect of EPA + DHA harder to detect. The Risk and Prevention Study set out to examine the effect of marine n-3 fatty acids on the composite primary outcome of death, non-fatal MI and non-fatal stroke; however, the event rate at one year was lower than anticipated and the primary outcome was revised to hospitalisation or death from cardiovascular causes over the follow-up period.

Unsurprisingly, several meta-analyses conducted over the last ten years reflect the inclusion of these null RCTs and report more mixed conclusions than earlier meta-analyses ([21,22,71–79]; Table 3). A meta-analysis from 2013 (representing 11 RCTs and 15,348 patients with CVD) reported a 32% reduction in cardiac death, 33% reduction in sudden death and 25% reduction in myocardial infarction, with no effect on all-cause mortality or stroke [75]. This meta-analysis included only those RCTs with EPA + DHA dosages of at least 1 g/d and with a duration of at least 1 year. Another meta-analysis published in 2014, which included a broader range of marine n-3 fatty acid dosages and durations and focused only on patients with ischaemic CHD, reported that whilst there were no effects on cardiovascular events, there was a 12% reduction in death from cardiac causes, 14% reduction in sudden cardiac death and 8% reduction in all-cause mortality in those taking EPA + DHA versus placebo [76]. Published in 2017, a meta-analysis focusing solely on cardiac death as the outcome examined 14 RCTs (involving 71,899 subjects in both mixed and secondary prevention settings) with marine n-3 fatty acid supplementation for a duration of at least 6 months [77]. The study found an 8% lower risk of cardiac death in the primary analysis and a 13%–29% lower risk of cardiac death in those participants with intakes of EPA + DHA of at least 1g/d and for certain subgroups, such as subjects with high plasma triglycerides or cholesterol, and where <40% subjects were taking statins.

Table 3. Meta-analyses published up to 2018 of RCTs investigating the effect of marine n-3 fatty acids on cardiovascular outcomes.

Study	Study Design	Form & Dosage of Marine-3 Fatty Acids	Duration of Treatment with Marine n-3 Fatty Acids	Pooled Effects of Marine n-3 Fatty Acids Versus Placebo
Bucher et al., 2002 [60]	11 RCTs (up to August 1999) representing 15,806 patients with CHD	Dietary (2 RCTs) and supplemental (9 RCTs) marine n-3 fatty acids with a dose range of 0.3–6.0 g/d EPA and 0.6–3.7 g/d DHA	6–46 months (mean: 20 months)	30% reduction in fatal MI 30% reduction in sudden death 20% reduction in overall mortality
Studer et al., 2005 [61]	14 RCTs (up to June 2003) representing 20,260 participants in primary and secondary prevention settings	Supplemental marine n-3 fatty acids; dose range not given	Mean: 1.9 ± 1.2 years	23% reduction in overall mortality 32% reduction in cardiovascular mortality
Zhao et al., 2009 [62]	8 RCTs (up to June 2008) representing 20,997 patients with CHD	Dietary (3 RCTs) and supplemental (5 RCTs) marine n-3 fatty acids with a dose range of 0.3–4.1 g/d EPA and 0.4–2.8 g/d DHA	9–108 months (mean: 33 months)	57% reduction in sudden death in patients with prior MI 39% increased risk of sudden death in patients with angina 29% reduction in cardiac death (NS) 23% reduction in all-cause mortality (NS)
Marik and Varon, 2009 [63]	11 RCTs (up to December 2008) representing 39,044 patients with all stages of CVD including high-risk and low-risk subjects	Supplemental marine n-3 fatty acids with a dose range of 0.7–4.8 g/d EPA + DHA (mean: 1.8 ± 1.2 g/d)	1–4.6 years (mean: 2.2 ± 1.2 years)	13% reduction in cardiovascular death in high-risk patients 13% reduction in sudden cardiac death in high-risk patients 8% reduction in all-cause mortality in high-risk patients 8% reduction in non-fatal cardiovascular events in moderate-risk patients.
Kotwal et al., 2012 [71]	20 RCTs (up to March 2011) representing 62,851 patients in primary and secondary prevention settings	Diet (3 RCTs) and supplemental (17 RCTs) marine n-3 fatty acids with a dose range of 0.8–3.4 g/d EPA + DHA	6 months–6 years	14% reduction in vascular death No effect on cardiovascular events, total mortality, coronary events, arrhythmia or cerebrovascular events
Kwak et al., 2012 [72]	14 RCTs (up to April 2011) representing 20,485 patients with CVD	Supplemental marine n-3 fatty acids with a dose range of 0.4–4.8 g/d EPA + DHA (mean: 1.7 g/d EPA + DHA)	1–4.7 years (mean: 2 years)	9% reduction in cardiovascular death No effect on cardiovascular events, all-cause mortality, sudden cardiac death, MI, congestive heart failure or stroke
Trikalinos et al., 2012 [73]	18 RCTs (up to May 2011) representing 51,264 patients	Supplemental marine n-3 fatty acids with a dose range of 0.27–6.0 g/d EPA + DHA	1–5 years	11% reduction in cardiovascular mortality
Rizos et al., 2012 [74]	20 RCTs (up to August 2012) representing 68,680 patients in primary and secondary prevention settings	Diet (2 RCTs) and supplemental (18 RCTs) marine n-3 fatty acids with a dose range of 0.53–1.80 g/d EPA + DHA (median EPA + DHA dose: 1 g/d)	1–6.2 years (median: 2 years)	No effect on all-cause mortality, cardiac death, sudden death, MI or stroke

Table 3. *Cont.*

Study	Study Design	Form & Dosage of Marine-3 Fatty Acids	Duration of Treatment with Marine n-3 Fatty Acids	Pooled Effects of Marine n-3 Fatty Acids Versus Placebo
Casula et al., 2013 [75]	11 RCTs (up to March 2013) representing 15,348 patients with CVD	Supplemental marine n-3 fatty acids with a dose range of 1–6 g/d EPA + DHA	≥ 1 year (duration ranged from 1–3.5 years)	32% reduction in cardiac death 33% reduction in sudden death 25% reduction in MI 11% reduction in all-cause mortality (NS) No effect on stroke
Wen et al., 2014 [76]	14 RCTs (up to May 2013) representing 32,656 patients with CHD	Supplemental marine n-3 fatty acids with a dose range of 0.4–6.9 g/d EPA + DHA	< 3 months to 4.6 years	12% reduction in death from cardiac causes 14% reduction in sudden cardiac death 8% reduction in all-cause mortality 7% reduction in cardiovascular events (NS)
Chowdhury et al., 2014 [21]	17 RCTs (up to June 2013) representing 76,580 participants	Supplemental marine n-3 fatty acids with a dose range of 0.3 g/d EPA to 6 g/d EPA + DHA.	0.1–8 years	7% reduction in coronary outcomes (NS)
Alexander et al., 2017 [22]	18 RCTs (up to November 2015)	Supplemental marine n-3 fatty acids with a dose range of 0.4–5.0 g/d EPA + DHA	0.5–7 years	14%–16% reduction in CHD in high-risk subgroups i.e., those with elevated triglycerides and LDL-cholesterol
Maki et al., 2017 [77]	14 RCTs (up to December 2016) representing 71,899 patients in a mixed/secondary prevention setting	Supplemental marine n-3 fatty acids with a dose range of 0.27–5.0 g/d EPA + DHA	≥ 6 months (range 0.5–6.2 years)	8% reduction in cardiac death ~13%–29% reduction in cardiac death in the subgroup with high-risk individuals (secondary prevention, high triglycerides, high LDL-cholesterol and <40% statin use) and with EPA+DHA > 1 g/d
Aung et al., 2018 [78]	10 RCTs representing 77,917 high-risk patients (prior CHD or stroke)	Supplemental marine n-3 fatty acids with a dose range of 0.2–1.8 g/d EPA and 0–1.7 g/d DHA	1–6.2 years (mean: 4.4 years)	7% reduction in CHD death (NS) No effect on non-fatal MI, CHD events or major vascular events
Abdelhamid et al., 2018 [79]	79 RCTs (up to April 2017) representing 112,059 participants in primary and secondary prevention settings	Dietary or supplemental marine n-3 fatty acids with a dose range from 0.5 g/d to ~5 g/d EPA + DHA	1–7 years	7% reduction in CHD events No effect on all-cause mortality, cardiovascular mortality, cardiovascular events, CHD mortality, stroke or arrhythmia.

Abbreviations: CHD, coronary heart disease; DHA, docosahexaenoic acid; EPA, eicosapentaenoic acid; LDL, low-density lipoprotein; MI, myocardial infarction; NS, not significant; RCT, randomised controlled trial.

5.3. An Important RCT and a New Meta-Analysis were Published in 2019

The Reduction of Cardiovascular Events with Icosapent Ethyl–Intervention Trial (REDUCE-IT), published in early 2019, included 8,179 participants (29% in a primary prevention cohort with diabetes plus another cardiovascular risk factor and 71% in a secondary prevention cohort) supplemented daily with 4 g of icosapent ethyl (a highly purified EPA ethyl ester) or mineral oil placebo and followed up for a median of 4.9 years [80]. All patients were being treated with statins and had triglyceride concentrations of 135–499 mg/dL (1.52–5.63 mmol/L). The primary outcome was a composite of cardiovascular death, non-fatal MI, non-fatal stroke, coronary revascularisation or unstable angina. The patients who received icosapent ethyl had a statistically significant reduction in the primary outcome compared to placebo (hazard ratio: 0.75; 95% CI: 0.68–0.83; $p < 0.001$), the pre-specified secondary outcome (composite of cardiovascular death, non-fatal MI or non-fatal stroke) (hazard ratio: 0.80; 95% CI: 0.66–0.98; $p = 0.03$) and a whole range of other pre-specified outcomes (Figure 2). This effect was greater in the secondary prevention cohort than in the primary prevention cohort [80]. Interestingly, as with JELIS, REDUCE-IT used EPA only, but at a much higher dose (4 g daily versus 1.8 g daily) and included participants with high triglyceride levels and on statin medication. Accordingly, the participants in the icosapent ethyl arm had a significant reduction in triglycerides (a decrease of 0.5 mmol/L; $p < 0.001$) and LDL-cholesterol (a decrease of 0.13 mmol/L; $p < 0.001$) relative to placebo at 1 year. Of note, the improvement in the primary outcome in the icosapent ethyl arm of the trial was not dependent on the baseline triglyceride level or the degree of subsequent triglyceride lowering, suggesting that the reduction in cardiovascular risk in this population may be via a different mechanism independent of (or in addition to) triglyceride lowering. REDUCE-IT is of key interest as it demonstrates that even in at-risk populations that are well managed with modern pharmacological treatments, a suitably high dosage of EPA (i.e., 4 g daily) can provide an additional benefit in reducing cardiovascular-related events and mortality.

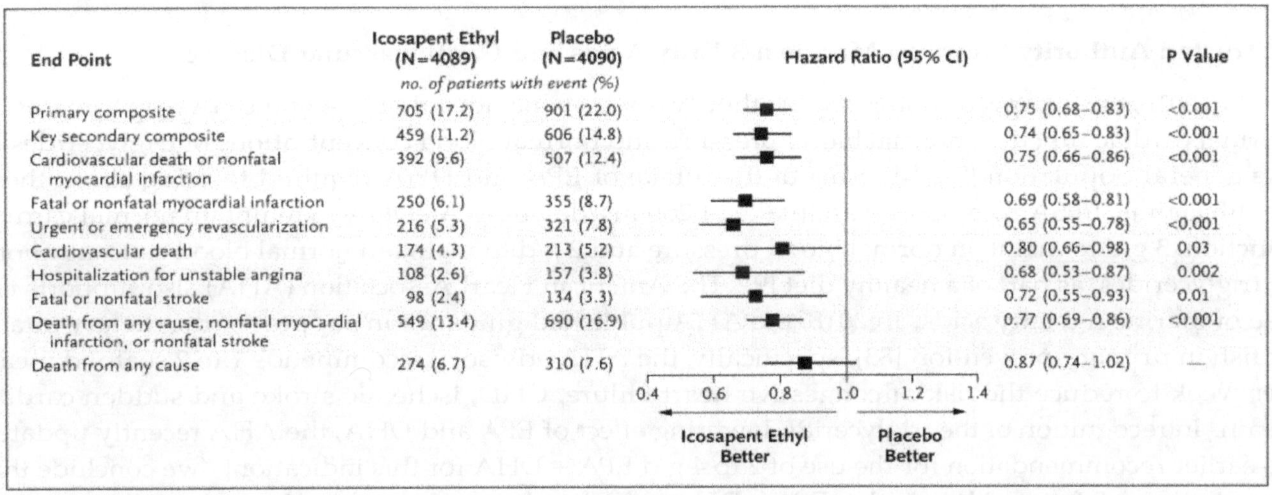

Figure 2. Effect of icosapent ethyl compared with placebo on different endpoints in REDUCE-IT [80]. "From New England Journal of Medicine, Bhatt D.L., Steg P.G., Miller M., Brinton E.A., Jacobson T.A., Ketchum S.B., Doyle R.T. Jr., Juliano R.A., Jiao L., Granowitz C., Tardif J.C., Ballantyne C.M.; REDUCE-IT Investigators, Cardiovascular Risk Reduction with Icosapent Ethyl for Hypertriglyceridemia, Volume No. 380, Page 11–22.

A recent meta-analysis, published in 2019, included data from 13 RCTs, including GISSI-Prevenzione, JELIS, GISSI-HF, SU.FOL.OM3, Alpha Omega, OMEGA, ORIGIN, VITAL, ASCEND and REDUCE-IT [81]. Trials had to have a sample size of at least 500 patients and a follow-up for at least one year to be included. The sample sizes ranged from 563 [82] to 25,871 [54], the mean duration of follow-up ranged from 1.0 [64] to 7.4 [53] years and the mean dose of EPA+DHA ranged from

0.37 [66] to 4.0 [80] g/d. The total sample size of the aggregated trials was 127,477, while the mean duration of follow-up was 5 years. The outcomes of interest included MI, CHD death, total CHD, total stroke, CVD death, total CVD and major vascular events. In the analysis excluding REDUCE-IT, marine n-3 fatty acid supplementation was associated with a significantly lower risk of MI, CHD death, CVD death and total CVD (Table 4). Inverse associations for all outcomes were strengthened after including REDUCE-IT (Table 4). Statistically significant linear dose–response relationships were found for several outcomes: for example, every 1 g/d EPA + DHA corresponded to 9% and 7% lower risk of MI and total CHD, respectively. The meta-analysis concluded that "marine [n-3 fatty acid] supplementation lowers risk for MI, CHD death, total CHD, CVD death, and total CVD, even after exclusion of REDUCE-IT. Risk reductions appeared to be linearly related to marine [n-3 fatty acid] dose."

Table 4. Summary of findings from the meta-analysis published by Hu et al. [81] in 2019.

Outcome	Number of Studies	Finding for Marine n-3 Fatty Acids Versus Placebo Rate Ratio [95% Confidence Interval] (p)	Finding if Data from REDUCE-IT Removed Rate Ratio [95% Confidence Interval] (p)
Myocardial infarction	13	0.88 [0.83, 0.94] (<0.001)	0.92 [0.86, 0.99] (0.020)
CHD death	12	0.92 [0.86, 0.98] (0.014)	Outcome not reported in REDUCE-IT
Total CHD	13	0.93 [0.89, 0.96] (<0.001)	0.95 [0.91, 0.99] (0.008)
Total stroke	13	1.02 [0.95, 1.10] (0.569)	1.05 [0.98, 1.14] (0.183)
CVD Death	12	0.92 [0.88, 0.97] (0.003)	0.93 [0.88, 0.99] (0.013)
Total CVD	13	0.95 [0.82, 0.98] (<0.001)	0.97 [0.94, 0.99] (0.015)
Major vascular events	13	0.95 [0.93, 0.98] (<0.001)	0.97 [0.94, 1.00] 90.058)

Abbreviations: CHD, coronary heart disease; CVD, cardiovascular disease.

6. Trusted Authority Views on Marine n-3 Fatty Acids and Cardiovascular Disease

In 2010, the European Food Safety Authority (EFSA) concluded that EPA and DHA help to maintain normal cardiac function, normal blood pressure and normal blood concentrations of triglycerides in the general population [9]. In terms of the intake of EPA and DHA required to bring about these health claims, EFSA recommend an intake of 250 mg/day of EPA+DHA to maintain normal cardiac function, 3 g/d to maintain normal blood pressure and 2 g/d to maintain normal blood concentrations of triglycerides, as part of a healthy diet [9]. The American Heart Association (AHA) also supports the use of marine n-3 fatty acids. In 2018, the AHA published guidance in support of the dietary intake of fish in primary prevention [83]; specifically, the AHA advisory recommends 1 to 2 seafood meals per week to reduce the risk of congestive heart failure, CHD, ischemic stroke and sudden cardiac death. In recognition of the triglyceride-lowering effect of EPA and DHA, the AHA recently updated its earlier recommendation for the use of 2 to 4 g/d EPA + DHA for this indication: "we conclude that prescription n-3 fatty acids, whether EPA + DHA or EPA-only, at a dose of 4 g/d, are clinically useful for reducing triglycerides, after any underlying causes are addressed and diet and lifestyle strategies are implemented, either as monotherapy or as an adjunct to other triglyceride-lowering therapies" [84]. On the basis of the positive outcomes of REDUCE-IT, the European Society of Cardiology and the European Atherosclerosis Society issued an update to the "Clinical Practice Guidelines for the Management of Dyslipidaemias" specifically recommending that "in high-risk patients with [triglyceride] levels between 1.5 and 5.6 mmol/L (135–499 mg/dL) despite statin treatment, n-3 polyunsaturated fatty acids (icosapent ethyl 2 × 2 g/day) should be considered with a statin" [85]. Furthermore, the American Diabetes Association makes a recommendation "that icosapent ethyl be considered for patients with diabetes and atherosclerotic cardiovascular disease or other cardiac risk factors on a statin with controlled low-density cholesterol, but with elevated triglycerides (135–499 mg/dL) to reduce cardiovascular risk" [86]. Finally, the National Lipid Association's position is "that for patients aged ≥45 years with clinical [atherosclerotic cardiovascular disease] ASCVD, or aged ≥50 years with diabetes mellitus requiring medication plus ≥1 additional risk factor, with fasting triglycerides 135 to 499 mg/dL on high-intensity or maximally tolerated statin therapy (±ezetimibe), treatment with icosapent ethyl is recommended for ASCVD risk reduction" [87]. In 2017, the AHA reinforced its earlier support for EPA+DHA in people with CVD [88] and extended [89] that "the recommendation for patients with prevalent CHD such as a recent MI remains essentially unchanged: Treatment with n-3 fatty acid supplements is reasonable for these patients. Even a potential modest reduction in CHD mortality (10%) in this clinical population would justify treatment with a relatively safe therapy. We now recommend treatment for patients with prevalent heart failure without preserved left ventricular function to reduce mortality and hospitalizations (9%) on the basis of a single, large RCT. Although we do not recommend treatment for patients with diabetes mellitus and prediabetes to prevent CHD, there was a lack of consensus on the recommendation for patients at high CVD risk. Because there are no reported RCTs related to the primary prevention of CHD, heart failure, and atrial fibrillation, we were not able to make recommendations for these indications." In contrast to these well thought out and carefully worded statements by the AHA, in 2014, the National Institute for Health and Clinical Excellence in the UK recommended not to use marine n-3 fatty acids for the primary prevention of CVD, for the secondary prevention of CVD or in people with diabetes [90].

7. Summary, Discussion and Conclusions

There is a large body of evidence gathered from long-term prospective cohort studies that consistently demonstrates an association between higher intakes of fish, fatty fish and marine n-3 fatty acids (EPA+DHA) or higher levels of EPA and DHA in the body and lower risk of developing CVD, especially CHD, having an MI and cardiovascular mortality in the general population. This cardioprotective effect of EPA and DHA is plausible considering the robust identification of mechanisms that show that EPA and DHA beneficially modulate a number of known risk factors for CVD, such as blood lipids, blood pressure, heart rate and heart rate variability, platelet aggregation, endothelial function and inflammation. Despite this, evidence for primary prevention of CVD through RCTs is relatively weak. In high-risk patients, especially in the secondary prevention setting (e.g., post-MI), a number of large RCTs support the use of EPA + DHA (or EPA alone) as confirmed through a very recent meta-analysis [81]. Surveying these trials serves to highlight a number of factors which may have contributed to the positive outcomes reported and why other trials have had less conclusive or even null findings. Such factors include a sufficiently high dose of EPA alone or of a combination of EPA + DHA; sufficient duration of supplementation; supplementation in post-MI patients to begin relatively soon post-MI; and the adequate powering of studies to detect an effect on the primary outcome which may have a low rate of occurrence. Given these considerations, it is unsurprising that studies of short duration or using low doses of EPA + DHA conducted in the setting of multiple pharmaceutical (and other) approaches to controlling risk have failed to demonstrate the effects of EPA + DHA. As discussed elsewhere [91,92], there are also other factors to consider when evaluating and interpreting the literature in this field. The first is that the marine n-3 fatty acid naive condition is unlikely to occur, such that any placebo-controlled trial of EPA and DHA is conducted against a certain background intake of those fatty acids in all participants, although that background intake may be very low [5,6]. Nevertheless, background intakes of EPA and DHA can be highly variable both within and between individuals, with significant changes occurring simply by eating a single meal of fatty fish. Finally, the bioavailability of EPA and DHA can vary [93] (a) among individuals due to physiological differences, (b) according to the intake of meals in relation to supplements and (c) perhaps according to the time of day, thus influencing how much of these bioactive fatty acids is actually available to exert their effects. Taken together, these factors highlight the challenges to conducting robust trials in humans with supplemental n-3 fatty acids, and they are likely to contribute to the variable outcomes from such trials, especially when low doses of EPA and DHA are used.

Recent AHA advisories support the use of marine n-3 fatty acids in the treatment of hypertriglyceridemia [84] and in a range of patients with CVD [89] and the use of fish for primary prevention of CVD [83]. Both EPA and DHA beneficially modify a range of risk factors, although DHA may be more effective [37]. Nevertheless, the highly successful REDUCE-IT used pure EPA, although at a high dose [80]. Differentiating the dose-dependent effects of EPA and DHA on cardiovascular risk factors and on clinical outcomes is going to be important. Furthermore, robust primary prevention trials are still needed. In the meantime, recent trials reviewed herein and the most recent meta-analysis support the use of marine n-3 fatty acids to reduce cardiovascular mortality.

Author Contributions: Conceptualization, P.C.C.; writing—original draft preparation, J.K.I.; writing—review and editing, J.K.I. and P.C.C. All authors have read and agreed to the published version of the manuscript.

Abbreviations

AHA	American Heart Association
ALA	alpha-linolenic acid
CHD	coronary heart disease
CI	confidence interval
CRP	C-reactive protein
CVD	cardiovascular disease
DHA	docosahexaenoic acid
DPA	docosapentaenoic acid
EFSA	European Food Safety Authority
EPA	eicosapentaenoic acid
HDL	high-density lipoprotein
IL	interleukin
LDL	low-density lipoprotein
MD	mean difference
MI	myocardial infarction
NS	not significant
RCT	randomised controlled trial
SMD	standard mean difference
TNF	tumour necrosis factor
WMD	weighted mean difference

References

1. Calder, P.C. Very long-chain n-3 fatty acids and human health: Fact, fiction and the future. *Proc. Nutr. Soc.* **2018**, *77*, 52–72. [CrossRef]
2. Kaur, G.; Cameron-Smith, D.; Garg, M.; Sinclair, A.J. Docosapentaenoic acid (22:5n-3): A review of its biological effects. *Prog. Lipid Res.* **2011**, *50*, 28–34. [CrossRef]
3. Arterburn, L.M.; Hall, E.B.; Oken, H. Distribution, interconversion, and dose response of n-3 fatty acids in humans. *Am. J. Clin. Nutr.* **2006**, *83*, 1467S. [CrossRef]
4. Baker, E.J.; Miles, E.A.; Burdge, G.C.; Yaqoob, P.; Calder, P.C. Metabolism and functional effects of plant-derived omega-3 fatty acids in humans. *Prog. Lipid Res.* **2016**, *64*, 30–56. [CrossRef]
5. Meyer, B.J.; Mann, N.J.; Lewis, J.L.; Milligan, G.C.; Sinclair, A.J.; Howe, P.R. Dietary intakes and food sources of omega-6 and omega-3 polyunsaturated fatty acids. *Lipids* **2003**, *38*, 391–398. [CrossRef]
6. Howe, P.; Meyer, B.; Record, S.; Baghurst, K. Dietary intake of long-chain omega-3 polyunsaturated fatty acids: Contribution of meat sources. *Nutrition* **2006**, *22*, 47–53. [CrossRef]

7. Scientific Advisory Committee on Nutrition/Committee on Toxicity. *Advice on Fish Consumption: Benefits and Risks*; TSO: London, UK, 2004.
8. Food and Agricultural Organisation of the United Nations. *Fat and Fatty Acids in Human Nutrition: Report of an Expert Consultation*; Food and Agricultural Organisation of the United Nations: Rome, Italy, 2010.
9. European Food Safety Authority. Panel on Dietetic Products, Nutrition and Allergies (NDA); Scientific Opinion on the substantiation of health claims related to eicosapentaenoic acid (EPA), docosahexaenoic acid (DHA), docosapentaenoic acid (DPA) and maintenance. *EFSA J.* **2010**, *8*, 1796. [CrossRef]
10. Kromann, N.; Green, A. Epidemiological studies in the Upernavik district, Greenland. *J. Intern. Med.* **1980**, *208*, 401–406. [CrossRef]
11. Bjerregaard, P.; Dyerberg, J. Mortality from ischaemic heart disease and cerebrovascular disease in Greenland. *Int. J. Epidemiol.* **1988**, *17*, 514–519. [CrossRef]
12. Bang, H.; Dyerberg, J.; Hjørne, N. The composition of food consumed by Greenland Eskimos. *J. Intern. Med.* **1976**, *200*, 69–73. [CrossRef]
13. Newman, W.; Middaugh, J.; Propst, M.; Rogers, D. Atherosclerosis in Alaska Natives and non-Natives. *Lancet* **1993**, *341*, 1056–1057. [CrossRef]
14. Yano, K.; MacLean, C.J.; Reed, D.M.; Shimizu, Y.; Sasaki, H.; Kodama, K.; Kato, H.; Kagan, A. A comparison of the 12-year mortality and predictive factors of coronary heart disease among Japanese men in Japan and Hawaii. *Am. J. Epidemiol.* **1988**, *127*, 476–487. [CrossRef]
15. Calder, P.C. n-3 Fatty acids and cardiovascular disease: Evidence explained and mechanisms explored. *Clin. Sci.* **2004**, *107*, 1–11. [CrossRef]
16. Hu, F.; Bronner, L.; Willett, W.; Stampfer, M.; Rexrode, K.M.; Albert, C.; Hunter, D.; Manson, J. Fish and omega-3 fatty acid intake and risk of coronary heart disease in women. *JAMA* **2002**, *287*, 1815–1821. [CrossRef]
17. Browning, L.M.; Walker, C.G.; Mander, A.P.; West, A.L.; Madden, J.; Gambell, J.M.; Young, S.; Wang, L.; Jebb, S.A.; Calder, P.C. Incorporation of eicosapentaenoic and docosahexaenoic acids into lipid pools when given as supplements providing doses equivalent to typical intakes of oily fish. *Am. J. Clin. Nutr.* **2012**, *96*, 748–758. [CrossRef]
18. Albert, C.; Campos, H.; Stampfer, M.; Ridker, P.; Manson, J.; Willett, W.; Ma, J. Blood levels of long-chain n–3 fatty acids and the risk of sudden death. *N. Engl. J. Med.* **2002**, *346*, 1113–1118. [CrossRef]
19. Zhang, Y.; Zhuang, P.; He, W.; Chen, J.N.; Wang, W.Q.; Freedman, N.D.; Abnet, C.C.; Wang, J.B.; Jiao, J.J. Association of fish and long-chain omega-3 fatty acids intakes with total and cause-specific mortality: Prospective analysis of 421 309 individuals. *J. Intern. Med.* **2018**, *284*, 399–417. [CrossRef]
20. Djoussé, L.; Akinkuolie, A.; Wu, J.; Ding, E.; Gaziano, J. Fish consumption, omega-3 fatty acids and risk of heart failure: A meta-analysis. *Clin. Nutr.* **2012**, *31*, 846–853. [CrossRef]
21. Chowdhury, R.; Warnakula, S.; Kunutsor, S.; Crowe, F.; Ward, H.; Johnson, L.; Franco, O.; Butterworth, A.; Forouhi, N.; Thompson, S.; et al. Association of dietary, circulating, and supplement fatty acids with coronary risk: A systematic review and meta-analysis. *Ann. Intern. Med.* **2014**, *160*, 398–406. [CrossRef]
22. Alexander, D.D.; Miller, P.E.; Van Elswyk, M.E.; Kuratko, C.N.; Bylsma, L.C. A meta-analysis of randomized controlled trials and prospective cohort studies of eicosapentaenoic and docosahexaenoic long-chain omega-3 fatty acids and coronary heart disease risk. *Mayo Clin. Proc.* **2017**, *92*, 15–29. [CrossRef]
23. Del Gobbo, L.C.; Imamura, F.; Aslibekyan, S.; Marklund, M.; Virtanen, J.K.; Wennberg, M.; Yakoob, M.Y.; Chiuve, S.E.; Dela Cruz, L.; Frazier-Wood, A.C.; et al. ω-3 Polyunsaturated fatty acid biomarkers and coronary heart disease: Pooling project of 19 cohort studies. *JAMA Intern. Med.* **2016**, *176*, 1155–1166. [CrossRef] [PubMed]
24. Harris, W.S.; Von Schacky, C. The Omega-3 Index: A new risk factor for death from coronary heart disease? *Prev. Med.* **2004**, *39*, 212–220. [CrossRef] [PubMed]
25. Harris, W.S.; Del Gobbo, L.; Tintle, N.L. The omega-3 index and relative risk for coronary heart disease mortality: Estimation from 10 cohort studies. *Atherosclerosis* **2017**, *262*, 51–54. [CrossRef] [PubMed]
26. AbuMweis, S.; Jew, S.; Tayyem, R.; Agraib, L. Eicosapentaenoic acid and docosahexaenoic acid containing supplements modulate risk factors for cardiovascular disease: A meta-analysis of randomised placebo-control human clinical trials. *J. Hum. Nutr. Diet.* **2018**, *31*, 67–84. [CrossRef]

27. Miller, P.E.; Van Elswyk, M.; Alexander, D.D. Long-chain omega-3 fatty acids eicosapentaenoic acid and docosahexaenoic acid and blood pressure: A meta-analysis of randomized controlled trials. *Am. J. Hypertens.* **2014**, *27*, 885–896. [CrossRef]
28. Mozaffarian, D.; Geelen, A.; Brouwer, I.A.; Geleijnse, J.M.; Zock, P.L.; Katan, M.B. Effect of fish oil on heart rate in humans: A meta-analysis of randomized controlled trials. *Circulation* **2005**, *112*, 1945–1952. [CrossRef]
29. Xin, W.; Wei, W.; Li, X. Short-term effects of fish-oil supplementation on heart rate variability in humans: A meta-analysis of randomized controlled trials. *Am. J. Clin. Nutr.* **2013**, *97*, 926–935. [CrossRef]
30. Hidayat, K.; Yang, J.; Zhang, Z.; Chen, G.-C.; Qin, L.-Q.; Eggersdorfer, M.; Zhang, W. Effect of omega-3 long-chain polyunsaturated fatty acid supplementation on heart rate: A meta-analysis of randomized controlled trials. *Eur. J. Clin. Nutr.* **2017**. [CrossRef]
31. Gao, L.; Cao, J.; Mao, Q.X.; Lu, X.X.; Zhou, X.L.; Fan, L. Influence of omega-3 polyunsaturated fatty acid-supplementation on platelet aggregation in humans: A meta-analysis of randomized controlled trials. *Atherosclerosis* **2013**, *226*, 328–334. [CrossRef]
32. Xin, W.; Wei, W.; Li, X. Effect of fish oil supplementation on fasting vascular endothelial function in humans: A meta-analysis of randomized controlled trials. *PLoS ONE* **2012**, *7*, e46028. [CrossRef]
33. Wang, Q.; Liang, X.; Wang, L.; Lu, X.; Huang, J.; Cao, J.; Li, H.; Gu, D. Effect of omega-3 fatty acids supplementation on endothelial function: A meta-analysis of randomized controlled trials. *Atherosclerosis* **2012**, *221*, 536–543. [CrossRef]
34. Pase, M.P.; Grima, N.A.; Sarris, J. Do long-chain n-3 fatty acids reduce arterial stiffness? A meta-analysis of randomised controlled trials. *Br. J. Nutr.* **2011**, *106*, 974–980. [CrossRef]
35. Li, K.; Huang, T.; Zheng, J.; Wu, K.; Li, D. Effect of marine-derived n-3 polyunsaturated fatty acids on C-reactive protein, interleukin-6 and tumor necrosis factor alpha: A meta-analysis. *PLoS ONE* **2014**, *9*, e88103. [CrossRef]
36. Jiang, J.; Li, K.; Wang, F.; Yang, B.; Fu, Y.; Zheng, J.; Li, D. Effect of marine-derived n-3 polyunsaturated fatty acids on major eicosanoids: A systematic review and meta-analysis from 18 randomized controlled trials. *PLoS ONE* **2016**, *11*, e0147351. [CrossRef] [PubMed]
37. Innes, J.K.; Calder, P.C. The differential effects of eicosapentaenoic acid and docosahexaenoic acid on cardiometabolic risk factors: A systematic review. *Int. J. Mol. Sci.* **2018**, *19*, 532. [CrossRef] [PubMed]
38. Grimsgaard, S.; Bonna, K.H.; Hansen, J.-B.; Nordøy, A. Highly purified eicosapentaenoic acid and docosahexaenoic acid in humans have similar triacylglycerol-lowering effects but divergent effects on serum fatty acids. *Am. J. Clin. Nutr.* **1997**, *66*, 649–659. [CrossRef] [PubMed]
39. Allaire, J.; Couture, P.; Leclerc, M.; Charest, A.; Marin, J.; Lépine, M.-C.; Talbot, D.; Tchernof, A.; Lamarche, B. A randomized, crossover, head-to-head comparison of eicosapentaenoic acid and docosahexaenoic acid supplementation to reduce inflammation markers in men and women: The Comparing EPA to DHA (ComparED) Study. *Am. J. Clin. Nutr.* **2016**, *104*, 280–287. [CrossRef]
40. Woodman, R.J.; Mori, T.A.; Burke, V.; Puddey, I.B.; Watts, G.F.; Beilin, L.J. Effects of purified eicosapentaenoic and docosahexaenoic acids on glycemic control, blood pressure, and serum lipids in type 2 diabetic patients with treated hypertension. *Am. J. Clin. Nutr.* **2002**, *76*, 1007–1015. [CrossRef]
41. Mori, T.A.; Burke, V.; Puddey, I.B.; Watts, G.F.; O'Neal, D.N.; Best, J.D.; Beilin, L.J. Purified eicosapentaenoic and docosahexaenoic acids have differential effects on serum lipids and lipoproteins, LDL particle size, glucose, and insulin in mildly hyperlipidemic men. *Am. J. Clin. Nutr.* **2000**, *71*, 1085–1094. [CrossRef]
42. Grimsgaard, S.; Bonaa, K.; Hansen, J.; Myhre, E. Effects of highly purified eicosapentaenoic acid and docosahexaenoic acid on hemodynamics in humans. *Am. J. Clin. Nutr.* **1998**, *68*, 52–59. [CrossRef]
43. Mori, T.; Bao, D.; Burke, V.; Puddey, I.; Beilin, L. Docosahexaenoic acid but not eicosapentaenoic acid lowers ambulatory blood pressure and heart rate in humans. *Hypertension* **1999**, *34*, 253–260. [CrossRef] [PubMed]
44. Mori, T.A.; Watts, G.F.; Burke, V.; Hilme, E.; Puddey, I.B.; Beilin, L.J. Differential effects of eicosapentaenoic acid and docosahexaenoic acid on vascular reactivity of the forearm microcirculation in hyperlipidaemic, overweight men. *Circulation* **2000**, *102*, 1264–1269. [CrossRef] [PubMed]
45. Nestel, P.; Shige, H.; Pomeroy, S.; Cehun, M.; Abbey, M.; Raederstorff, D. The n-3 fatty acids eicosapentaenoic acid and docosahexaenoic acid increase systemic arterial compliance in humans. *Am. J. Clin. Nutr.* **2002**, *76*, 326–330. [CrossRef] [PubMed]
46. Park, Y.; Harris, W. EPA, but not DHA, decreases mean platelet volume in normal subjects. *Lipids* **2002**, *37*, 941–946. [CrossRef] [PubMed]

47. Woodman, R.J.; Mori, T.A.; Burke, V.; Puddey, I.B.; Barden, A.; Watts, G.F.; Beilin, L.J. Effects of purified eicosapentaenoic acid and docosahexaenoic acid on platelet, fibrinolytic and vascular function in hypertensive type 2 diabetic patients. *Atherosclerosis* **2003**, *166*, 85–93. [CrossRef]
48. Vors, C.; Allaire, J.; Marin, J.; Lepine, M.C.; Charest, A.; Tchernof, A.; Couture, P.; Lamarche, B. Inflammatory gene expression in whole blood cells after EPA vs. DHA supplementation: Results from the ComparED study. *Atherosclerosis* **2017**, *257*, 116–122. [CrossRef] [PubMed]
49. Mori, T.A.; Puddey, I.B.; Burke, V.; Croft, K.D.; Dunstan, D.W.; Rivera, J.H.; Beilin, L.J. Effect of omega 3 fatty acids on oxidative stress in humans: GC-MS measurement of urinary F-2-isoprostane excretion. *Redox Rep.* **2000**, *5*, 45–46. [CrossRef]
50. Mas, E.; Woodman, R.J.; Burke, V.; Puddey, I.B.; Beilin, L.J.; Durand, T.; Mori, T.A. The omega-3 fatty acids EPA and DHA decrease plasma F2-isoprostanes: Results from two placebo-controlled interventions. *Free Radic. Res.* **2010**, *44*, 983–990. [CrossRef]
51. Mori, T.A.; Woodman, R.J.; Burke, V.; Puddey, I.B.; Croft, K.D.; Beilin, L.J. Effect of eicosapentaenoic acid and docosahexaenoic acid on oxidative stress and inflammatory markers in treated-hypertensive type 2 diabetic subjects. *Free Radic. Biol. Med.* **2003**, *35*, 772–781. [CrossRef]
52. Yokoyama, M.; Origasa, H.; Matsuzaki, M.; Matsuzawa, Y.; Saito, Y.; Ishikawa, Y.; Oikawa, S.; Sasaki, J.; Hishida, H.; Itakura, H.; et al. Effects of eicosapentaenoic acid on major coronary events in hypercholesterolaemic patients (JELIS): A randomised open- label, blinded endpoint analysis. *Lancet* **2007**, *369*, 1090–1098. [CrossRef]
53. Bowman, L.; Mafham, M.; Wallendszus, K.; Stevens, W.; Buck, G.; Barton, J.; Murphy, K.; Aung, T.; Haynes, R.; Cox, J.; et al. Effects of n-3 fatty acid supplements in diabetes mellitus. *N. Engl. J. Med.* **2018**, *379*, 1540–1550. [CrossRef] [PubMed]
54. Manson, J.A.E.; Cook, N.R.; Lee, I.M.; Christen, W.; Bassuk, S.S.; Mora, S.; Gibson, H.; Albert, C.M.; Gordon, D.; Copeland, T.; et al. Marine n-3 fatty acids and prevention of cardiovascular disease and cancer. *N. Engl. J. Med.* **2019**, *380*, 23–32. [CrossRef] [PubMed]
55. Burr, M.L.; Gilbert, J.F.; Holliday, R.M.; Elwood, P.C.; Fehily, A.M.; Rogers, S.; Sweetnam, P.M.; Deadman, N.M. Effects of changes in fat, fish, and fibre intakes on death and myocardial reinfarction: Diet and reinfarction trial (DART). *Lancet* **1989**, *344*, 757–761. [CrossRef]
56. The GISSI-Prevenzione Investigators. Dietary supplementation with n-3 polyunsaturated fatty acids and vitamin E after myocardial infarction: Results of the GISSI-Prevenzione trial. *Lancet* **1999**, *354*, 447–455. [CrossRef]
57. Marchioli, R.; Barzi, F.; Bomba, E.; Chieffo, C.; Di Gregorio, D.; Di Mascio, R.; Franzosi, M.G.; Geraci, E.; Levantesi, G.; Maggioni, A.; et al. Early protection against sudden death by n-3 polyunsaturated fatty acids after myocardial infarction: Time-course analysis of the results of the Gruppo Italiano per lo Studio della Sopravvivenza nell'Infarto Miocardico (GISSI)-Prevenzione. *Circulation* **2002**, *105*, 1897–1903. [CrossRef]
58. Romagna, E. The GISSI-HF Investigators Effect of n-3 polyunsaturated fatty acids in patients with chronic heart failure (the GISSI-HF trial): A randomised, double-blind, placebo-controlled trial. *Lancet* **2008**, *372*, 1223–1230. [CrossRef]
59. Itakura, H.; Yokoyama, M.; Matsuzaki, M.; Saito, Y.; Origasa, H.; Ishikawa, Y.; Oikawa, S.; Sasaki, J.; Hishida, H.; Kita, T.; et al. Relationships between plasma fatty acid composition and coronary artery disease. *J. Atheroscler. Thromb.* **2011**, *18*, 99–107. [CrossRef]
60. Bucher, H.C.; Hengstler, P.; Schindler, C.; Meier, G. N-3 polyunsaturated fatty acids in coronary heart disease: A meta-analysis of randomized controlled trials. *Am. J. Med.* **2002**, *112*, 298–304. [CrossRef]
61. Studer, M.; Briel, M.; Leimenstoll, B.; Glass, T.R.; Bucher, H.C. Effect of different antilipidemic agents and diets on mortality: A systematic review. *Arch. Intern. Med.* **2005**, *165*, 725–730. [CrossRef]
62. Zhao, Y.-T.; Chen, Q.; Sun, Y.-X.; Li, X.-B.; Zhang, P.; Xu, Y.; Guo, J.-H. Prevention of sudden cardiac death with omega-3 fatty acids in patients with coronary heart disease: A meta-analysis of randomized controlled trials. *Ann. Med.* **2009**, *41*, 301–310. [CrossRef]
63. Marik, P.E.; Varon, J. Omega-3 dietary supplements and the risk of cardiovascular events: A systematic review. *Clin. Cardiol.* **2009**, *32*, 365–372. [CrossRef] [PubMed]
64. Rauch, B.; Schiele, R.; Schneider, S.; Diller, F.; Victor, N.; Gohlke, H.; Gottwik, M.; Steinbeck, G.; Del Castillo, U.; Sack, R.; et al. OMEGA, a randomized, placebo-controlled trial to test the effect of highly purified omega-3

fatty acids on top of modern guideline-adjusted therapy after myocardial infarction. *Circulation* **2010**, *122*, 2152–2159. [CrossRef] [PubMed]

65. Galan, P.; Kesse-Guyot, E.; Czernichow, S.; Briancon, S.; Blacher, J.; Hercberg, S. Effects of B vitamins and omega 3 fatty acids on cardiovascular diseases: A randomised placebo controlled trial. *BMJ* **2010**, *341*, c6273. [CrossRef] [PubMed]
66. Kromhout, D.; Giltay, E.J.; Geleijnse, J.M. n–3 Fatty acids and cardiovascular events after myocardial infarction. *N. Engl. J. Med.* **2010**, *363*, 2015–2026. [CrossRef]
67. Bosch, J.; Gerstein, H.; Dagenais, G.; Diaz, R.; Dyal, L.; Jung, H.; Maggiono, A.; Probstfield, J.; Ramachandran, A.; Riddle, M.; et al. n–3 Fatty acids and cardiovascular outcomes in patients with dysglycemia (ORIGIN). *N. Engl. J. Med.* **2012**, *367*, 309–318. [CrossRef]
68. Roncaglioni, M.; Tombesi, M.; Avanzini, F.; Barlera, S.; Caimi, V.; Longoni, P.; Marzona, I.; Milani, V.; Silletta, M.; Tognoni, G.; et al. n–3 Fatty acids in patients with multiple cardiovascular risk factors (Risk and Prevention Study). *N. Engl. J. Med.* **2013**, *368*, 1800–1808. [CrossRef]
69. Calder, P.C.; Yaqoob, P. Marine omega-3 fatty acids and coronary heart disease. *Curr. Opin. Cardiol.* **2012**, *27*, 412–419. [CrossRef]
70. Calder, P.C. Limited impact of omega-3 fatty acids in patients with multiple cardiovascular risk factors. *Evid. Based Med.* **2014**, *19*, 18. [CrossRef]
71. Kotwal, S.; Jun, M.; Sullivan, D.; Perkovic, V.; Neal, B. Omega 3 fatty acids and cardiovascular outcomes: Systematic review and meta-analysis. *Circ. Cardiovasc. Qual. Outcomes* **2012**, *5*, 808–818. [CrossRef]
72. Kwak, S.M.; Myung, S.K.; Lee, Y.J.; Seo, H.G. Efficacy of omega-3 fatty acid supplements (eicosapentaenoic acid and docosahexaenoic acid) in the secondary prevention of cardiovascular disease: A meta-analysis of randomized, double-blind, placebo-controlled trials. *Arch. Intern. Med.* **2012**, *172*, 686–694. [CrossRef]
73. Trikalinos, T.; Lee, J.; Moorthy, D.; Yu, W.; Lau, J.; Lichtenstein, A.; Chung, M. Effects of eicosapentanoic acid and docosahexanoic acid on mortality across diverse settings: Systematic review and meta-analysis of randomized trials and prospective cohorts. *Tech. Rev.* **2012**, *17*, 4.
74. Rizos, E.; Ntzani, E.; Bika, E.; Kostapanos, M.; Elisaf, M. Association between omega-3 fatty acid supplementation and risk of major cardiovascular disease events: A systematic review and meta-analysis. *JAMA* **2012**, *308*, 1024–1033. [CrossRef] [PubMed]
75. Casula, M.; Soranna, D.; Catapano, A.L.; Corrao, G. Long-term effect of high dose omega-3 fatty acid supplementation for secondary prevention of cardiovascular outcomes: A meta-analysis of randomized, double blind, placebo controlled trials. *Atheroscler. Suppl.* **2013**, *14*, 243–251. [CrossRef]
76. Wen, Y.T.; Dai, J.H.; Gao, Q. Effects of omega-3 fatty acid on major cardiovascular events and mortality in patients with coronary heart disease: A meta-analysis of randomized controlled trials. *Nutr. Metab. Cardiovasc. Dis.* **2014**, *24*, 470–475. [CrossRef]
77. Maki, K.C.; Palacios, O.M.; Bell, M.; Toth, P.P. Use of supplemental long-chain omega-3 fatty acids and risk for cardiac death: An updated meta-analysis and review of research gaps. *J. Clin. Lipidol.* **2017**, *11*, 1152–1160.e2. [CrossRef]
78. Aung, T.; Halsey, J.; Kromhout, D.; Gerstein, H.C.; Marchioli, R.; Tavazzi, L.; Geleijnse, J.M.; Rauch, B.; Ness, A.; Galan, P.; et al. Associations of omega-3 fatty acid supplement use with cardiovascular disease risks. *JAMA Cardiol.* **2018**, *3*, 225–234. [CrossRef]
79. Abdelhamid, A.; Brown, T.; Brainard, J.; Biswas, P.; Thorpe, G.; Moore, H.; Deane, K.; AlAbdulghafoor, F.; Summerbell, C.; Worthington, H.; et al. Omega-3 fatty acids for the primary and secondary prevention of cardiovascular disease. *Cochrane Database Syst. Rev.* **2018**, CD003177. [CrossRef]
80. Bhatt, D.L.; Steg, P.G.; Miller, M.; Brinton, E.A.; Jacobson, T.A.; Ketchum, S.B.; Doyle, R.T.; Juliano, R.A.; Jiao, L.; Granowitz, C.; et al. Cardiovascular risk reduction with icosapent ethyl for hypertriglyceridemia. *N. Engl. J. Med.* **2019**, *380*, 11–22. [CrossRef]
81. Hu, Y.; Hu, F.B.; Manson, J.E. Marine omega-3 supplementation and cardiovascular disease: An updated meta-analysis of 13 randomized controlled trials involving 127,477 participants. *J. Am. Heart Assoc.* **2019**, *8*, e013543. [CrossRef]
82. Einvik, G.; Ole Klemsdal, T.; Sandvik, L.; Hjerkinn, E.M. A randomized clinical trial on n-3 polyunsaturated fatty acids supplementation and all-cause mortality in elderly men at high cardiovascular risk. *Eur. J. Cardiovasc. Prev. Rehabil.* **2010**, *17*, 588–592. [CrossRef]

83. Rimm, E.B.; Appel, L.J.; Chiuve, S.E.; Djoussé, L.; Engler, M.B.; Kris-Etherton, P.M.; Mozaffarian, D.; Siscovick, D.S.; Lichtenstein, A.H. Seafood long-chain n-3 polyunsaturated fatty acids and cardiovascular disease: A science advisory from the American Heart Association. *Circulation* **2018**, *138*, 35–47. [CrossRef] [PubMed]
84. Skulas-Ray, A.C.; Wilson, P.W.F.; Harris, W.S.; Brinton, E.A.; Kris-Etherton, P.M.; Richter, C.K.; Jacobson, T.A.; Engler, M.B.; Miller, M.; Robinson, J.G.; et al. Omega-3 fatty acids for the management of hypertriglyceridemia: A science advisory from the American Heart Association. *Circulation* **2019**, *140*, e673–e691. [CrossRef] [PubMed]
85. Mach, F.; Baigent, C.; Carapano, A.L.; Koskinas, K.C.; Casula, M.; Badimon, L.; Chapman, M.J.; de Backer, G.G.; Delgado, V.; Ference, B.A.; et al. 2019 ESC/EAS guidelines for the management of dyslipidaemias: Lipid modification to reduce cardiovascular risk. *Eur. Heart J.* **2020**, *41*, 111–188. [CrossRef] [PubMed]
86. The Living Standards of Medical Care in Diabetes—Updates to the standards of medical care in diabetes. Available online: https://care.diabetesjournals.org/living-standards#March%2027,%202019 (accessed on 7 February 2020).
87. Orringer, C.E.; Jacobson, T.A.; Maki, K.C. National Lipid Association Scientific Statement on the use of icosapent ethyl in statin-treated patients with elevated triglycerides and high or very-high ASCVD risk. *J. Clin. Lipidol.* **2019**, *13*, 860–872. [CrossRef]
88. Kris-Etherton, P.M.; Harris, W.S.; Appel, L.J. Fish consumption, fish oil, omega-3 fatty acids, and cardiovascular disease. *Circulation* **2002**, *106*, 2747–2757. [CrossRef]
89. Siscovick, D.S.; Barringer, T.A.; Fretts, A.M.; Wu, J.H.Y.; Lichtenstein, A.H.; Costello, R.B.; Kris-Etherton, P.M.; Jacobson, T.A.; Engler, M.B.; Alger, H.M.; et al. Omega-3 polyunsaturated fatty acid (fish oil) supplementation and the prevention of clinical cardiovascular disease: A Science Advisory from the American Heart Association. *Circulation* **2017**, *135*, e867–e884. [CrossRef]
90. NICE Cardiovascular disease: Risk assessment and reduction, including lipid modification (clinical guideline CG181). Available online: https://www.nice.org.uk/guidance/cg181 (accessed on 14 July 2014).
91. Von Schacky, C. Omega-3 fatty acids in cardiovascular disease—An uphill battle. *Prostagland. Leukot. Essent Fatty Acids* **2015**, *92*, 41–47. [CrossRef]
92. Rice, H.B.; Bernasconi, A.; Maki, K.C.; Harris, W.S.; von Schacky, C.; Calder, P.C. Conducting omega-3 clinical trials with cardiovascular outcomes: Proceedings of a Workshop held at ISSFAL 2014. *Prostagland. Leukot. Essent. Fatty Acids* **2016**, *107*, 30–42. [CrossRef]
93. Schuchardt, J.P.; Hahn, A. Bioavailability of long-chain omega-3 fatty acids. *Prostagland. Leukot. Essent. Fatty Acids* **2013**, *89*, 1–9. [CrossRef]

7

Mitochondrial DNA Mutations and Rheumatic Heart Diseases

Fatou Balla Wade *, Marie Parsine Sall, Fatimata Mbaye and Mbacké Sembene

Genetics and Population Management Team, Department of Animal Biology, Faculty of Sciences and Techniques, Cheikh Anta Diop University, Dakar 5005, Senegal; mparsine@yahoo.fr (M.P.S.); fatimata.mbaye@ucad.edu.sn (F.M.); mbacke.sembene@ucad.edu.sn (M.S.)

* Correspondence: fatouballa.wade@ucad.edu.sn

Abstract: Acute rheumatic fever (ARF) is an autoimmune disease affecting the heart-valve endocardium in its final stage. Although rare in developing countries, ARF persists in third-world countries, particularly Senegal, where rheumatic heart diseases (RHDs) are the most common pediatric cardiovascular pathology. This study aimed to investigate mutations in *MT-CYB* in ARF and RHD in Senegalese patients. *MT-CYB* was amplified from blood samples from ARF patients at the Clinical of Thoracic and Cardiovascular Surgery of Fann National University Hospital Centre, Dakar, Senegal (control group, healthy individuals) and sequenced. More than half of the *MT-CYB* mutations (58.23%) were heteroplasmic. Transitions (61.67%) were more frequent than transversions (38.33%), and non-synonymous substitutions represented 38.33% of mutations. Unoperated RHD patients harbored frequent *MT-CYB* polymorphisms (7.14 ± 14.70 mutations per sample) and accounted for 72.73% of mutations. Paradoxically, subjects undergoing valvular replacement harbored infrequent polymorphisms (1.39 ± 2.97 mutations per patient) and lacked 36 mutations present in unoperated subjects. A genetic differentiation was observed between these two populations, and the mutations in operated subjects were neutral, while those in unoperated subjects were under positive selection. These results indicate a narrow link (perhaps even causal) between *MT-CYB* mutations and ARF and its complications (i.e., RHDs) and that these mutations are largely deleterious.

Keywords: acute rheumatic fever; rheumatic heart diseases; *MT-CYB*; mutation; Senegal

---

1. Introduction

Acute rheumatic fever (ARF) is a major cause of cardiac disease and premature death in numerous regions worldwide [1]. ARF and rheumatic heart disease (RHD) have a high prevalence in developing countries in contrast with developed countries where these diseases have largely regressed [2]. ARF results in high morbidity and mortality rates worldwide and its incidence is the highest in Sub-Saharan Africa [3]. ARF incidence in developing countries exceeds 50 per 100,000 children [4]. In Senegal, RHD is the most prominent pediatric cardiovascular pathology [5].

Mutations in numerous genes, particularly those encoding immunity-related factors, are associated with ARF and RHD [6]. Genes encoding pattern recognition receptors belonging to the innate immune system, including ficolin [7], have been investigated. Genes encoding several cytokines including TNF-α or IL-6/-10 were reported to promote or aggravate ARF in studies in Mexico [8,9], Turkey [10], and Egypt [11].

On the other hand, it has been shown that the decrease in oxidative phosphorylation [12] Khatami mainly affects energy-intensive tissues, such as muscles, brain, heart, liver, and kidneys. This mechanism allows the production of ATP by the mitochondrial respiratory chain [13]. *MT-CYB* encodes the cytochrome b protein, which is the only subunit of the respiratory complex III (one of the five complexes of the respiratory chain), encoded by mitochondrial DNA, the others being of nuclear origin [13]. Cytochrome b plays a central role in the production of ATP [12] and as a catalytic subunit binding to the substrate of quinone and facilitating the transmission of electrons to cytochrome c [14]. Many mutations of *MT-CYB*, identified so far, are related to diseases such as stress intolerance, myopathies, cardiomyopathies, and neuropathies. These mutations generally show a deficit of enzymatic activity and a decrease in the number of certain subunits of complex III [13]. Mitochondrial dysfunction is characteristic of heart failure [15].

Thus far, no study on the mitochondrial genome has focused on ARF and RHD, and genetic investigations of these pathologies has not been carried out in Senegal. Hence, we hypothesized that mitochondrial *MT-CYB* mutations influence the occurrence and/or complications in ARF. This study aimed to investigate mutations in *MT-CYB* in ARF and RHD in Senegalese patients. The following were the objectives of our study: (1) To investigate *MT-CYB* polymorphisms in ARF; (2) to evaluate the genetic diversity of *MT-CYB* in ARF; (3) to determine the genetic structure of *MT-CYB* based on populations; (4) to identify the type of *MT-CYB* mutations in ARF.

2. Materials and Methods

2.1. Study Population

Patients with ARF undergoing follow-up examination at the Clinic of Thoracic and Cardiovascular Surgery of Fann National University Hospital Centre in Dakar, Senegal, were included herein. The study was approved by the ethics and research committee of Cheikh Anta Diop University (reference number: Protocol 0274/2018/CER/UCAD), and patients provided written informed consent prior to their participation in the study in accordance with the tenets of the Declaration of Helsinki. Some of these patients had undergone valvular replacement surgery, while others did not receive surgical intervention. Healthy individuals were recruited as controls.

Patients were divided into three groups: First group, healthy individuals (control group); second group, unoperated ARF patients; third group, operated ARF patients (n = 42 per group). In total, 126 blood samples obtained from each patient were stored in EDTA and labeled as Sg1, Sg2, etc.

2.2. Genetic Analysis

2.2.1. DNA Extraction and Amplification and Sequencing of MT-CYB

Genomic DNA was extracted using the DNase Blood Kit (Qiagen, South Korea) in accordance with the manufacturer's instructions. Polymerase chain reaction (PCR) was carried out to amplify *MT-CYB*, since it is reportedly involved in cardiovascular pathologies [12,15–19]. PCR amplification of *MT-CYB* was carried out at a reaction volume of 50 µL containing 2 µL of concentrated DNA and 48 µL of the PCR mix comprising 29.8 µL of MilliQ water, 5 µL of buffer, 1 µL of supplementary $MgCl_2$, 2 µL of dATP, dCTP, dGTP, and dTTP, 5 µL of H15915, 5 µL of L14723, and 0.2 µL of Tap polymerase. L14723 (5′-ACCAATGACATGAAAAATCATGGTT-3′) and H15915 (5′-TCTCCATTTCTGGTTTACAAGAC-3′) were the forward and reverse primers, respectively. The PCR program included the following conditions: 94 °C for 3 min; 40 cycles (94 °C for 45 s; 52 °C for 1 min; 72 °C 1 min for 30 s); 72 °C for 10 min. PCR products were purified and sequenced. Sequencing reactions were performed using an MJ Research PTC-225 Peltier thermocycler with the ABI PRISM kit and electrophoresed in an ABI 3730 XL sequencer.

2.2.2. Molecular Analyses

The chromatograms obtained after sequencing were submitted to the Mutation Surveyor software (https://softgenetics.com) version 5.0 to identify mutations and to determine their nature (homoplasmic or heteroplasmic) and their status (transition or transversion). Sequences of ARF with those of the controls. Mutation Surveyor assigned a score for each mutation, thus indicating the level of confidence regarding the accuracy of the cited base. Only those mutations with a score of ≥20 were retained (the probability that a cited base is false was 0.001; accuracy, 99%).

To determine the appropriate nucleotide position of our mutations in the mitochondrial genome, we performed BLASTn analysis (NCBI; https://ncbi.nlm.nih.gov/) with our raw control sequence. The position of each mutation and the corresponding amino acid was determined using BLASTx 2.8.0 [20], thus facilitating the identification of putative conserved domains [21].

To highlight the potential pathogenicity of non-synonymous mutations, we performed prediction analysis using three different software for transparency and reliability:

- POLYPHEN-2 [22], which yields the following putative results: Probably damaging ($p \leq 5\%$), potentially damaging ($5 < p \leq 10\%$), and benign ($p > 10\%$);
- SIFT [23], which assigns a score between zero and one. Amino acid substitutions are predicted to affect protein function when the score is ≤0.05 and to be tolerable when the score is >0.05;
- PROVEAN [24] wherein variants with a score of ≤–2.5 are predicted as deleterious and those with a score of >–2.5 are considered neutral.

Non-synonymous *MT-CYB* mutations have been considered pathogenic if thus stipulated by at least two prediction software; if these mutations are not reported as neutral polymorphisms and if they are present in a conserved domain; heteroplasmy indicates high pathogenicity [25].

For further molecular analysis, we corrected and aligned sequences of ARF patients with those of the controls, using BioEdit version 7.1.9 [26] using the CLUSTALW algorithm [27]. Thereafter, we determined the following parameters underlying the genetic diversity of *MT-CYB* relative to each population, on the basis of which the groups were assessed and differentiated:

- The population size n corresponding to the number of individuals;
- The number of sites N that define the size of sequences;
- The variable sites, invariable sites, non-informative variables, and informative variables, the number of total mutations (Eta), thus elucidating *MT-CYB* polymorphisms in the study population;
- The number of haplotypes and the haplotype diversity (Hd), to analyze the distribution of individuals within a population;
- The nucleotide diversity (Pi) and the average number of nucleotide differences (k) that reflect genetic differences within a population.

These parameters were determined using DNAsp 5.10.01 [28]. Other parameters elucidating the genetic diversity are the following:

- The nucleotide frequencies: General and at each codon position;
- The nature of mutations (transitions and transversions);
- The rate of mutations (R);
- The rate of substitutions: Ks (synonymous) and Kns (non-synonymous).

These parameters were determined using Mega7 software version 7.0.26 [29], and the frequencies of amino acids was determined at the best reading frame (no stop codon).

For analysis using Mega7, it was necessary to determine the model describing the best pattern of substitution; hence, we used the following models:

- The HKY model [30] to control the population;
- The JC model [31] for unoperated ARF patients;
- The JC+G model [31] for operated ARF patients a gamma value of 0.06.

We used the Kimura 2-parameter model [32] to determine the rate of mutations because preferential models were unavailable for this analysis. The Nei-Gojobori modified model was used to estimate substitution rates.

Thereafter, we defined the parameters of genetic diversity among populations, thus highlighting *MT-CYB* polymorphisms in ARF patients. Using the DNAsp software, we estimated the following:

- The rate of nucleotide divergence representing the percentage of nucleotide-level differences in each generation;
- The nucleotide diversity between two populations;
- The average number of nucleotide-level differences at each site between pairwise sequences.

Further, we evaluated genetic differences and structural differences in *MT-CYB* in accordance with the study population. Using Mega7 version 7.0.26 [29], the genetic distances were determined, which facilitated the estimation of the rates of allele replacement among the compared entities, using the JC+G model (with G = 0.36), which was the most suitable model. To estimate genetic distances within populations, we used the K2 model, which is suitable for this analysis, while the JC+G model was not. Furthermore, we estimated the genetic distance between the control population and ARF patients (operated and unoperated). For all analyses of genetic distances, the bootstrap method was used with 1000 replicates and all reading frames were accounted for. Using Arlequin version 3.1 [33], we estimated the genetic differentiation factor (Fst) between populations and performed analysis of molecular variance (AMOVA) to determine the origin of the variants. These analyses were performed considering polymorphic loci only and with 1023 permutations.

The Z-test for selection was performed using Mega7 in accordance with three different alternative hypotheses, the null hypothesis being that H0: dN = dS. We then assessed the neutral selection (H_1: dN ≠ dS), the positive selection (dN > dS), and the negative selection (dN < dS). We used the Nei-Gojobori modified model [34], which differs from the original method of Nei-Gojobori in that transitional and transversional substitutions were no longer considered to occur at the same frequency. Thus, we calculated the ratio of transitions/transversions with the following formula [30]:

$$\kappa = \frac{(\pi t \pi c + \pi a \pi g)}{\pi y \pi r} \alpha / \beta \quad (1)$$

where πa, πc, πg, and πt are the nucleotide frequencies (of a, c, g, and t, respectively) estimated by their proportions in all sequences: πy = πt + πc and πr = πa + πg; α and β are the number of transitions and transversions, respectively, observed by considering all sequences in a pairwise manner.

2.3. Statistical Analyses

Data normality was assessed using XLSTAT 2018.3.50896 with the Shapiro-Wilk test with a rate of significance level set to 5%. We then performed the Fisher test (for non-normally distributed data) to establish an association between mutations and the state of the disease, always at a threshold of 5%. Mean and standard deviation values for mutations were determined using MS Excel 2010 and compared using R commander (Rcmdr) implemented in RGui version 3.3.4 to assess differences between operated and unoperated ARF patients.

Average amino acid frequencies of the controls and unoperated AFR patients and between the controls and operated ARF patients were compared using the chi-square test in Rstudio version 1.1.447. Since chi-square analysis is only feasible when the number of groups is <5, we used complementary values (100-effective).

3. Results

3.1. Evaluation of MT-CYB Polymorphisms

3.1.1. Analysis of MT-CYB Mutations

BLASTn analysis revealed 97% identity with *MT-CYB* and 5 gaps. BLASTx analysis revealed 98% identity (without gaps) with the cytochrome b (mitochondrion) [*Homo sapiens*] [35] and [*Homo sapiens subsp. 'Denisova'*] [36] and 97% identity (without gaps) with cytochrome b (mitochondrion) [*Homo heidelbergensis*] [37] and [*Homo sapiens neanderthalensis*] [38].

Alignment of the chromatograms of ARF patients (operated and unoperated) with those of the controls (Sg97) revealed 165-point mutations with a score of ≥20 or 60 different variants, in the overall study population. Among them, 41.67% corresponded with homoplasmic mutations and 58.23% corresponded with heteroplasmic mutations. Transitions largely surpassed the transversions (respectively 61.67% and 38.33%). Most mutations were present in unoperated ARF patients (72.73%) wherein 7.14 ± 14.70 mutations on average were harbored per individual. Indeed, seven mutations were present at high frequencies in ARF patients (G15849A, T15824C, A15784G, A15362T, A15323C, G15314C, and A15308T). Synonymous (A15362T and A15323C) and missense (G15314C and A15308T) mutations were exclusively present in unoperated ARF patients at frequencies of 67.86%, 67.86%, 42.86%, and 57.14%, respectively. The Fisher test revealed significant results for these mutations, thus indicating their association with ARF. Overall, 36 mutations were absent in the operated ARF patients. Thus, operated ARF patients harbored 1.39 ± 2.97 mutations on average. Differences in the average mutation frequencies were significant (p = 0.031). The frequency for synonymous mutations was 38.33% among the ARF patients. Among these amino acid substitutions, nine were pathogenic according to the predictions of Polyphen-2, SIFT, and PROVEAN. All the pathogenic mutations were absent in the operated patients, except for the missense substitutions K287P and N286P, present in all positions of their corresponding codons and present in only one subject (Sg56). Most mutated sites were detected through MITOMAP (https://www.mitomap.org/MITOMAP); however, the corresponding bases differed from the those in the present sequences (Table 1).

3.1.2. Variability of Amino Acids

Transcription was carried out based on the second reading frame. Gly and Leu were the most frequent amino acids in the protein. Asn and His were absent in the ARF patients and the controls. Pro and Thr were absent in the controls but present at low frequencies in the ARF patients. However, none of the P-values is significant (Table 2).

3.1.3. Determination of Genetic Diversity of MT-CYB

The analysis of the genetic diversity of the study population is summarized in Table 3. In the study population, 12, 28, and 54 individuals belonged to the control, unoperated, and operated groups, respectively. The sizes of the sequences were the same for each individual (492 bp). The unoperated group differed from the other two groups and displayed the highest *MT-CYB* polymorphism frequency. The nucleotide frequencies were similar in all groups. Cytosine was the least represented base with a minimal frequency at the third codon position in contrast with thymine and guanine, which were more frequent at this position. Adenine occurred mostly at the first codon position. In position 1, no transversions occurred, and all mutations were transitions (conservation of the mutated base); hence, the mutation rate (R) tended towards infinity.

Table 1. Characteristics of *MT-CYB* mutations.

Mutations	Rate	p. rCRS	Proportions of Mutations			Status	Nature	p. AA	CD	PolyPhen-2 Prediction	Sift Prediction	Provean Prediction	Conclusion	References
			S %	NO %	O%									
T69C	**91**	**15851**	**1.22**	**3.57**	**0.00**	**Homo**	**T**	**I369V**	**Yes**	**Benign 0**	TOL	Neutral	N.P	+ (A > C) (1)
G71A	142	15849	9.76	10.71	9.26 *	Homo	T	T368I	Yes	Benign 0	TOL	Neutral	N.P	+ (C > T)
G81GC	20	15839	1.22	3.57	0.00	Hetero	T	L365L	Yes					+ (C > T)
A89AT	22	15831	1.22	3.57	0.00	Hetero	T	I362I	Yes					
T94TA	83	15826	1.22	3.57	0.00	Hetero	T	T360T	Yes					
T96C	101	15824	15.85	21.43	12.96 *	Homo	T	T360A	Yes	Benign 0	TOL	Neutral	N.P	+ (A > G)
T121C	119	15799	1.22	0.00 *	1.85	Homo	T	Q352Q	Yes					+ (A > G)
G130A	103	15790	2.44	0.00	3.70 *	Homo	T	T348T	Yes					+ (C > T)
A133AC	21	15787	1.22	0.00 *	1.85	Hetero	T	F347F	Yes					+ (C > T)
A136G	86	15784	14.63	10.71 *	16.67 *	Homo	T	P346P	Yes					+ (C > T) (3)
A136AG	45	15784	1.22	0.00 *	1.85	Hetero	T	P346P	Yes					+ (C > T) (3)
A141AT	25	15779	1.22	3.57	0.00	Hetero	T	Y345Y	Yes					+ (T > C)
C143G	150	15777	1.22	3.57	0.00	Homo	T	S344T	Yes	p.D	AFP	Neutral	P	+ (G > C)
T162C	146	15758	2.44	0.00	3.70 *	Homo	T	I338V	Yes	Benign	AFP	Neutral	N.P	+ (A > G) (1)
G171GC	25	15749	3.66	3.57	3.70	Hetero	T	L335L	Yes					+ (C > T)
G177GC	23	15743	1.22	3.57	0.00	Hetero	t	L333L	Yes					+ (C > T)
C186T	119	15734	1.22	3.57	0.00	Homo	T	A330T	Yes	Benign	AFP	Neutral	N.P	+ (G > A)
G187GC	28	15733	1.22	0.00 *	1.85	Hetero	t	A330A	Yes					+ (C > A)
A250G	99	15670	2.44	7.14	0.00 *	Homo	T	H308H	Yes					+ (T > C)
A254AT	36	15666	1.22	0.00 *	1.85	Hetero	t	L307L	Yes					

Table 1. *Cont.*

Mutations	Rate	p. rCRS	Proportions of Mutations			Status	Nature	p. AA	CD	PolyPhen-2 Prediction	Sift Prediction	Provean Prediction	Conclusion	References
			S %	NO %	O%									
G256A	151	15664	1.22	3.57	0.00	Homo	T	I306I	Yes					+ (C > A)
A257AG	40	15663	1.22	3.57	0.00	Hetero	T	I306I	Yes					+ (T > C)
T267TG	24	15653	1.22	0.00 *	1.85	Hetero	t	M303M	Yes					+ (A > G)
G279GA	40	15641	2.44	7.14	0.00 *	Hetero	T	L299F	Yes	P.D	AFP	Neutral	P	+ (C > T)
A281AG	**44**	**15639**	**1.22**	**3.57**	**0.00**	**Hetero**	**T**	**I298T**	**Yes**	**P.D**	AFP	Del	P	+ (T > C)
A287AC	32	15633	1.22	0.00 *	1.85	Hetero	T	L296L	Yes					
G288GA	24	15632	1.22	3.57	0.00	Hetero	T	L296L	Yes					+ (C > T)
A291AG	22	15629	1.22	3.57	0.00	Hetero	T	L295L	Yes					+ (T > C)
G294A	41	15626	1.22	0.00 *	1.85	Homo	T	L294L	Yes					+ (C > T)
G304C	23	15616	1.22	0.00 *	1.85	Homo	T	G290G	Yes					+ (C > T)
T307C	48	15613	1.22	0.00 *	1.85	Homo	T	G289G	Yes					+ (A > G)
T313C	70	15607	1.22	0.00 *	1.85	Homo	T	K287P	Yes	P.D	AFP	Del	P	(1)(2)(3)
T314TC	50	15606	1.22	0.00 *	1.85	Hetero	T	K287P	Yes	P.D	AFP	Del	P	
T315TC	50	15605	1.22	0.00 *	1.85	Hetero	T	K287P	Yes	P.D	AFP	Del	P	
G316GC	44	15604	1.22	0.00 *	1.85	Hetero	T	N286P	Yes	P.D	TOL	Del	P	+ (C > T)
T317TC	45	15603	1.22	0.00 *	1.85	Hetero	T	N286P	Yes	P.D	TOL	Del	P	+ (A > G)
T318TC	38	15602	1.22	0.00 *	1.85	Hetero	T	N286P	Yes	P.D	TOL	Del	P	
A319G	128	15601	1.22	3.57	0.00	Homo	T	P285P	Yes					+ (T > C)
A319AG	58	15601	2.44	7.14	0.00 *	Hetero	T	P285P	Yes					
G320GC	22	15600	1.22	0.00 *	1.85	Hetero	T	P285P	Yes					

Table 1. *Cont.*

Mutations	Rate	p. rCRS	Proportions of Mutations			Status	Nature	p. AA	CD	PolyPhen-2 Prediction	Sift Prediction	Provean Prediction	Conclusion	References
			S %	NO %	O%									
G321GC	106	15599	1.22	0.00 *	1.85	Hetero	T	P285P	Yes					
A323AG	24	15597	1.22	3.57	0.00	Hetero	T	V284V	Yes					
A342G	23	15578	1.22	3.57	0.00	Hetero	T	Y278Y	Yes					
G343GC	35	15577	1.22	3.57	0.00	Hetero	T	A277A	Yes					
A390AG	73	15530	1.22	3.57	0.00	Hetero	T	L262L	Yes					+ (T > C) (1)
C454CT	31	15466	2.44	7.14	0.00 *	Hetero	T	M240M	Yes					+ (G > A)
G460GA	44	15460	1.22	3.57	0.00	Hetero	T	S238L	Yes	Benign	TOL	Neutral	N.P	+ (C > T)
A466AG	24	15454	2.44	7.14	0.00 *	Hetero	T	L236L	Yes					+ (T > C)
G487GA	24	15433	1.22	3.57	0.00	Hetero	T	A229A	Yes					+ (C > T)
G534C	**149**	**15386**	**1.22**	**3.57**	**0.00**	**Homo**	**T**	**H214D**	**Yes**	**Benign**	TOL	Neutral	N.P	+ (C > A)
G539A	148	15381	1.22	3.57	0.00	Homo	T	T212I	Yes	Benign	TOL	Neutral	N.P	+ (C > T)
A558T	80	15362	23.17	67.86 *	0.00 *	Homo	T	Y206Y	Yes					
A597C	128	15323	23.17	67.86 *	0.00 *	Homo	T	S193S	No					+ (G > A)
G606C	32	15314	14.63	42.86 *	0.00 *	Homo	T	T190A	No					+ (G > A)
T609C	49	15311	3.66	10.71	0.00 *	Homo	T	L189V	No	Benign	TOL	-	N.P	+ (A > G)
A610AC	21	15310	1.22	3.57	0.00	Hetero	T	F188I	No					+ (T > C)
A610GA	66	15310	1.22	3.57	0.00	Homo	T	F188I	No					+ (T > C)
A612T	42	15308	19.51	57.14 *	0.00 *	Homo	T	F188I	No					+ (A > G)
G616GA	43	15304	1.22	3.57	0.00	Hetero	T	P186P	No					+ (C > T)
T619C	45	15301	3.66	10.71	0.00 *	Homo	T	I185L	No					+ (G > A) (3)

Rate: Mutation rates determined via Mutation Surveyor; **p. rCRS**: Position according to the Cambridge reference sequence; **S**: ARF patients; **NO**: Unoperated; **O**: Operated; **p.AA**: Amino acid position according to the protein reference sequence (UniProt accession number: P00156); **CD**: Conserved domain [MT-CYB (52-570) preserved in mammals; Cytochrom_B_C (97-399) preserved in cellular organisms; QcrB (97-564) preserved in cellular organisms; cytochrome_b_C (115-555) containing the redox sites of quinol and the polypeptide binding site, preserved in cellular organisms; MT-CYB6/f-IV (301-435) preserved in cellular organisms]; **Homo**: Homoplasmic mutation; **Hetero**: Heteroplasmic mutation; **T**: Transition; **t**: Transversion; **(1)**: [14] (A > G); **(2)**: [39] (T > C); **(3)**: [16] (A > G); **NP**: Not pathogenic; **P**: Pathogenic; **P.D**: Probably damaging; **p.D**: Potentially damaging; **TOL**: Tolerable; **Del**: Deleterious; *: Significant Fisher; **+**: Listed in MITOMAP, the letters in parentheses represent the referenced substitutions.

Table 2. Frequencies of amino acids according to populations.

Amino Acids	Controls	Operated	Non-Operated	P-Value C vs. O	P-Value C vs. NOP	P-Value O vs. NOP
Ala	0.67	0.68	0.69	0.999	0.999	0.999
Cys	4.72	4.68	4.74	0.997	0.999	0.996
Asp	0.00	0.00	0.00	1	1	1
Glu	3.89	3.96	3.96	0.996	0.997	0.999
Phe	2.67	2.70	2.69	0.998	0.999	0.999
Gly	21.40	21.20	21.06	0.987	0.978	0.999
His	0.00	0.00	0.00	1	1	1
Ile	2.67	2.68	2.67	0.999	1	0.992
Lys	2.00	1.93	2.07	0.996	0.996	0.998
Leu	20.68	20.73	20.71	0.997	0.998	1
Met	6.00	6.01	6.00	0.999	0.999	1
Asn	2.67	2.67	2.67	1	1	1
Pro	0.00	0.04	0.07	0.998	0.996	0.998
Gln	1.33	1.34	1.43	1	0.995	0.995
Arg	7.34	7.52	7.46	0.989	0.993	0.996
Ser	3.34	3.36	3.34	0.998	1	0.998
Thr	0.00	0.01	0.05	0.999	0.997	0.999
Val	10.01	9.91	9.89	0.994	0.993	0.999
Trp	8.62	8.57	8.58	0.997	0.998	0.999
Tyr	2.00	2.00	1.93	1	0.996	0.996

C: Controls, O: Operated, NOP: Unoperated.

Table 3. Parameters for genetic diversity of the study population.

Parameters		Controls				Unoperated				Operated			
Size of population n		12				28				54			
Number of sites N		492				492				492			
Non-variables sites		485				441				450			
Variables sites		7				51				42			
Non-informative variables sites		5				43				25			
Informative variables sites		2				8				17			
Number of total mutations Eta		7				52				52			
Number of haplotypes		7				17				29			
Haplotypic diversity hd		0.833 ± 0.100				0.923 ± 0.037				0.883 ± 0.039			
Nucleotide diversity Pi		0.00314 ± 0.00071				0.00996 ± 0.00336				0.00645 ± 0.00129			
The average number of nucleotide differences k		1.545				4.902				3.173			
Nucleotide frequencies		T	C	A	G	T	C	A	G	T	C	A	G
General		29.5	9.3	25.2	36.0	29.4	9.5	25.3	35.8	29.5	9.5	25.2	35.9
Position 1		21	9.8	27.4	21	9.7	42.1	27.4	21	9.8	42.0	27.3	42.1
Position 2		29	17.1	20.8	32.9	29	17.4	20.9	32.5	29	17.3	20.8	32.6
Position 3		38	1.2	12.7	47.7	38	1.4	12.8	47.5	38	1.3	12.7	47.6
Nature of mutations	Transitions	100				46.92				34.91			
	Transversions	0				53.08				65.09			
Rate of mutations R		∞				0.88				0.54			
Rate of synonymous substitutions Ks		0.002 ± 0.001				0.011 ± 0.003				0.006 ± 0.003			
Rate of non-synonymous substitutions Kns		0.003 ± 0.002				0.007 ± 0.002				0.005 ± 0.002			

3.1.4. Evaluation of the Differentiation and Genetic Structuring of MT-CYB in Accordance with the Study Population

The genetic distance was the largest among unoperated ARF patients (0.011 ± 0.002) and the lowest in the controls (0.003 ± 0.001). Genetic distances were greater between unoperated and operated

ARF patients (0.009 ± 0.001) than between the controls and operated ARF patients (0.005 ± 0.001) (Table 4).

Analysis of the genetic differentiation factor (Fst) revealed no genetic differentiation of *MT-CYB* between the controls and patients (p = 0.58559). However, a genetic differentiation of *MT-CYB* between operated and unoperated subjects was observed (p = 0.01466) (Table 5). Nevertheless, AMOVA (Table 6) revealed that more than 98% of genetic variability between unoperated and operated ARF patients is of an intra-population origin.

Table 4. Genetic distances within and among groups.

	Controls	Non-Operated	Operated
Controls	0.003 ± 0.001		
Non-operated	0.007 ± 0.001	**0.011 ± 0.002**	
Operated	0.005 ± 0.001	0.009 ± 0.001	0.007 ± 0.001

In boldface: The highest genetic distances.

Table 5. Genetic differentiation factor.

	Controls	Unoperated	Operated
Controls		*0.87195*	*0.38416*
Unoperated	0		***0.01466***
Operated	0.00128	0.01419	

In italics, the p-values and in bold the significant p-value.

Table 6. Analysis of molecular variance.

Source of Variation	Percentage Variation
Inter-populations	1.41855
Intra-population	98.58145

3.1.5. Evolution of MT-CYB Mutations

As shown in Table 7, the results of the Z selection test among groups were recorded. The non-significant p-values (0.965, 0.483, and 1.000) among operated ARF patients indicate that their mutations follow a neutral evolution. However, among unoperated ARF patients, the p-value, highly significant under the neutrality hypothesis (0.015), highly significant under the hypothesis of positive selection, and not significant under the hypothesis of negative selection, shows that *MT-CYB* mutations in the unoperated patients are under positive selection.

Table 7. Results of the Z selection test (p-values).

	Neutrality	Positive Selection	Negative Selection
Operated	0.965	0.483	1.000
Non-operated	**0.015**	**0.008**	1.000

In boldface: Significant p-values.

4. Discussion

This study attempted to identify *MT-CYB* mutations in Senegalese ARF patients. Since cardiac tissues were not available for molecular analysis, mutations in this region were assessed in peripheral blood. The present results show a high rate of *MT-CYB* polymorphisms in unoperated subjects (72.73% of mutations). Unoperated ARF patients developed a cardiopathy following ARF; however, since they did not undergo valvular replacement, the disease was seemingly induced in them, and *MT-CYB* mutations were detected in the cells involved in the autoimmune response in blood, similar to T and B lymphocytes, and macrophages, since self-reactive T cells migrate from peripheral blood to the heart and proliferate in the valves in response to stimulation by specific cytokines [6].

Two synonymous substitutions (Y206Y and S193S) associated with ARF (according to the Fisher test) were observed at high frequencies (67.86%) and exclusively in the operated subjects. Despite the absence of amino acid substitutions, the corresponding positions (A15362T and A15323C) may serve as potential molecular markers if consistently present in individuals with ARF. Non-synonymous substitutions T190A, F188I, and I185L, frequent in the unoperated group, are also associated with the pathology. These sites were polymorphic in comparison with the control but monomorphic in comparison with the Caucasian reference sequence. These mutations were detected on MITOMAP but matched with different substitutions. The mutation T15301C (I185L) is associated with idiopathic dilated cardiomyopathy [14] as being a synonymous substitution Leu-Leu. Three missense mutations (S344T, L299F, and I298T), predicted to be pathogenic, have been reported in unoperated patients 2 and 1. The substitution of an aliphatic Leu with an aromatic Phe and that of nonpolar Ile with a polar Thr affected protein structure and function. The substitution of Ser with Thr could have been inconsequential, since they are both thiolated/hydroxylated and polar amino acids and the mutation is homoplasmic (the predictions of this mutation are not formal; thus, mutation may be benign). However, these mutations are in a conserved domain, playing a crucial role in cytochrome b function and thus in the activity of complex III. The C-terminal domain contains the binding sites for ubiquinone/ubiquinol [40,41] and is responsible for proton translocation outside the mitochondrial membrane [42]. Furthermore, the L299F mutation has been reported in breast cancer; however, it was a substitution from cytosine to thymine (according to the reference sequence) at position 15641, whereas the mutation detected herein corresponds to the heteroplasmic substitution of guanine by adenine (according to our control sequence). Both mutations were transitions occurring in the same position. Several mutations were present in both unoperated and operated patients, including G15849A and T15824C synonymous substitutions and the A15784G sense mutation. G15849A and T15824C corresponding to substitutions T368I and T360A have been predicted to be non-pathogenic, although they are polar Thr substitutions by non-polar Ile and Ala. These point mutations occur in a conserved domain in mammals, but are outside the C-terminal domain, thus probably accounting for their benign state. T15824C is present in breast cancer as A15824G, and A15784G has been reported in patients with dilated idiopathic cardiomyopathy [16]. Most (60%) of the mutations were absent in operated patients. Mutations present only in the latter were either synonymous or non-pathogenic, except for those present in one patient (Sg56). More than half of the *MT-CYB* mutations were heteroplasmic (58.23%), probably because polymorphonuclear mitochondrial genomes do not contain *MT-CYB* mutations leading to a mixture of wildtype and mutated genomes or heteroplasmy in immune cells. Cells were not isolated for DNA extraction; either of the hypotheses cannot be considered accurate. However, the current speculation that heteroplasmic mutations are more likely to occur in pathogenic mutations rather than in normal polymorphisms [16] is consistent with the present pathogenic mutations.

Amino acid frequencies did not differ significantly upon pairwise group comparisons. However, Pro and Thr were absent in the controls but present in ARF patients at low frequencies, indeed because of the presence of missense mutations.

Differences in the degree of *MT-CYB* polymorphisms between operated and unoperated patients suggest that valvular replacement suppressed gene mutations. This is corroborated by the results of the genetic diversity of the study population, which facilitated the characterization and analysis of differences between unoperated ARF patients and the other two groups in the study population. Similarly, group comparisons in the study population revealed the genetic proximity of operated subjects and the controls (Pi, k, and the genetic distances were low) and those genetic differences between the operated and unoperated patients. These results may have been obtained because surgery eliminates diseased valvular cells and simultaneously the source of the pathology. The proteins of valvular cells similar to those of *Streptococcus pyogenes* [43] are the targets of immune cells. Eradication of the source of the pathology would lead to a correction between the mechanism underlying autoimmunity, and the cells involved in the defense against *Streptococcus* of Group A and autoimmunity would become functional again in the next generation. Selection analyses have indicated that mutations in the operated subjects follow a neutral evolution, while those present in the unoperated patients are under positive selection. These results are concurrent with previous findings; non-synonymous *MT-CYB* mutations tend to consistently occur in unoperated patients. These variants have a deleterious effect on the protein, and an increase in their frequency would further cause protein damage and simultaneously aggravate the disease. Since these mutations generally do not occur in operated patients and those persisting after valvular replacement are neutral (neither beneficial nor deleterious), the involvement of *MT-CYB* mutations in ARF complications can be considered (RHD).

5. Conclusions

This study used a population genetics approach to investigate the association of *MT-CYB* mutations with ARF and RHD in Senegalese patients. The present results confirmed our initial hypothesis. Indeed, sixty polymorphic variants of *MT-CYB* were identified herein. Some of these mutations were neutral, while other mutations were pathogenic, as revealed through their effects on cytochrome b structure and function. Furthermore, the absence of more than half of these mutations in patients with valvular replacement and genetic differentiation between the latter and unoperated patients indicates *MT-CYB* polymorphisms, which are closely associated with ARF and RHD. These mutations cause or result from abnormal activation of immune cells against autoantigens. A study combining both immune assessment with a genetics approach would be interesting to clarify why only some individuals infected with group A streptococcus develop an inadequate immune response leading to ARF. A subsequent analysis of the protein would also provide useful insights into the role of cytochrome b in ARF and RHD. In addition, DNA extraction in the same patient before and after surgery could validate our results.

Author Contributions: Conceptualization, F.B.W. and F.M.; Data curation, F.B.W.; Formal analysis, F.B.W.; Investigation, F.B.W. and M.P.S.; Methodology, F.B.W.; Project administration, F.M.; Resources, M.S.; Software, F.B.W.; Supervision, F.M. and M.S.; Validation, F.M. and M.S.; Visualization, F.B.W. and F.M.; Writing—original draft, F.B.W.; Writing—review and editing, F.M.

References

1. Bryant, P.A.; Robins-Browne, R.; Carapetis, J.R.; Curtis, N. Some of the People, Some of the Time: Susceptibility to Acute Rheumatic Fever. *Circulation* **2009**, *119*, 742–753. [CrossRef] [PubMed]
2. Templeton, C.G.; Cooper, A.R.; Human, D.G.; Rahman, P. Rhumatisme articulaire aigu. *Le Programme Canadien de Surveillance Pédiatrique*, Unpublished. 2007; 4p.
3. Venter, M.; Van der Westhuizen, F.H.; Elson, J.L. The aetiology of cardiovascular disease: A role for mitochondrial DNA? *Cardiovasc. J. Afr.* **2017**, *29*, 122–132. [CrossRef] [PubMed]
4. Carapetis, J.R.; Steer, A.; Mulholland, E.; Weber, M. The global burden of group A streptococcal disease. *Lancet Infect. Dis.* **2005**, *5*, 685–694. [CrossRef]
5. Fall, A.L.; Ndiaye, O.; Lavou, I.; Sow, H.D. La cardiopathie rhumatismale à l'Hôpital d'Enfants Albert Royer de Dakar: À propos de 76 cas. In Proceedings of the Conférence IVème Congrès de l'Association des Pédiatres d'Afrique Noire Francophone (APANF) et IIème Congrès de la Société Sénégalaise de Pédiatrie (SOSEPED), Dakar, Senegal, November 2007. Résumé.
6. Guilherme, L.; Köhler, K.F.; Postol, E.; Kalil, J. Genes, autoimmunity and pathogenesis of rheumatic heart disease. *Ann. Paediatr. Cardiol.* **2011**, *4*, 13–21. [CrossRef] [PubMed]
7. Messias-Reason, I.J.; Schafranski, M.D.; Kremsner, P.G.; Kun, J.F. Ficolin 2 (FCN2) functional polymorphisms and the risk of rheumatic fever and rheumatic heart disease. *Clin. Exp. Immunol.* **2009**, *157*, 395–399. [CrossRef] [PubMed]

8. Hernández-Pacheco, G.; Flores-Domínguez, C.; Rodríguez-Pérez, J.M.; Pérez-Hernández, N.; Fragoso, J.M.; Saul, A.; Vargas-Alarcón, G. Tumour necrosis factor-alpha promoter polymorphisms in Mexican patients with rheumatic heart disease. *J. Autoimmun.* **2003**, *21*, 59–63. [CrossRef]
9. Sallakci, N.; Akcurin, G.; Köksoy, S.; Kardelen, F.; Uguz, A.; Coskun, M.; Yegin, O. TNF-alpha G-308A polymorphism is associated with rheumatic fever and correlates with increased TNF-alpha production. *J. Autoimmun.* **2005**, *25*, 150–154. [CrossRef]
10. Yeğin, O.; Coşkun, M.; Ertuğ, H. Cytokines in acute rheumatic fever. *Eur. J. Paediatr.* **1997**, *156*, 25–29. [CrossRef]
11. Settin, A.; Abdel-Hady, H.; El-Baz, R.; Saber, I. Gene polymorphisms of TNF-alpha^{-308}, IL-10^{-108}, IL-6^{-174}, and IL-1Ra^{VNTR} related to susceptibility and severity of rheumatic heart disease. *Paediatr. Cardiol.* **2007**, *28*, 363–371. [CrossRef]
12. Marin-Garcia, J.; Ananthakrishnan, R.; Gonzalvo, A.; Goldenthal, M.J. Novel mutations in mitochondrial cytochrome b in fatal post-partum cardiomyopathy. *J. Inherit. Metab. Dis.* **1995**, *18*, 77–78. [CrossRef]
13. Ekiert, R.; Borek, A.; Kuleta, P.; Czernek, J.; Osyczka, A. Mitochondrial disease-related mutations at the cytochrome b-iron–sulfur protein (ISP) interface: Molecular effects on the large-scale motion of ISP and superoxide generation studied in Rhodobacter capsulatus cytochrome bc1. *Biochim. Biophys. Acta* **2016**, *1857*, 1102–1110. [CrossRef] [PubMed]
14. Andreu, A.L.; Bruno, C.; Hadjigeorgiou, G.M.; Shanske, S.; DiMauro, S. Polymorphic Variants in the Human Mitochondrial Cytochrome b Gene. *Mol. Genet. Metab.* **1999**, *67*, 49–52. [CrossRef]
15. Hagen, C.H.; Aidt, F.H.; Havndrup, O.; Hedley, P.L.; Jespersgaard, C.; Jensen, M.; Christiansen, M. MT-CYB mutations in hypertrophic cardiomyopathy. *Mol. Genet. Genom. Med.* **2013**, *1*, 54–65. [CrossRef] [PubMed]
16. Marin-Garcia, J.; Goldenthal, M.J.; Ananthakrishnan, R.; Pierpont, M.E. The Complete Sequence of mtDNA Genes in Idiopathic Dilated Cardiomyopathy Shows Novel Missense and tRNA Mutations. *J. Card. Fail.* **2000**, *6*, 321–329. [CrossRef] [PubMed]
17. Andreu, A.L.; Checcarelli, N.; Iwata, S.; Shanske, S.; Dimauro, S. Missense Mutation in the Mitochondrial Cytochrome b Gene in a Revisited Case with Histiocytoid Cardiomyopathy. *Pediatr. Res.* **2000**, *48*, 311–314. [CrossRef] [PubMed]
18. Wang, J.; Lin, F.; Guo, L.; Xiong, X.; Fan, X. Cardiovascular Disease, Mitochondria, and Traditional Chinese Medicine. *Evidence-Based Complement. Med.* **2015**, *2015*, 1–7. [CrossRef]
19. Khatami, M.; Heidari, M.M.; Karimian, N.; Hadadzadeh, M. Mitochondrial Mutations in tRNAGlu and Cytochrome b Genes Associated with Iranian Congenial Heart Disease. *Int. Cardiovasc. Res. J.* **2016**, *10*, 193–198.
20. Altschul, S.F.; Madden, T.L.; Schäffer, A.A.; Zhang, J.; Zhang, Z.; Miller, W.; Lipman, D.J. Gapped BLAST and PSI-BLAST: A new generation of protein database search programs. *Nucleic Acids Res.* **1997**, *25*, 3389–3402. [CrossRef]
21. Geer, L.Y.; Domrachev, M.; Lipman, D.J.; Bryant, S.H. CDART: Protein homology by domain architecture. *Genome Res.* **2002**, *12*, 1619–1623. [CrossRef]
22. Adzhubei, I.; Jordan, D.; Sunyaev, S. Predicting functional effect of human missense mutations using PolyPhen-2. *Curr. Protoc. Hum. Genet.* **2013**, *7*, 1–52. [CrossRef]
23. Pauline, C.N.; Steven, H. Predicting Deleterious Amino Acid Substitutions. *Genome Res.* **2001**, *11*, 863–874.
24. Choi, Y.; Sims, G.E.; Murphy, S.; Miller, J.R.; Chan, A.P. Predicting the Functional Effect of Amino Acid Substitutions and Indels. *PLoS ONE* **2012**, *7*, 1–13. [CrossRef] [PubMed]
25. Chinnery, P.F.; Howell, N.; Andrews, R.M.; Turnbull, D.M. Mitochondrial DNA analysis: Polymorphisms and pathogenicity. *J. Med. Genet.* **1999**, *36*, 505–510. [CrossRef] [PubMed]
26. Hall, T.A. BioEdit: A user-friendly biological sequence alignment editor and analysis program for Windows 95/98/NT. *Nucleic Acids Symp. Ser.* **1999**, *41*, 95–98.
27. Thompson, J.D.; Higgins, D.G.; Gibson, T.J. CLUSTAL W: Improving the sensitivity of progressive multiple sequence alignment through sequence weighting, position-specific gap penalties and weight matrix choice. *Nucleic Acids Res.* **1994**, *22*, 4673–4680. [CrossRef] [PubMed]
28. Librado, P.; Rozas, J. DnaSP v5: A software for comprehensive analysis of DNA polymorphism data. *Bioinformatics* **2009**, *25*, 1451–1452. [CrossRef] [PubMed]

29. Kumar, S.; Stecher, G.; Tamura, K. MEGA7: Molecular Evolutionary Genetics Analysis version 7.0 for bigger datasets. *Mol. Biol. Evol.* **2016**, *33*, 1870–1874. [CrossRef] [PubMed]
30. Hasegawa, M.; Kishino, H.; Yano, T. Dating the human-ape split by a molecular clock of mitochondrial DNA. *J. Mol. Evol.* **1985**, *22*, 160–174. [CrossRef]
31. Jukes, T.; Cantor, C. Evolution of protein molecules. In *Mammalian Protein Metabolism*; Munro, H.N., Ed.; Academic Press: New York, NY, USA, 1969; p. 21.
32. Kimura, M. A simple method for estimating evolutionary rate of base substitutions through comparative studies of nucleotide sequences. *J. Mol. Evolut.* **1980**, *16*, 111–120. [CrossRef]
33. Excoffier, L. *Computational and Molecular Population Genetics Lab CMPG*; Zoological Institute, University of Berne: Bern, Switzerland, 2006.
34. Nei, M.; Gojobori, T. Simple methods for estimating the numbers of synonymous and nonsynonymous nucleotide substitutions. *Mol. Biol. Evolut.* **1986**, *3*, 418–426.
35. Andrews, R.M.; Kubacka, I.; Chinnery, P.F.; Lightowlers, R.N.; Turnbull, D.M.; Howell, N. Reanalysis and revision of the Cambridge reference sequence for human mitochondrial DNA. *Nat. Genet.* **1999**, *23*, 147. [CrossRef] [PubMed]
36. Krause, J.; Fu, Q.; Good, J.M.; Viola, B.; Shunkov, M.V.; Derevianko, A.P.; Pääbo, S. The complete mitochondrial DNA genome of an unknown hominin from southern Siberia. *Nature* **2010**, *464*, 894–897. [CrossRef] [PubMed]
37. Meyer, M.; Fu, Q.; Aximu-Petri, A.; Glocke, I.; Nickel, B.; Arsuaga, J.L.; Pääbo, S. A mitochondrial genome sequence of a hominin from Sima de los Huesos. *Nature* **2014**, *505*, 403–419. [CrossRef] [PubMed]
38. Green, R.E.; Malaspinas, A.S.; Krause, J.; Briggs, A.W.; Johnson, P.L.; Uhler, C.; Prüfer, K. A complete Neandertal mitochondrial genome sequence determined by high-throughput sequencing. *Cell* **2008**, *134*, 416–426. [CrossRef] [PubMed]
39. Sazonova, M.A.; Zhelankin, A.V.; Barinova, V.A.; Sinyov, V.V.; Khasanova, Z.B.; Postnov, A.Y.; Orekhov, A.N. Dataset of mitochondrial genome variants associated with asymptomatic atherosclerosis. *Data Brief.* **2016**, *7*, 1570–1575. [CrossRef] [PubMed]
40. Schultz, B.; Chan, S. Structures and proton-pumping strategies of mitochondrial respiratory enzymes. *Ann. Rev. Biophys. Biomol. Struct.* **2001**, *30*, 23–65. [CrossRef]
41. Hunte, C.; Koepke, J.; Lange, C.; Roßmanith, T.; Michel, H. Structure at 2.3 A resolution of the cytochrome bc (1) complex from the yeast *Saccharomyces cerevisiae* co-crystallized with an antibody Fv fragment. *Structure* **2000**, *8*, 669–684. [CrossRef]
42. Dasgupta, S.; Hoque, M.O.; Upadhyay, S.; Sidransky, D. Forced Cytochrome B gene mutation expression induces mitochondrial proliferation and prevents apoptosis in human uroepithelial SV-HUC-1 cells. *Int. J. Cancer* **2009**, *15*, 2829–2835. [CrossRef]
43. Mirabel, M.; Ferreira, B.; Sidi, D.; Lachaud, M.; Jouven, X.; Marijon, E. Rhumatisme articulaire aigu-Perspectives. *Med. Sci.* **2012**, *28*, 633–638.

8

Arterial Structural and Functional Characteristics at End of Early Childhood and Beginning of Adulthood: Impact of Body Size Gain during Early, Intermediate, Late and Global Growth

Juan M. Castro [1,†], Victoria García-Espinosa [1], Agustina Zinoveev [1], Mariana Marin [1], Cecilia Severi [2], Pedro Chiesa [3], Daniel Bia [1,†] and Yanina Zócalo [1,*,†]

1 Departamento de Fisiología, Facultad de Medicina, Centro Universitario de Investigación, Innovación y Diagnóstico Arterial, Universidad de la República, General Flores 2125, 11800 Montevideo, Uruguay

2 Departamento de Medicina Preventiva y Social, Instituto de Higiene, Facultad de Medicina, Universidad de la República, Alfredo Navarro 3051, 11600 Montevideo, Uruguay

3 Servicio de Cardiología Pediátrica, Centro Hospitalario Pereira-Rossell, ASSE-Facultad de Medicina, Universidad de la República, Bulevar Artigas 1550, 11600 Montevideo, Uruguay

* Correspondence: yana@fmed.edu.uy

† These authors contributed equally to this work.

Abstract: An association between nutritional characteristics in theearlylife stages and the state of the cardiovascular (CV) system in early childhood itself and/or at the beginning of adulthood has been postulated. It is still controversial whether changes in weight, height and/or body mass index (BMI) during childhood or adolescence are independently associated with hemodynamics and/or arterial properties in early childhood and adulthood. Aims: First, to evaluate and compare the strength of association between CVproperties (at 6 and 18 years (y)) and (a) anthropometric data at specific growth stages (e.g., birth, 6 y, 18 y) and (b) anthropometric changes during early (0–2 y), intermediate (0–6 y), late (6–18 y) and global (0–18 y) growth. Second, to determine whether the associations between CVproperties and growth-related body changes depend on size at birth and/or at the time of CVstudy. Third, to analyze the capacity of growth-related body size changes to explain hemodynamic and arterial properties in early childhood and adulthood before and after adjusting for exposure to CV risk factors. Anthropometric, hemodynamic (central, peripheral) and arterial parameters (structural, functional; elastic, transitional and muscular arteries) were assessed in two cohorts (children, n = 682; adolescents, n = 340). Data wereobtained and analyzed following identical protocols. Results: Body-size changes in infancy (0–2 y) and childhood (0–6 y) showed similar strength of association with CV properties at 6 y. Conversely, 0–6, 6-18 or 0–18 ychanges were not associated with CV parameters at 18 y. The association between CV properties at 6 yand body-size changes during growth showed: equal or greater strength than the observed for body-size at birth, and lower strength compared to that obtained for current z-BMI. Conversely, only z-BMI at 18 y showed associations with CV z-scores at 18 y. Body size at birth showed almost no association with CVproperties at 6 or 18 y. Conclusion: current z-BMI showed the greatest capacity to explain variations in CV properties at 6 and 18 y. Variations in some CV parameters were mainly explained by growth-related anthropometric changes and/or by their interaction with current z-BMI. Body size at birth showed almost no association with arterial properties at 6 or 18 y.

Keywords: adolescents; arterial stiffness; birth weight; body-size trajectories; cardio-metabolic health; children; growth; intima-media thickness; blood pressure

1. Introduction

Childhood overweight or obesity have beenshown to be associated with an increase in the prevalence of cardiovascular risk factors (CRFs), cardiovascular (CV) risk and development of CV and metabolic diseases later in life [1–3]. This, together with the observed increase in the prevalence of obesity during childhood has led to an increased interest in knowing the factors associated with increased adiposity gain and the link between adiposity gain in early life-stages and future CV alterations; fundamental steps to enable the development of adequate prevention, control and/or treatment strategies. Several studies have been carried out in children and adolescents mainly with the aim of analyzing the association between hemodynamic or arterial characteristics in childhood or adolescence and: (1) body size at birth, (2) growth-related increases in body weight (BW), height (BH), BW-for-BH (BWH), and/or body mass index (BMI), and/or (3) body size at the time of CV evaluation. Results have been heterogeneous. Up to now the factors associated with body size gain as well as the mechanisms underlying the association (impact) of body characteristics and their growth-related changes with CV parameters are not fully known. The controversial findings and lack of a clear understanding of the problem could be attributed to its inherent complexity (e.g., age-related differential impact of body size gain, interaction among co-factors, dependence on prior anthropometric conditions), as well as to characteristics and differences between studies designed to address it (e.g., methodological approaches, publication bias, statistical analyses) [4–6].

Early accelerated BW gain (e.g., defined as an increase in BW-for-age z-score of at least 0.67 units between 0 and 2 years old (y)) would be associated with detrimental CV changes in children and adolescents [7,8]. In this regard, at least five interrelated issues should be clarified. First, the strength of the association between CV characteristics (i.e., hemodynamic and arterial) and anthropometric changes (e.g., early BW gain), along with their independence from birth weight and current body conditions.An association between low birth weight (LBW) and CV alterationshas been described, which would be reinforced by (or could even depend on) an accelerated BW gain in the postnatal period and/or by associated excessive subsequent adipose gain expressed by an elevated BMI at the time of CV evaluation [9]. Second, the magnitude of the interactions of anthropometric and CV parameters respect to body size at birth and current BMI should be addressed [10]. Third, the association between BW gain and CV parameters should be analyzed considering that it may depend on the timing of growth-related body changes (e.g., acceleration) [7,8] and/or on thesubject'sage (i.e., at the time of CVassessment) [6,11]. Fourth, as previous works reported that early growthpatterns could be associated with the development or exposure to factors associated with increased CV risk (CRFs' clustering) [12], the real (independent) clinical meaning or CV impact of BW gain should be determined, taking into account the exposure to CRFs. Fifth, the association between body size gain, birth-size and/or current anthropometric conditions with hemodynamic or arterial parameters could vary, depending on the: (a) arterial type (e.g., muscular vs. elastic); (b) site of evaluation and hemodynamic parameters considered (e.g., peripheral vs. central); and (c) arterial pathway considered (e.g., conductance vs. resistance) [13,14]. Recently, our group demonstrated that z-BMI variations in children and adolescents are positively associated with peripheral (brachial) and central (aortic) blood pressure levels (pBP and cBP, respectively); carotid, femoral and brachial artery diameters; carotid (but not femoral or brachial) intima-media thickness (IMT); arterial stiffness and stiffness gradient. Moreover, we found a "hierarchical order" among hemodynamic and arterial variations associated with z-BMI. pBP was the variable with the greatest variations associated with z-BMI (particularly pBP rather than cBP was associated with z-BMI). The stiffness of central (but not peripheral) arteries was associated with z-BMI (a pBP-dependent association). In turn, variations in arterial diameters were associated with z-BMI, without differences between the elastic and muscular arteries [13]. The above highlights the importance of a comprehensive, multiparametric approach when evaluating the CV system. If results obtained in an arterial segment and/or for a given parameter were generalized, significant errors (biases) could be made.

This work's aims were: (1) to evaluate and compare the strength of association between hemodynamic and arterial characteristics and (a) anthropometric data at specific growth stages (e.g., birth, 6 y, 18 y) and (b) body size changes during early (e.g., 0–2 y), intermediate (0–6 y), late (6–18 y) and global (0–18 y) growth; (2) to determine whether the association between CV characteristics and growth-related body size changes depends on size at birth and/or at the time of CV evaluation; and (3) to analyze the explanatory capacity of growth-related body size changes for hemodynamic and arterial characteristics in early childhood (6 y) and at the beginning of adulthood (18 y), before and after adjusting for body-size at birth, current BMI and/or exposure to CRFs.

2. Materials and Methods

2.1. Study Population

The study was carried out in the context of the Centro Universitario de Investigación, Innovación y Diagnóstico Arterial (CUiiDARTE) Project [13–16]. The protocol was approved by the Institutional Ethics Committee. Both parents' consent and child's assent were received before data collection. Participants (or their guardians) signed a written consent prior to the evaluation. Subjects from two cohorts, one of children (n = 682) and the other of adolescents (n = 340) were included (Table 1). The children cohort, defined based on probabilistic, bi-stage and stratified sampling of subjects attending public kindergartens in Montevideo, is part (subsample) of the longitudinal study "Patrón de crecimiento, estadonutricional y calidad de la alimentaciónen la primerainfancia: análisis de suimpactosobre la estructura y función vascular y el riesgo cardiovascular relativoenniñosuruguayos (CUiiDARTE-Agencia Nacional de Investigación e Innovación(ANII), Ministerio de Desarrollo Social (MIDES), United Nations Children's Fund(UNICEF) that started in 2010 (first phase) and had in 2016 a second phase [15,16]. In turn, the adolescent cohort (subsample from Montevideo) belongs to a longitudinal (four stages) study called "Estudio Longitudinal del Bienestaren Uruguay" (ELBU) aimed at investigating multidimensional well-being [17] working with a national representative sample of children (and their families) attending in 2004 the first grade of primary public schools in urban areas, which account for 87% of the Uruguayan population.

Similar approaches were carried out on children and adolescents: clinical and anthropometric evaluation, compilation (questionnaires) of data about lifestyle and family history (e.g., educational level, socioeconomic conditions, nutritional factors) and non-invasive CV evaluation.

2.2. Anthropometric Evaluation

Anthropometric data (BW and BH) corresponding to ages ≤36 months (mos.) were obtained from registers of the obligatory health-controlsfor children within those ages, established by the Ministry of Health (Children cohort). BW and length at birth in the adolescent cohort were obtained by documented self-report, during parents' interviews. In turn, following standard procedures, trained technicians obtained anthropometric data from children and adolescents (at participants' home, school and/or during the CV evaluation). BW and BH were measured with lightweight clothing and without shoes. Standing BH was measured (subject's head in the Frankfurt Plane position) using a portable stadiometer and recorded to the nearest 0.1 cm. BW was measured with an electronic scale (model 841/843, Seca Inc., Hamburg, Germany; model HBF-514C, Omron Inc., Chicago, Illinois, USA) and recorded to the nearest 0.1 kg. Two measurements were made and a third measurement was obtained in case the first two readings differed by more than 0.5 cm or 0.5 kg. After aggregating records from our technicians and those from health-controls, we obtained BW and BH data corresponding to: (1) birth, 6, 12, 18, 24, 36 and ~72 mos (~6 y) in the children cohort, and (2) birth, ~6 y, ~8 y, ~12 y and ~18 y in the adolescents' cohort. BMI was calculated as BW-to-squared BH ratio and converted into z-scores (z-BMI). Standardized z-scores for BMI and BWH (up to 2 y), BW-for-age, BH-for-age and BMI-for-age were obtained using World Health Organization software (Anthro-v.3.2.2; Anthro-Plus-v.1.0.4). The changes or differences (Δ) in BWH z-score (ΔBWH z-score) between birth (0 y) and 24 mos. (0–2y, children cohort) were determined. In turn, the changes in z-BMI (ΔBMI z-score) between 0 and 6 y (0–6y, both cohorts), 0 and 18 y (0–18y, adolescents cohort) and 6 and 18 y (6–18y, adolescents cohort) were calculated. Changes were always determined as the difference between the latest (e.g., 18 y) and the earliest (e.g., 0 y) z-score.

Table 1. Clinical, anthropometric and arterial parameters, of children and adolescent cohorts.

	Children Cohort (n = 632)						Adolescent Cohort (n = 340)					
	MV	STD	Min.	p25th	p75th	Max.	MV	STD	Min.	p25th	p75th	Max.
Demographic, anthropometric and cardiovascular risk factors												
Age (years)	6.02	0.3	5.07	5.80	6.26	6.66	18.2	0.50	17.0	17.8	18.5	20.7
Subjects (n, %female)			632 (49.5)						340 (53.2)			
Body weight (kg)	22.31	4.67	14.00	19.20	24.35	46.50	64.4	14.2	40.2	55.0	70.0	120.0
Body height (m)	1.14	0.05	0.99	1.10	1.17	1.33	1.66	0.09	1.32	1.60	1.73	1.94
BMI (Kg/m^2)	17.03	2.48	12.10	15.37	18.06	27.15	23.17	4.47	15.1	20.2	24.7	48.2
z-BMI (STD)	0.96	1.47	−2.60	0.06	1.62	7.37	0.36	1.16	-3.4	−0.4	1.0	4.8
z-BW for age (STD)	0.45	1.30	−2.39	−0.45	1.18	6.15	-	-	-	-	-	-
z-BH for age (STD)	−0.33	1.04	−3.43	−1.05	0.29	3.55	−0.41	0.88	−4.73	-0.90	0.13	2.39
Obesity (n, %)			108 (17.1)						26 (7.4)			
Dyslipidemia (n, %)			1 (0.2)						18 (5.3)			
Diabetes (n, %)			1 (0.2)						0 (0.0)			
Hypertension (n, %)			27 (4.3)						18 (5.3)			
CV Family background (n, %)			0 (0.0)						13 (3.9)			
Current Smoke (n, %)			0 (0.0)						35 (10.4)			
Anthropometric z-scores												
z-BW for age at birth (STD)	0.02	0.95	−5.24	−0.56	0.68	2.95	−0.18	1.24	-5.19	−0.89	0.57	2.87
z-BH for age at birth (STD)	−0.27	1.13	−4.91	−1.00	0.46	4.75	−0.35	1.52	-5.75	−1.15	0.46	4.82
z-BMI for age at birth (STD)	0.27	1.06	−3.59	−0.38	0.93	3.65	−0.01	1.72	−6.31	−1.00	0.96	5.56
z-BW for height 24 m. (STD)	0.59	1.26	−3.86	−0.20	1.29	4.76	-	-	-	-	-	-
z-BW for age 24 m. (STD)	0.38	1.14	−2.83	−0.44	1.08	4.54	-	-	-	-	-	-
z-BH for age 24 m. (STD)	−0.15	1.11	−4.12	−0.92	0.60	3.30	-	-	-	-	-	-
z-BMI for age 24 m. (STD)	0.66	1.29	−4.07	−0.15	1.40	5.42	-	-	-	-	-	-
1st Wave: anthropometry												
Age (years)	-	-	-	-	-	-	6.7	0.5	5.42	6.32	6.92	8.98
z-BW for age (STD)	-	-	-	-	-	-	0.39	1.01	−1.93	−0.27	1.06	3.56
z-BH for age (STD)	-	-	-	-	-	-	−0.13	0.93	−3.19	−0.72	0.53	2.10
z-BMI for age (STD)	-	-	-	-	-	-	0.65	0.99	−1.81	−0.08	1.27	4.63
2nd Wave: anthropometry												
Age (years)	-	-	-	-	-	-	8.1	0.4	6.82	7.77	8.38	10.27
z-BW for age (STD)	-	-	-	-	-	-	0.44	1.14	−2.40	−0.36	1.24	4.05
z-BH for age (STD)	-	-	-	-	-	-	−0.10	0.98	−4.53	−0.69	0.51	2.07
z-BMI for age (STD)	-	-	-	-	-	-	0.66	1.16	−3.12	−0.17	1.36	4.99
3rd Wave: anthropometry												
Age (years)	-	-	-	-	-	-	12.2	0.5	10.74	11.83	12.46	14.80
z-BW for age (STD)	-	-	-	-	-	-	-	-	-	-	-	-
z-BH for age (STD)	-	-	-	-	-	-	−0.03	1.12	−3.46	−0.87	0.71	2.98
z-BMI for age (STD)	-	-	-	-	-	-	0.47	1.14	−3.17	−0.37	1.23	3.12
Aortic and peripheral blood pressure, hemodynamic and wave reflection parameters												
Heart rate (beats/min)	91	11	66	84	99	134	69	12	43	61	76	132
pSBP (mmHg)	100	8	80	94	105	126	120	11	90	113	127	156
pDBP (mmHg)	59	7	50	54	62	86	64	7	48	60	68	100
pPP (mmHg)	41	7	24	36	46	77	56	11	21	48	63	90
pMBP (mmHg)	72	7	31	68	77	96	83	7	65	78	87	118
cSBP (mmHg)	83	6	64	78	87	100	102	9	83	96	107	135
cPP (mmHg)	22	4	7	19	25	43	37	8	18	31	43	61
CO (liter/min)	4.4	0.3	3.2	4.1	4.8	5.7	5.4	0.7	3.9	4.9	5.9	7.1
C.I. (liter/min/m^2)	4.9	0.6	3.5	4.4	5.4	5.9	3.2	0.8	1.8	2.9	3.5	16.0
SVR (s.mmHg/mL)	1.10	0.10	0.86	1.04	1.19	1.41	1.05	0.15	0.78	0.93	1.16	1.47
AIx (%)	9.7	9.7	−16	3	17	37	−0.7	9.1	−28.0	−6	5	25
AIx@75 (%)	17.0	9.3	−10	11	23	43	−3.3	10.0	−34.0	−10	2	27
AP (mmHg)	2	2	−5	1	4	9	−1	4	−15	−2	2	8
PF (mmHg)	20	5	7	17	23	43	36	10	9	29	42	82
PB (mmHg)	10	4	3	9	11	78	14	3	4	12	16	26

Table 1. *Cont.*

	Children Cohort (n = 632)						Adolescent Cohort (n = 340)					
	MV	STD	Min.	p25th	p75th	Max.	MV	STD	Min.	p25th	p75th	Max.
Structural arterial parameters, local and regional arterial stiffness												
R-CCA SD (mm)	6.04	0.50	4.83	5.70	6.39	7.41	6.82	0.51	5.20	6.48	7.11	8.82
R-CCA DD (mm)	5.38	0.47	4.21	5.03	5.71	6.91	6.16	0.47	4.53	5.88	6.46	7.90
R-CCA IMT (mm)	0.421	0.028	0.370	0.405	0.431	0.537	0.494	0.039	0.380	0.473	0.512	0.631
L-CCA SD (mm)	5.92	0.46	4.84	5.59	6.22	7.48	6.75	0.46	5.46	6.41	7.07	8.18
L-CCA DD (mm)	5.25	0.43	4.25	4.96	5.53	6.99	6.11	0.44	4.90	5.76	6.40	7.56
L-CCA IMT (mm)	0.420	0.027	0.316	0.405	0.431	0.567	0.492	0.042	0.343	0.472	0.508	0.722
R-CFA SD (mm)	4.74	0.53	3.44	4.42	5.05	6.50	7.20	0.99	5.42	6.44	7.94	9.76
R-CFA DD (mm)	4.42	0.51	3.13	4.11	4.72	6.11	6.87	0.93	5.22	6.13	7.52	9.44
R-CFA IMT (mm)	0.331	0.032	0.282	0.313	0.346	0.411	0.409	0.063	0.320	0.373	0.448	0.645
L-CFA SD (mm)	4.72	0.50	3.51	4.36	5.01	6.37	7.30	1.02	4.69	6.48	8.08	10.26
L-CFA DD (mm)	4.40	0.50	3.29	4.06	4.71	5.98	6.97	0.98	4.48	6.18	7.68	9.75
L-CFA IMT (mm)	0.335	0.026	0.271	0.319	0.355	0.398	0.393	0.060	0.313	0.355	0.417	0.585
R-CCA EM (mmHg)	187	45	71	156	216	304	360	89	181	292	416	643
L-CCA EM (mmHg)	179	46	54	146	205	314	358	88	186	300	397	670
R-CFA EM (mmHg)	618	267	237	417	724	1555	1317	530	533	944	1565	3411
L-CFA EM (mmHg)	592	219	219	427	711	1561	1349	535	529	962	1639	3497
cfPWV (m/s)	4.81	0.76	2.88	4.28	5.25	7.72	6.10	0.75	4.02	5.61	6.57	8.20

MV: mean value. STD: standard deviation. Min., Max.: minimum and maximum values. z: z-score. p25th, p75th: percentile 25 and 75. BW, BH: body weight and height. BMI: body mass index. CV: cardiovascular. pSBP, pDBP, pPP, pMBP: peripheral systolic, diastolic, pulse and mean pressure. CO, C.I.: cardiac output and index. cSBP, cPP: central systolic and pulse pressure. SVR: systemic vascular resistances. AIx, AIx@75: aortic augmentation index without and with heart rate adjustment. AP: augmented pressure. PF and PB: forward and backward aortic pressure component. R: Right. L: Left. CCA, CFA: common carotid and femoral artery. DD, SD: diastolic and systolic diameter. EM: elastic modulus. IMT: intima-media thickness. cfPWV: carotid-femoral pulse wave velocity.

2.3. *Clinical Evaluation*

None of the included subjects were taking medications, had congenital, chronic or infectious diseases at the moment of the CV study A brief clinical interview, together with the anthropometric evaluation enabled to assess CRFs exposure. Hypertension, dyslipidemia and diabetes were considered present if they had been previously diagnosed, in agreement with reference guidelines [18]. Subjects <16 y who had brachial systolic and/or diastolic pBP (pSBP and pDBP) >95th percentile for sex, age and BH during the study were considered with high BP levels (HBP); regardless previous diagnosis of hypertension. For subjects aged ≥16 y, HBP levels were defined using cutoff values similar to those for adults (pSBP ≥ 140 mmHg, pDBP ≥ 90 mmHg) [18]. Smokingwas defined as at least one cigarette/week for as long as a month. A family history of CV disease (CVD) was defined by presence of first-degree relatives with premature (<55 y in males; <65 y in females) CVD.

2.4. *Cardiovascular Evaluation*

CV studies were performed in children and adolescents (6 and 18 y, respectively) at the educational centers and/or in CUiiDARTE non-invasive vascular laboratories. The same protocol was applied in both cohorts (Figure 1) and was performed by experienced technicians using the same equipment. In order to reach steady hemodynamic conditions, before starting CV evaluation the subjects hada 10 min rest in a supine position in a quiet, temperature-controlled room.

2.5. *Peripheral and Central Pressure and Aortic Wave-Derived Parameters*

Heart rate (HR), pSBP and pDBP were obtained at 5 min intervals (Hem-4030, OmronInc., Illinois, USA). Peripheral pulse pressure (pPP = pSBP − pDBP) and mean BP (MBP = pDBP + pPP/3) were calculated. To assess cBP and aortic wave-derived parameters, radial artery BP waveforms were recorded using applanation tonometry (SphygmoCor-CvMS, AtCor-Medical, Sidney Australia) (Figure 1). Pressure signals were calibrated topDBP and MBP. A generalized transfer-function (GTF) enabled us to obtain the correspondingcBP waves and central systolic, diastolic and pulse pressure levels (cSBP, cDBP, cPP) [15,19] (Figure 1).

Only adequate waveforms (visual inspection) and high-quality recordings (operator index ≥85) were considered. By means of pulse wave analysis (PWA) the first (P1) and second (P2) peaks in cBP wave were identified and their height (amplitude) and time were determined. Then, the difference between P2 and P1 was computed as central augmented pressure (AP) and used to quantify central aortic augmentation index (Aix = AP/cPP). Since AIx depends on HR, AIx adjusted to a 75 beats/minHR (AIx@75) was calculated. Forward and backward (Pf and Pb) components of the aortic pulse wave were also quantified (Figure 1). AIx is a measure of the contribution of reflections to cBP wave amplitude. It depends on the timing and magnitude of the reflected (backward) wave and is influenced by the compliance and structure of vessels distal to the site of measurement, as well as by the distance to the reflection sites. Greater Pb and/or AIx values indicate increased reflections and/or earlier return of reflected waves due to increased arterial stiffness and/or closer reflection sites. Systemic vascular resistance, cardiac output and index were quantified from brachial pulse contour analysis (Mobil-O-Graph, I.E.M.-GmbH, Stolberg, Germany) [15,19]. Only high quality records (index ≤2) and satisfactory waves (visual inspection) were considered. Subjects' values are the average of at least six consecutive records obtained in a single visit.

2.6. *Arterial Beat-to-Beat Diameter and Intima-Media Thickness (IMT)*

Left and right common carotid and femoral arteries (CCA, CFA) were analyzed using ultrasound (6–13 MHz, M-Turbo, SonoSite Inc., Bothell, WA, USA) and image sequences (30 s, B-Mode, longitudinal views) were stored for off-line analysis. Beat-to-beat diameter waves were obtained using border detection software. Systolic (SD) and end-diastolic (DD) diameters and IMT (far wall, end-diastolic) values were obtained averaging at least 20 beats (Figure 1). CCA diameter and IMT were measured one centimeter proximal to the bulb; CFA diameter and IMT were measured in the straight segment of the penultimate centimeter proximal to the arterial bifurcation (Figure 1) [13].

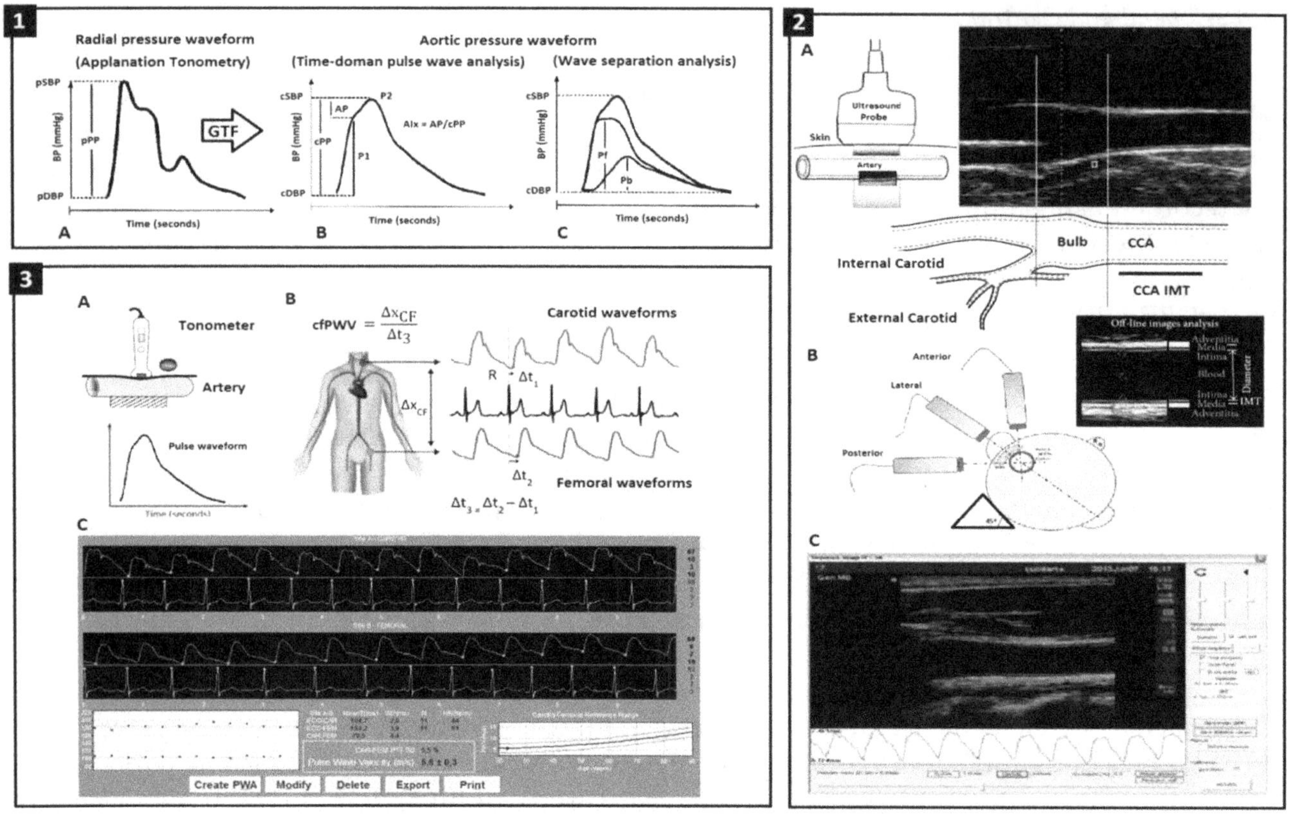

Figure 1. 1-A: Radial pulse wave obtained by applanation tonometry (SphygmoCor device); pSBP, pDBP, pPP: peripheral systolic, diastolic and pulse pressure. GTF: general transfer function. 1-B: Aortic wave derived using a GTF; augmented pressure (AP) and augmentation index (AIx) quantified from time-domain pulse wave analysis (PWA). cSBP, cDBP, cPP: central systolic, diastolic and pulsepressure. P1, P2: first and second pressure wave peaks. 1-C: Forward (Pf) and backward (Pb) components' amplitude obtained from wave separation analysis (WSA). 2-A, 2-B: Methodological approach used to assess common carotid (CCA) and femoral (CFA) artery diameter and intima-media thickness (IMT). Z: acoustic impedance. 2-C: Software for IMT and diameter measurement (Hemodyn-4M). 3-A, 3-B: Methodological approach used to assess carotid-femoral pulse wave velocity (cfPWV). Δx: CCA-to-CFA distance. Δt1, Δt2: time delay between R (ECG) and CCA and CFA foot wave. Δt3: time delay between arterial waves. 3-C: Software for cfPWV measurement (SphygmoCor device).

2.7. Local and Regional Arterial Stiffness

CCA and CFA pressure-strain elastic modulus (EM; local stiffness) were calculated as EM = PP/(SD − DD)/DD; cPP and pPP were considered to quantify CCA EM and CFA EM, respectively. Aortic regional stiffness was assessed by means of carotid-femoral pulse wave velocity (cfPWV) (SphygmoCor-CvMS) (Figure 1). The SphygmoCor allowed us to obtain cfPWV from sequential CCA and CFA wave recordings. cfPWV was calculated as the quotient between pulse wave travel distanceand pulse transit time. Real cfPWV was obtained multiplying measured cfPWV by 0.8. cfPWV values were obtained as the mean of three measurements.

2.8. Data Analysis and Statistics

A step-wise analysis was performed. First, CV variables were standardized and expressed as z-scores. To this end, subjects not exposed to CRFs (i.e., hypertension, HBP, dyslipidemia, smoking, diabetes, obesity or family history of CVD) were selected from each cohort (reference subgroups: 400 children, 153 adolescents) (Supplementary (S) Table S1). Working with the reference subgroups, mean value (MV) and standard deviation (STD) were determined for each variable (considering age and sex). Then, individual data were converted into z-scores (dimensionless numbers obtained by subtracting the reference MV from an observation, dividing the result by the reference STD) (Table S2) [13].

Second, Pearson product-moment correlations were obtained to quantify the strength of association between CVz-scores and anthropometric variables: (1) at birth: BWH z-score (both cohorts); (2) at the time of the CVstudy: current z-BMI (6 y for children, 18 y for adolescents); (3) growth-related changes: (a) early: ΔBWHz-score 0–2y, (b) intermediate: ΔBMI z-score 0–6y, (c) late: ΔBMI z-score 6–18y and (d) global: ΔBMI z-score 0–18y (Tables 2 and 3).

Third, statistical comparisons of the correlations' strengths were done using two-tailed William's test, making statistical corrections for dependent (same cohort) and overlapping (correlations have a variable in common) variables (e.g., when comparing the correlations "ΔBMI z-score 0–6y and z-pSBP" and "current z-BMI and z-pSBP" in the children cohort) [20] (Tables 2 and 3). Comparisons between cohorts were made considering William's test for non-overlapping (no variables in common) and independent (different cohort) variables (e.g., when comparing the R obtained for ΔBMI z-score 0–6y and z-pSBP in children and adolescents) (Table 4).

Fourth, the association between CV z-scores and anthropometric changes during growth was analyzed after statistical adjustment (partial correlations) for: (a) BWH z-score at birth; (b) BWH z-score at birth and current z-BMI and (c) BWH z-score at birth and ΔBMI z-score 6-18y (Tables 5–8). Multiple linear regression models (MLR; input: enter and forward), enabled to analyze the association between standardized CV data (dependent variables) and (1) single, specific anthropometric changes (ΔBWH z-score 0–2y, Δz-BMI 0–6y, Δz-BMI 0–18y and Δz-BMI 6–18y); (2) BWH z-score at birth; (3) current z-BMI, and (4) the interactions between growth-related changes and birth size or current z-BMI (e.g., (Δz-BMI 0–6y*BWH at birth) and (Δz-BMI 0–6y*current z-BMI)). In other words, since an association between postnatal growth and CV properties might be modified by birth or current body size, interaction between these conditions and growth-related body size changes on CV characteristics was tested adding two product terms (as continuous variables) to the model [21] (Tables S3–S12).

Fifth, using MLR models (input: enter and forward) we analyzed the association between standardized CV variables at 6 and 18 y and anthropometric variables and CRFs (independent variables) (Tables 8 and 9, Tables S13 and 14). A variance inflation factor (VIF) <5 was selected to evaluate (discard) significant collinearity.

Analyses were done using MedCalc Statistical Software (v.18.5. MedCalc Inc., Ostend, Belgium); Cocor Statistical Package (http://comparingcorrelations.org/) and IBM-SPSS Software (v.20, IBM-SPSS Inc., Chicago, IL, USA). A $p < 0.05$ was considered statistically significant.

3. Results

3.1. Arterial System at 6 and 18 y: Comparative Analysis of the Association between Birth or Current Body Size and Early, Intermediate, Late or Global Growth-Related Body Size Changes

The association between CV z-scores at 6 y and (a) body size at birth and 6 y or (b) body size changes during growing-up (0–2 or 0–6y) are shown in Table 2 (children cohort). Both, ΔBWH z-score 0–2y and Δz-BMI 0–6y, were associated with structural and hemodynamic parameters. Positive associations were found between z-pSBP, z-pMBP, z-cSBP, z-cDBP and the ΔBWH z-score 0–2y and Δ z-BMI 0-6y ($p < 0.05$). Negative associations were observed when z-AP, z-AIx and z-AIx@75 were considered. z-Pf was positively associated with Δz-BMI 0-6y (statistical threshold, $p = 0.053$), but the association with ΔBWH z-score 0–2 y did not reach significance ($p = 0.09$). The characteristics and statistical significance of the associations between anthropometric changes and structural properties varied, depending (among on other factors) on the structural parameter considered. No significant associations were found between stiffness z-scores and ΔBWH z-score 0-2 y and Δz-BMI 0–6 y (Table 2)

Table 2. Comparative analysis CV variables' association with anthropometric characteristics at birth, at 6 y and with anthropometric changes within that period (0–2 and 0–6 y) (children cohort, $n = 632$).

	Zero-OrderCorrelations								William Test (Comparison of Correlations)				
	Δ z-BWH (0–2y) [1]		Δ z-BMI (0–6y) [2]		z-BWH (at Birth) [3]		z-BMI (at 6 y) [4]		1–2	1–3	1–4	2–3	2–4
	R	*p*	*R*	*p*	*R*	*p*	*R*	*p*	*p*	*p*	*P*	*p*	*p*
Aortic and peripheral blood pressure, hemodynamic and wave reflection parameters													
z-pSBP	0.16	0.026	0.20	0.003	0.08	0.228	0.32	<0.001	0.408	0.469	0.019	0.245	0.009
z-pDBP	0.13	0.064	0.16	0.019	0.05	0.437	0.22	<0.001	0.538	0.476	0.182	0.299	0.174
z-pPP	0.05	0.474	0.06	0.389	0.03	0.613	0.13	0.034	0.839	0.883	0.236	0.805	0.110
z-pMBP	0.16	0.027	0.19	0.005	0.07	0.304	0.28	<0.001	0.514	0.425	0.062	0.243	0.038
z-cSBP	0.18	0.008	0.20	0.003	0.05	0.391	0.29	<0.001	0.663	0.253	0.079	0.138	0.042
z-cDBP	0.14	0.040	0.16	0.017	0.04	0.501	0.23	<0.001	0.665	0.355	0.150	0.237	0.091
z-cPP	0.06	0.396	0.07	0.312	0.04	0.579	0.10	0.106	0.831	0.831	0.549	0.726	0.534
z-AIx	–0.16	0.017	–0.17	0.009	0.11	0.078	–0.16	0.009	0.828	0.008	0.964	0.005	0.762
z-AIx@75	–0.16	0.020	–0.16	0.014	0.03	0.648	–0.23	<0.001	0.949	0.073	0.291	0.063	0.106
z-AP	–0.15	0.027	–0.14	0.030	0.12	0.054	–0.11	0.064	0.829	0.009	0.576	0.008	0.502
z-Pf	0.11	0.092	0.13	0.053	–0.02	0.791	0.17	0.006	0.667	0.208	0.427	0.143	0.395
z-Pb	0.01	0.938	0.00	0.949	0.04	0.494	0.03	0.609	0.850	0.709	0.701	0.634	0.427
Structural arterial parameters, local and regional arterial stiffness													
z-R-CCA SD	0.08	0.455	0.24	0.016	0.03	0.785	0.29	0.001	0.026	0.758	0.036	0.168	0.430
z-R-CCA DD	0.07	0.506	0.22	0.024	0.03	0.744	0.29	0.002	0.002	0.820	0.033	0.225	0.311
z-R-CCA IMT	–0.29	0.004	0.28	0.005	–0.05	0.631	0.29	<0.001	<0.001	0.018	<0.001	0.001	0.833
z-L-CCA SD	0.12	0.092	0.15	0.027	0.13	0.039	0.19	0.037	0.532	0.911	0.476	0.923	0.545
z-L-CCA DD	0.09	0.206	0.14	0.035	0.16	0.012	0.29	<0.001	0.298	0.469	0.003	0.812	<0.001
z-L-CCA IMT	0.11	0.115	0.14	0.043	0.07	0.178	0.18	0.004	0.695	0.735	0.312	0.513	0.390
z-R-CFA SD	0.32	0.003	0.36	<0.001	–0.16	0.118	0.36	<0.001	0.807	0.004	0.708	0.001	0.952
z-R-CFA DD	0.34	0.001	0.35	<0.001	–0.18	0.077	0.33	<0.001	0.827	0.002	0.890	0.001	0.765
z-R-CFA IMT	–0.23	0.338	–0.25	0.296	0.14	0.552	–0.40	0.065	0.674	0.335	0.470	0.294	0.323
z-L-CFA SD	0.11	0.123	0.14	0.034	0.09	0.194	0.29	<0.001	0.767	0.838	0.086	0.610	<0.001
z-L-CFA DD	0.09	0.198	0.12	0.071	0.08	0.208	0.26	<0.001	0.690	0.948	0.014	0.730	0.002
z-L-CFA IMT	0.08	0.617	0.17	0.250	–0.12	0.379	–0.01	0.919	0.101	0.372	0.542	0.173	0.001
z-R-CCA EM	0.05	0.620	0.12	0.226	–0.02	0.822	0.13	0.162	0.205	0.650	0.463	0.028	0.864
z-L-CCA EM	–0.03	0.746	0.06	0.405	0.11	0.161	0.12	0.080	0.242	0.280	0.057	0.697	0.213
z-R-CFA EM	0.15	0.179	0.07	0.493	–0.08	0.422	0.00	0.981	0.103	0.177	0.189	0.353	0.343
z-L-CFA EM	–0.04	0.596	–0.06	0.407	0.04	0.579	–0.01	0.863	0.115	0.993	0.703	0.360	0.287
z-cfPWV	0.00	0.991	–0.03	0.775	–0.02	0.790	0.00	1.00	0.649	0.876	0.989	0.959	0.610

z: z-score. BW, BH: body weight and height. Δ: change in the analyzed period. BMI: body mass index. SBP, DBP, PP, MBP: systolic, diastolic, pulse and mean pressure (p: peripheral, c: central). AIx, AIx@75: aortic augmentation index without and with heart rate adjustment. AP: augmented pressure. Pf, Pb: forward and backward pressure components. R: Right. L: Left. CCA, CFA: common carotid and femoral artery. EM: elastic modulus. IMT: intima-media thickness. DD, SD: diastolic and systolic diameter. cfPWV: carotid-femoral pulse wave velocity. *R*: Pearson coefficient. $p < 0.05$ (red text) was considered significant. In Zero-order correlations columns, the numbers in square brackets define de groups. Then in "William Test (Comparison of Correlations)" (also in columns in the same table), groups are compared in pairs cnsidering groups numbers. Identical comment for next Tables.

Unlike BWH at birth, current z-BMI (6y) was associated with hemodynamic and structural parameters. Furthermore, whereas BWH at birth did not show significant associations with hemodynamic variables, current z-BMI was associated ($p < 0.05$) with almost all of them (pBP, cBPandwave-derived parameters) (Table 2).

Compared to ΔBWH z-score 0–2y and Δz-BMI 0–6y, current z-BMI levels (at 6 y) were more strongly associated with CV z-scores. For example, R coefficients for the association between z-pSBP and ΔBWH z-score 0–2y, Δz-BMI 0–6y and current z-BMI (6 y) were 0.16, 0.20 and 0.32, respectively ($p < 0.05$). When compared, the association was stronger in case of z-BMI at 6 y ($p = 0.019$ and $p = 0.009$) (Table 2). The strength of association between arterial parameters at 6 y and ΔBWH z-score 0–2y and Δz-BMI 0–6y did not show statistical differences, with the only exception of z-Right CCA SD, DD and IMT that showed stronger association with 0–6y changes ($p = 0.026$, $p = 0.002$ and $p < 0.01$, respectively).

In adolescents, CVz-scores showed associations with current z-BMI, while almost no association was observed between arterial parameters at 18 y and prior body size characteristics (i.e., BWH at birth and Δz-BMI 0-6y) (Table 3). On the other hand, in case of variables associated with Δz-BMI 0–18y (z-pSBP, z-pPP, z-CCA SD and DD) or BWH z-score at birth (z-Right CCA EM and z-Left CCA EM), the comparative analysis (William's test) showed that the strongest associations were obtained when considering current z-BMI (18 y) (Table 3).

Jointly analyzing data from both cohorts it was observed that the strength of the associations between CV z-scores and current z-BMI (6 or 18 y), were always greater than those obtained for any change in body size between birth and the time of the study (0–2, 0–6 or 6–18 y) (Tables 2 and 3).

As mentioned, arterial properties at 6 y were associated with body size changes in that life period (i.e., 0–2 and 0–6 y) whereas the CV properties in subjects 18 y showed almost no association with prior (i.e., Δz-BMI 0–6, 6–18 and 0–18 y) anthropometric conditions (Table 4). When the cohorts were statistically compared, it was observed that for the same "body change" (Δz-BMI 0–6 y), associations were significant for almost all the studied variables when subjects were 6 y, but not when they were 18 y (Table 4).

Thus, as the subject's age increases, the association between CV z-scores and prior anthropometric changes (i.e., during childhood) decreases (Table 4).

3.2. Arterial Structure and Function at 6 y: Independent Association with ΔBWH z-Score 0–2 y

Associations between hemodynamic and structural parameters at 6 y and ΔBWH z-score 0–2 y kept significant after controlling for BWH z-score at birth (Table 5). After adjusting for BWH z-score at birth and current z-BMI only associations with z-cSBP (but not with z-pSBP, $p = 0.103$) remained significant ($R = 0.14$, $p = 0.041$) (Table 5). Thus, the association between ΔBWH z-score 0-2 y and cSBP, while weak, is independent of size at birth and at the time of CV study. AIx@75 ($p = 0.009$) and Pf ($p = 0.052$) showed significant associations after controlling for body size at birth (Table 5).

As mentioned, significant positive associations were found between ΔBWH z-score 0–2 y and structural parameters. Disregarding BWH z-scores at birth, ΔBWH z-score 0-2y values were positively associated with z-IMT (both CCA) and z-diameters (both CFA, left CCA). Then, the greater the body size change within the first 2 y, the higher the diameters and wall thickness (Table 5). The associations between ΔBWH z-score 0–2 y and z-IMT remained significant after adjusting for BWH at birth and current z-BMI (6 y). Then, regardless of nutritional status at birth and at the time of arterial evaluation, z-IMT levels at 6 y are influenced by ΔBWH z-score 0–2y (Table 5).

There were no significant associations between ΔBWH z-score 0–2 y and stiffness z-scores, before (zero-order correlations) and after (partial correlations) adjusting for BWH z-scores at birth and/or current z-BMI (Table 5).

Table 3. Comparative analysis CV variables' association with anthropometric characteristics at birth, at 18 y and with anthropometric changes within that period (0–6, 0–18, 6–18 y) [adolescent cohort, $n = 340$].

	Zero-Ordercorrelations										William Test (Comparison of Correlations)								
	Δ z-BMI (0–6y) [1]		Δ z-BMI (0–18y) [2]		Δ z-BMI (6–18y) [3]		z-BWH (at Birth) [4]		z-BMI (18y) [5]		1–2	1–3	1–4	1–5	2–3	2–4	2–5	3–4	3–5
	R	*p*	*R*	*p*	*R*	*p*	*R*	*p*	*R*	*p*	*p*	*p*	*p*	*p*	*p*	*p*	*p*	*p*	*p*
Aortic and peripheral blood pressure, hemodynamic and reflection parameters																			
z-pSBP	0.08	0.234	0.14	0.021	0.09	0.172	0.01	0.931	0.25	<0.001	0.411	0.905	0.488	0.010	0.421	0.203	0.040	0.458	0.009
z-pDBP	−0.02	0.757	0.02	0.798	0.07	0.286	0.03	0.581	0.17	0.002	0.623	0.283	0.609	0.004	0.424	0.922	0.006	0.711	0.107
z-pPP	0.10	0.111	0.14	0.016	0.04	0.478	−0.02	0.715	0.15	0.007	0.541	0.473	0.002	0.460	0.108	0.118	0.854	0.579	0.077
z-pMBP	0.02	0.732	0.08	0.206	0.09	0.162	0.03	0.660	0.24	<0.001	0.438	0.403	0.954	0.001	0.873	0.283	0.003	0.577	0.014
z-cSBP	0.02	0.765	0.07	0.226	0.05	0.461	0.10	0.081	0.27	<0.001	0.464	0.721	0.421	<0.001	0.749	0.775	<0.001	0.641	0.000
z-cDBP	0.002	0.977	0.03	0.613	−0.01	0.818	0.09	0.135	0.14	0.011	0.692	0.886	0.396	0.038	0.523	0.568	0.050	0.353	0.016
z-cPP	0.02	0.773	0.05	0.394	0.06	0.301	0.04	0.504	0.18	0.001	0.663	0.634	0.844	0.017	0.873	0.924	0.020	0.853	0.053
z-AIx	0.02	0.744	0.02	0.682	0.03	0.602	−0.01	0.931	−0.02	0.774	0.944	0.906	0.495	0.008	0.874	0.772	0.471	0.714	0.428
z-AIx@75	−0.05	0.416	0.004	0.948	0.09	0.159	0.07	0.265	0.01	0.918	0.451	0.287	0.266	0.110	0.172	0.523	0.970	0.853	0.204
z-AP	0.02	0.735	0.02	0.741	0.02	0.744	0.001	0.996	−0.02	0.693	1.000	0.987	0.850	<0.001	0.992	0.849	0.470	0.398	0.526
z-PF	0.06	0.397	0.06	0.308	0.02	0.707	−0.02	0.755	0.11	0.047	0.967	0.643	0.459	0.432	0.535	0.449	0.376	0.719	0.161
z-PB	0.11	0.096	0.06	0.309	−0.08	0.211	0.05	0.402	0.06	0.289	0.519	0.028	0.578	0.484	0.030	0.925	0.990	0.243	0.030
Structural arterial parameters, local and regional arterial stiffness																			
z-R-CCA SD	0.09	0.146	0.15	0.015	0.10	0.123	−0.02	0.692	0.26	<0.001	0.437	0.905	0.273	0.012	0.423	0.098	0.041	0.269	0.009
z-R-CCA DD	0.08	0.208	0.14	0.021	0.09	0.129	−0.003	0.962	0.26	<0.001	0.413	0.905	0.291	0.006	0.424	0.164	0.026	0.392	0.006
z-R-CCA IMT	0.04	0.501	0.03	0.604	0.12	0.060	0.002	0.967	0.12	0.032	0.900	0.341	0.716	0.238	0.153	0.787	0.104	0.277	0.949
z-L-CCA SD	0.11	0.077	0.13	0.034	0.10	0.100	−0.01	0.883	0.25	<0.001	0.811	0.905	0.248	0.034	0.632	0.174	0.026	0.312	0.015
z-L-CCA DD	0.10	0.121	0.12	0.054	0.09	0.136	0.03	0.597	0.28	<0.001	0.822	0.905	0.513	0.007	0.632	0.382	0.003	0.581	0.002
z-L-CCA IMT	0.12	0.069	0.06	0.283	0.09	0.150	−0.01	0.868	0.13	0.020	0.440	0.721	0.212	0.860	0.634	0.772	0.205	0.359	0.524
z-R-CFA SD	0.12	0.233	0.08	0.418	0.18	0.057	0.02	0.840	0.34	<0.001	0.708	0.647	0.537	0.036	0.309	0.712	0.002	0.345	0.133
z-R-CFA DD	0.11	0.281	0.08	0.437	0.18	0.069	0.01	0.957	0.32	<0.001	0.755	0.593	0.522	0.046	0.309	0.667	0.004	0.316	0.140
z-R-CFA IMT	0.15	0.496	0.17	0.390	0.19	0.363	−0.16	0.423	0.27	0.149	0.936	0.886	0.380	0.607	0.924	0.343	0.582	0.339	0.697
z-L-CFA SD	0.11	0.292	0.11	0.244	0.11	0.273	−0.02	0.870	0.26	0.003	0.986	0.988	0.440	0.148	0.960	0.422	0.077	0.446	0.120
z-L-CFA DD	0.09	0.407	0.10	0.307	0.10	0.322	0.01	0.951	0.26	0.003	0.943	0.940	0.607	0.100	0.984	0.578	0.059	0.597	0.097
z-L-CFA IMT	0.01	0.967	−0.15	0.445	−0.26	0.190	0.27	0.162	0.33	0.068	0.160	0.328	0.437	0.151	0.589	0.215	0.005	0.136	0.002
z-R-CCA EM	−0.05	0.485	0.02	0.788	0.06	0.317	0.12	0.043	0.21	<0.001	0.360	0.196	0.102	<0.001	0.528	0.327	0.003	0.581	0.016
z-L-CCA EM	0.02	0.787	0.06	0.296	0.06	0.345	0.13	0.029	0.31	<0.001	0.551	0.639	0.288	<0.001	0.954	0.498	0.003	0.520	<0.001
z-R-CFA EM	−0.03	0.793	0.02	0.821	−0.10	0.308	−0.09	0.364	−0.07	0.443	0.648	0.601	0.725	0.721	0.230	0.503	0.306	0.953	0.764
z-L-CFA EM	−0.14	0.175	−0.05	0.630	−0.09	0.351	0.12	0.223	0.09	0.309	0.408	0.706	0.118	0.032	0.689	0.298	0.109	0.222	0.070
z-cfPWV	0.01	0.912	0.01	0.802	−0.03	0.621	0.03	0.632	0.03	0.599	0.944	0.633	0.862	0.770	0.523	0.845	0.716	0.579	0.337

z: z-score. BW, BH: body weight and height. Δ: change in the studied period. BMI: body mass index. SBP, DBP, PP, MBP: systolic, diastolic, pulse and mean pressure (p: peripheral, c: central). AIx, AIx@75: augmentation index without and with heart rate adjustment. AP: augmented pressure. Pf, Pb: forward and backwardpressure components. R: Right. L: Left. CCA, CFA: common carotid and femoral artery. EM: elastic modulus. IMT: intima-media thickness. DD, SD: diastolic and systolic diameter. cfPWV: carotid-femoral pulse wave velocity. R: Pearson coefficient. $p < 0.05$ (red) was considered significant.

Table 4. Comparative analysis of the associations between CV and anthropometric parameters: children vs. adolescents.

	Zero-OrderCorrelations										Comparison of Correlations					
	ChildrenCohort (n = 632)				AdolescentCohort (n = 340)											
	ΔBWH (0–2y) [1]		Δ z-BMI (0–6y) [2]		Δ z-BMI (0–6y) [3]		Δ z-BMI (0–18y) [4]		Δ z-BMI (6–18y) [5]		1–3	1–4	1–5	2–3	2–4	2–5
	R	p	R	p	R	p	R	p	R	p	p	P	p	P	p	p
Aortic and peripheral blood pressure, hemodynamic and wave reflection parameters																
z-pSBP	0.16	0.026	0.20	0.003	0.08	0.234	0.14	0.021	0.09	0.172	0.320	0.802	0.384	0.613	0.449	0.169
z-pDBP	0.13	0.064	0.16	0.019	−0.02	0.757	0.02	0.798	0.07	0.286	0.065	0.175	0.458	0.708	0.084	0.264
z-pPP	0.05	0.474	0.06	0.389	0.10	0.111	0.14	0.016	0.04	0.478	0.538	0.266	0.624	0.902	0.322	0.806
z-pMBP	0.16	0.027	0.19	0.005	0.02	0.732	0.08	0.206	0.09	0.162	0.083	0.320	0.383	0.705	0.170	0.211
z-cSBP	0.18	0.008	0.20	0.003	0.02	0.765	0.07	0.226	0.05	0.461	0.047	0.159	0.097	0.794	0.095	0.055
z-cDBP	0.14	0.040	0.16	0.017	0.002	0.977	0.03	0.613	−0.01	0.818	0.080	0.163	0.058	0.797	0.098	0.031
z-cPP	0.06	0.396	0.07	0.312	0.02	0.773	0.05	0.394	0.06	0.301	0.614	0.900	0.930	0.899	0.801	0.899
z-AIx	−0.16	0.017	−0.17	0.009	0.02	0.744	0.02	0.682	0.03	0.602	0.023	0.023	0.016	0.897	0.016	0.011
z-AIx@75	−0.16	0.020	−0.16	0.014	−0.05	0.416	0.004	0.948	0.09	0.159	0.169	0.041	0.002	0.962	0.041	0.002
z-AP	−0.15	0.027	−0.14	0.030	0.02	0.735	0.02	0.741	0.02	0.744	0.035	0.032	0.032	0.898	0.043	0.043
z-Pf	0.11	0.092	0.13	0.053	0.06	0.397	0.06	0.308	0.02	0.707	0.534	0.534	0.263	0.802	0.383	0.063
z-Pb	0.01	0.938	−0.004	0.949	0.11	0.096	0.06	0.309	−0.08	0.211	0.215	0.537	0.266	0.883	0.429	0.347
Structural arterial parameters, local and regional arterial stiffness																
z-R-CCA SD	0.08	0.455	0.24	0.016	0.09	0.146	0.15	0.015	0.10	0.123	0.924	0.503	0.248	0.121	0.377	0.173
z-R-CCA DD	0.07	0.506	0.22	0.024	0.08	0.208	0.14	0.021	0.09	0.129	0.924	0.404	0.849	0.148	0.435	0.208
z-R-CCA IMT	−0.29	0.004	0.28	0.005	0.04	0.501	0.03	0.604	0.12	0.060	0.001	0.002	<0.001	<0.001	0.015	0.115
z-L-CCA SD	0.12	0.092	0.15	0.027	0.11	0.077	0.13	0.034	0.10	0.100	0.900	0.900	0.803	0.706	0.801	0.530
z-L-CCA DD	0.09	0.206	0.14	0.035	0.10	0.121	0.12	0.054	0.09	0.136	0.901	0.708	0.940	0.531	0.802	0.531
z-L-CCA IMT	0.11	0.115	0.14	0.043	0.12	0.069	0.06	0.283	0.09	0.150	0.900	0.535	0.803	0.708	0.318	0.531
z-R-CFA SD	0.32	0.003	0.36	<0.001	0.12	0.233	0.08	0.418	0.18	0.057	0.100	0.050	0.244	0.725	0.021	0.129
z-R-CFA DD	0.34	0.001	0.35	0.001	0.11	0.281	0.08	0.437	0.18	0.069	0.058	0.033	0.180	0.930	0.026	0.153
z-R-CFA IMT	−0.23	0.338	−0.25	0.296	0.15	0.496	0.17	0.390	0.19	0.363	0.173	0.151	0.131	0.942	0.131	0.113
z-L-CFA SD	0.11	0.123	0.14	0.034	0.11	0.292	0.11	0.244	0.11	0.273	0.992	0.977	0.992	0.773	0.773	0.773
z-L-CFA DD	0.09	0.198	0.12	0.071	0.09	0.407	0.10	0.307	0.10	0.322	0.970	0.924	0.924	0.774	0.848	0.848
z-L-CFA IMT	0.08	0.617	0.17	0.250	0.01	0.967	−0.15	0.445	−0.26	0.190	0.751	0.296	0.118	0.679	0.145	0.048
z-R-CCA EM	0.05	0.620	0.12	0.226	−0.05	0.485	0.02	0.788	0.06	0.317	0.355	0.781	0.926	0.515	0.353	0.576
z-L-CCA EM	−0.03	0.746	0.06	0.405	0.02	0.787	0.06	0.296	0.06	0.345	0.570	0.306	0.306	0.306	0.991	0.955
z-R-CFA EM	0.15	0.179	0.07	0.493	−0.03	0.793	0.02	0.821	−0.10	0.308	0.160	0.309	0.051	0.530	0.698	0.186
z-L-CFA EM	−0.04	0.596	−0.06	0.407	−0.14	0.175	−0.05	0.630	−0.09	0.351	0.343	0.925	0.637	0.851	0.925	0.777
z-cfPWV	−0.001	0.991	−0.03	0.775	0.01	0.912	0.01	0.802	−0.03	0.621	0.908	0.9082	0.761	0.761	0.753	0.95

z: z-score. BW, BH: body weight and height. Δ: change in the analyzed period. BMI: body mass index. SBP, DBP, PP, MBP: systolic, diastolic, pulse and mean pressure (p: peripheral, c: central). AIx, AIx@75: aortic augmentation index without and with heart rate adjustment. AP: augmented pressure. Pf, Pb: forward and backward pressure components. R: Right. L: Left. CCA, CFA: common carotid and femoral artery. EM: elastic modulus. IMT: intima-media thickness. DD, SD: diastolic and systolic diameter. cfPWV: carotid-femoral pulse wave velocity. R: Pearson coefficient. $p < 0.05$ (red) was considered significant.

3.3. Arterial Structure and Function at 6 and 18 y: Independent Association with Δz-BMI(Body Mass Index) 0–6 y

Table 6 shows correlations between CV z-scores (at 6 and 18 y) and Δz-BMI 0-6y. In children, z-pSBP, z-pDBP, z-pMBP, z-cSBP, z-cDPB and z-cMBP correlated (positively) with Δz-BMI 0–6 y. Associations remained significant after controlling for BWH at birth, but showed dependence on current z-BMI. AIx and AIx@75 showed significant negative associations when controlling for BWH at birth but when controlling for z-BMI at 6 y, positive correlations were observed (R=0.14, p = 0.034; R=0.19, p = 0.005). Both z-CCA IMT were associated with Δz-BMI 0–6 y, with independence of BWH at birth and current z-BMI. Similar results were observed for right and left CFA IMT and DD.

CV parameters (z-scores) at 18 ywere not associated (zero-order correlation) with Δz-BMI 0–6 y. However, several correlations became significant after adjusting for BWH z-scores at birth. Then, body size changes within 0–6 y would contribute to explain CV characteristics at 18 y. Unlike the observed at 6 y, CVparameters at 18 ywere not associated with Δz-BMI 0–6 y (except z-Pb and z-left CCA IMT) after adjusting for body size at birth and current z-BMI (Table 6)

3.4. Arterial Structure and Function at 18 y: Independent Association with Δz-BMI 0–18 y and 6–18 y

Tables 7 and 8 show the association between CV z-scores and Δz-BMI 0–18 and 6–18 y. There were no independent associations between CV properties at 18 y and overall (0–18 y) or late (6–18 y) anthropometric (z-BMI) changes, being the only exceptions z-pPP (for Δz-BMI 0–18 y; p = 0.017) and z-Right CCA SD (for Δz-BMI 6–18 y; p = 0.035). Then, global changes in body size from birth (0–18 y) or childhood (6–18 y) until late in adolescence would not contribute to explain CV characteristics at the beginning of adulthood, with independence of birth size or current z-BMI.

3.5. Hemodynamic and Arterial Properties at 6 and 18 y: Hierarchical Impact of Anthropometric Variables

MLRmodels allowed analyzing whether growth-related body size changes contribute to explain CV properties, considering and comparing BWH z-score at birth, current z-BMI and the interaction of variables (Supplementary Tables S3–S12). In children, cBP and pBP variables (z-SBP, z-DBP, z-PP, z-MBP) were only explained by z-BMI, while wave-derived parameters were explained by z-BMI (z-AIx@75, z-Pf, z-Pb), ΔBWH z-score 0–2 y (z-AIx, z-AP), Δz-BMI 0–6 y (z-AIx) and by Δz-BMI 0–6 y and z-BMI interaction (z-AP). Structural variables were mainly explained by z-BMI; arterial stiffness showed no association with body size parameters (Supplementary Tables S3–S6).

In the adolescents: (1) Δz-BMI 0–6 y showed explanatory capacity when interacting with current z-BMI (both z-CFA IMT) (Supplementary Tables S7 and S8); (2) Δz-BMI 0–18 y showed explanatory capacity when interacting with current z-BMI (z-cDBP, z-Right CFA diameters) or BWH z-score at birth (z-cDBP, z-cPP) (Supplementary Tables S9 and S10) and (3) Δz-BMI 6–18 ydid not showsignificant explanatory capacity for the studied variables (Supplementary Tables S11 and S12). Current z-BMI was always the variable with the greatest explanatory power. The explanatory capacity of the interactions between z-BMI (or z-BWH at birth) and Δz-BMI 0-6, 0–18 or 6–18 y was limited. Compared to current z-BMI, intermediate (0–6 y), late (6–18 y) or global (0–18 y) body-size changes showed almost no explanatory capacityfor interindividual variations in CV properties at 18 y.

The joint analysis of both cohorts showed that CV variables were mainly associated with current (i.e., 6 or 18 y) z-BMI. Body-size changes showed little individual explanatory power and their contribution was mainly relatedto the interaction with z-BMI at the time of CVevaluation.

3.6. Arterial Function at 6 and 18 y: Impact of Body Size Changes vs. Anthropometric and Cardiovascular Risk Factors (CRFs)

Table 9 and Supplementary Table S13 show explanatory models for CV parameters in children. pBP parameters were explained by current z-BMI, while cBP parameters and wave-derivedindexes were mainly associated with z-pSBP. Then, early (0–2 y) or intermediate (0–6 y) body size changes contributed little to explain cBP or pBPvariations found at 6 y compared to the conditions associated with CV risk (i.e., BMI and pSBP) at the time of the CV study.

Table 5. Associations between CV z-scores and z-BWHvariations between 0–2y (childrencohort, $n = 632$).

	Δ z-BWH (0–2y)					
	Zero-Order		Partial [1]		Partial [2]	
	R	*p*	*R*	*p*	*R*	*p*
Aortic and peripheral blood pressure, hemodynamic and wave reflection parameters						
z-pSBP	0.16	0.026	0.26	<0.001	0.11	0.103
z-pDBP	0.13	0.064	0.21	0.003	0.10	0.136
z-pPP	0.05	0.474	0.09	0.197	0.02	0.756
z-pMBP	0.16	0.027	0.25	<0.001	0.12	0.082
z-cSBP	0.18	0.008	0.27	<0.001	0.14	0.041
z-cDBP	0.14	0.040	0.21	0.002	0.10	0.136
z-cPP	0.06	0.396	0.10	0.135	0.06	0.379
z-AIx	−0.16	0.017	−0.12	0.085	−0.02	0.797
z-AIx@75	−0.16	0.020	−0.18	0.009	−0.06	0.419
z-AP	−0.15	0.027	−0.09	0.167	−0.02	0.762
z-Pf	0.11	0.092	0.13	0.052	0.04	0.528
z-Pb	0.01	0.938	0.04	0.545	0.03	0.619
Structural arterial parameters, local and regional arterial stiffness						
z-R-CCA SD	0.08	0.455	0.12	0.250	−0.06	0.595
z-R- CCA DD	0.07	0.506	0.11	0.277	−0.06	0.569
z-R-CCA IMT	−0.29	0.004	0.34	0.001	0.27	0.008
z-L-CCA SD	0.12	0.092	0.26	<0.001	0.13	0.058
z-L-CCA DD	0.09	0.206	0.24	<0.001	0.12	0.088
z-L-CCA IMT	0.11	0.115	0.20	0.004	0.13	0.048
z-R-CFA SD	0.32	0.003	0.28	0.008	0.08	0.472
z-R-CFA DD	0.34	0.001	0.30	0.005	0.12	0.288
z-R-CFA IMT	−0.23	0.338	−0.19	0.451	0.07	0.777
z-L-CFA SD	0.11	0.123	0.21	0.003	0.07	0.353
z-L-CFA DD	0.09	0.198	0.18	0.009	0.05	0.453
z-L-CFA IMT	0.08	0.617	0.00	0.991	−0.01	0.956
z-R-CCA EM	0.05	0.620	0.05	0.644	−0.03	0.750
z-L-CCA EM	−0.03	0.746	0.05	0.528	−0.01	0.888
z-R-CFA EM	0.15	0.179	0.12	0.270	0.13	0.223
z-L-CFA EM	−0.04	0.596	−0.02	0.796	−0.01	0.888
z-cfPWV	0.00	0.991	−0.02	0.827	−0.03	0.766

z: z-score. BW, BH: body weight and height. BMI: body mass index. SBP, DBP, PP, MBP: systolic, diastolic, pulse and mean pressure (p: peripheral, c: central). AIx, AIx@75: aortic augmentation index without and with heart rate adjustment. AP: augmented pressure. Pf, Pb: forward and backward pressure components. CCA, CFA: common carotid and femoral artery. EM: elastic modulus. IMT: intima-media thickness. DD, SD: diastolic and systolic diameter. cfPWV: carotid-femoral pulse wave velocity. *R*: Pearson coefficient. $p < 0.05$ (red) was considered significant. Partial correlations controlling for: [1] BW-for-BH (length) z-score at birth; [2] BW-for-BH (length) z-score at birth and z-BMI at the time of measurement (6 y).

Table 6. Associations between CV z-scores and z-BMIvariations between 0–6 y(both cohorts).

	Δ z-BMI (0–6y)													
	ChildrenCohort (n = 632)						AdolescentCohort (n = 340)							
	Zero-order		Partial [1]		Partial [2]		Zero-order		Partial [1]		Partial [2]		Partial [3]	
	R	p	R	p	R	p	R	p	R	p	R	p	R	p
Aortic and peripheral blood pressure, hemodynamic and wave reflection parameters														
z-pSBP	0.20	**0.003**	0.28	**<0.001**	−0.04	0.588	0.08	0.234	0.13	**0.049**	0.02	0.805	0.18	**0.008**
z-pDBP	0.16	**0.019**	0.22	**0.001**	0.03	0.621	−0.02	0.757	0.01	0.890	−0.08	0.239	0.04	0.558
z-pPP	0.06	0.389	0.09	0.195	−0.11	**0.095**	0.10	0.111	0.14	**0.037**	0.08	0.245	0.17	**0.013**
z-pMBP	0.19	**0.005**	0.26	**<0.001**	0.00	0.961	0.02	0.732	0.07	0.302	−0.05	0.483	0.11	**0.097**
z-cSBP	0.20	**0.003**	0.26	**<0.001**	−0.04	0.529	0.02	0.765	0.16	0.014	0.05	0.483	0.20	**0.003**
z-cDBP	0.16	**0.017**	0.21	**0.001**	−0.04	0.567	0.00	0.977	0.11	**0.083**	0.06	0.380	0.12	**0.074**
z-cPP	0.07	0.312	0.10	0.135	0.03	0.624	0.02	0.773	0.08	0.228	0.00	0.977	0.11	**0.088**
z-cMBP	0.18	**0.005**	0.24	**<0.001**	−0.02	0.718	−0.04	0.556	−0.03	0.636	−0.09	0.158	0.06	0.406
z-AIx	−0.17	**0.009**	−0.13	**0.045**	0.14	**0.034**	0.02	0.744	0.03	0.676	0.04	0.555	0.04	0.519
z-AIx@75	−0.16	**0.014**	−0.17	**0.009**	0.19	**0.005**	−0.05	0.416	0.00	0.984	0.00	0.976	0.04	0.562
z-AP	−0.14	**0.030**	−0.09	0.161	0.12	**0.056**	0.02	0.735	0.04	0.590	0.05	0.439	0.05	0.485
z-Pf	0.13	**0.053**	0.14	0.036	−0.09	0.173	0.06	0.397	0.07	0.322	0.02	0.820	0.08	0.228
z-Pb	0.00	0.949	0.02	0.747	0.00	0.956	0.11	**0.096**	0.24	**<0.001**	0.24	**<0.001**	0.23	**0.001**
Structural arterial parameters, local and regional arterial stiffness														
z-R-CCA SD	0.24	**0.016**	0.29	**0.003**	0.05	0.639	0.09	0.146	0.12	**0.066**	0.00	0.968	0.17	**0.011**
z-R-CCA DD	0.22	**0.024**	0.28	**0.005**	0.02	0.838	0.08	0.208	0.13	**0.054**	0.01	0.917	0.18	**0.008**
z-R-CCA IMT	0.28	**0.005**	0.29	**0.003**	0.33	**0.001**	0.04	0.501	0.07	0.268	0.02	0.763	0.13	**0.054**
z-L-CCA SD	0.15	**0.027**	0.25	**<0.001**	−0.02	0.779	0.11	**0.077**	0.17	**0.009**	0.06	0.321	0.23	**0.001**
z-L-CCA DD	0.14	**0.035**	0.26	**<0.001**	0.03	0.623	0.10	0.121	0.20	**0.002**	0.09	0.189	0.26	**<0.001**
z-L-CCA IMT	0.14	**0.043**	0.20	**0.002**	0.13	**0.044**	0.12	**0.069**	0.17	**0.007**	0.13	**0.048**	0.24	**<0.001**
z-R-CFA SD	0.36	**<0.001**	0.33	**0.002**	−0.17	0.105	0.12	0.233	0.22	**0.032**	0.08	0.428	0.32	**0.002**
z-R-CFA DD	0.35	**0.001**	0.31	**0.003**	−0.18	**0.094**	0.11	0.281	0.18	**0.075**	0.05	0.645	0.28	**0.007**
z-R-CFA IMT	−0.25	0.296	−0.21	0.397	0.74	**<0.001**	0.15	0.496	0.04	0.865	−0.10	0.645	0.12	0.607
z-L-CFA SD	0.14	**0.034**	0.22	**0.001**	−0.15	**0.033**	0.11	0.292	0.16	0.136	0.04	0.685	0.22	**0.039**
z-L-CFA DD	0.12	**0.071**	0.19	**0.004**	−0.15	**0.032**	0.09	0.407	0.15	0.164	0.03	0.769	0.20	**0.056**
z-L-CFA IMT	0.17	0.250	0.12	0.413	0.36	**0.013**	0.01	0.967	0.36	**0.073**	0.26	0.218	0.30	0.149
z-R-CCA EM	0.12	0.226	0.13	0.203	0.00	0.977	−0.05	0.485	0.08	0.229	−0.01	0.850	0.12	0.080
z-L-CCA EM	0.06	0.405	0.14	**0.073**	0.12	0.130	0.02	0.787	0.19	**0.003**	0.07	0.320	0.24	**<0.001**
z-R-CFA EM	0.07	0.493	0.04	0.741	0.06	0.581	−0.03	0.793	−0.15	0.144	−0.14	0.184	−0.21	**0.042**
z-L-CFA EM	−0.06	0.407	−0.04	0.524	−0.09	0.214	−0.14	0.175	−0.08	0.436	−0.14	0.205	−0.12	0.241
z-cfPWV	−0.03	0.775	−0.04	0.625	−0.15	**0.083**	0.01	0.912	0.05	0.475	0.04	0.560	0.04	0.566

z: z-score. BMI: body mass index. SBP, DBP, PP, MBP: systolic, diastolic, pulse and mean pressure (p: peripheral, c: central). AIx, AIx@75: augmentation index without and with heart rate adjustment. AP: augmented pressure. Pf,Pb: forward and backward pressure components. R: Right. L: Left. CCA, CFA: common carotid and femoral artery. EM: elastic modulus. IMT: intima-media thickness. DD, SD: diastolic and systolic diameter. cfPWV: carotid-femoral pulse wave velocity. R: Pearson coefficient. $p < 0.05$ (red text) was considered significant. Partial correlations controlling for: [1] BW-for-BHz-score at birth; [2] BWH z-score at birth and z-BMI at the time of CV study; [3] BWH z-score at birth and z-BMI variation between 6 and 18 y.

Table 7. Associations between CVz-scores and z-BMI variations between 0–18y(adolescent cohort, n = 340).

	Δ z-BMI (0–18y)					
	Zero-Order		Partial [1]		Partial [2]	
	R	P	R	p	R	p
Aortic and peripheral blood pressure, hemodynamic and wave reflection parameters						
z-pSBP	0.14	0.021	−0.14	0.682	−0.19	0.595
z-pDBP	0.02	0.798	−0.03	0.923	0.37	0.291
z-pPP	0.14	0.016	−0.13	0.712	−0.73	0.017
z-pMBP	0.08	0.206	−0.07	0.836	0.21	0.558
z-cSBP	0.07	0.226	0.27	0.419	0.31	0.388
z-cDBP	0.03	0.613	−0.10	0.777	0.02	0.962
z-cPP	0.05	0.394	0.61	0.045	0.57	0.084
z-AIx	0.02	0.682	−0.06	0.851	0.23	0.527
z-AIx@75	0.00	0.948	−0.13	0.704	0.13	0.720
z-AP	0.02	0.741	−0.08	0.818	0.16	0.668
z-Pf	0.06	0.308	0.05	0.895	0.16	0.660
z-Pb	0.06	0.309	0.15	0.658	0.15	0.679
	Δ z-BMI (0–18y)					
	Zero-Order		Partial [1]		Partial [2]	
	R	P	R	p	R	p
Structural arterial parameters, local and regional arterial stiffness						
z-R-CCA SD	0.15	0.015	0.07	0.846	0.23	0.517
z-R-CCA DD	0.14	0.021	0.04	0.902	0.25	0.494
z-R-CCA IMT	0.03	0.604	0.15	0.667	−0.26	0.468
z-L-CCA SD	0.13	0.034	0.11	0.755	0.07	0.844

Table 7. *Cont.*

z-L-CCA DD	0.12	0.054	0.08	0.820	0.10	0.789
z-L-CCA IMT	0.06	0.283	−0.05	0.895	0.06	0.878
z-R-CFA SD	0.08	0.418	0.01	0.967	0.20	0.575
z-R-CFA DD	0.08	0.437	−0.08	0.806	0.18	0.615
z-R-CFA IMT	0.17	0.390	0.31	0.354	−0.16	0.656
z-L-CFA SD	0.11	0.244	−0.02	0.948	0.12	0.750
z-L-CFA DD	0.10	0.307	−0.17	0.622	0.10	0.784
z-L-CFA IMT	−0.15	0.445	0.08	0.813	0.13	0.731
z-R-CCA EM	0.02	0.788	0.38	0.254	0.33	0.359
z-L-CCA EM	0.06	0.296	0.37	0.267	0.44	0.208
z-R-CFA EM	0.02	0.821	−0.31	0.358	−0.37	0.298
z-L-CFA EM	−0.05	0.630	−0.52	0.105	−0.29	0.409
z-cfPWV	0.01	0.802	−0.29	0.387	0.32	0.367

z: z-score. BW, BH: body weight and height. BMI: body mass index. SBP, DBP, PP, MBP: systolic, diastolic, pulse and mean pressure (p: peripheral, c: central). AIx, AIx@75: augmentation index without and with heart rate adjustment. AP: augmented pressure. Pf, Pb: forward and backward pressure components. CCA, CFA: common carotid and femoral artery. EM: elastic modulus. IMT: intima-media thickness. DD, SD: diastolic and systolic diameter. cfPWV: carotid-femoral pulse wave velocity. *R*: Pearson coefficient. $p < 0.05$ (red) was considered significant. Partial correlations controlling for: [1] BW-for-BH (length) z-score at birth; [2] BW-for-BH z-score at birth and z-BMI at the time of CV study.

Table 8. Associations between CV z-scores and z-BMI variations between 6–18 y (adolescent cohort, $n = 340$).

	Δ z-BMI (6–18y)					
	Zero-Order		**Partial [1]**		**Partial [2]**	
	R	*p*	*R*	*p*	*R*	*p*
Aortic and peripheral blood pressure, hemodynamic and wave reflection parameters						
z-pSBP	0.09	0.172	−0.29	0.453	−0.24	0.566
z-pDBP	0.07	0.286	−0.31	0.419	−0.23	0.591
z-pPP	0.04	0.478	0.04	0.918	0.01	0.980
z-pMBP	0.09	0.162	−0.35	0.357	−0.27	0.521
z-cSBP	0.05	0.461	−0.22	0.565	−0.65	**0.079**
z-cDBP	−0.01	0.818	−0.42	0.260	−0.42	0.305
z-cPP	0.06	0.301	0.12	0.749	−0.51	0.193
z-AIx	0.03	0.602	−0.56	0.114	−0.51	0.200
z-AIx@75	0.09	0.159	−0.53	0.142	−0.45	0.264
z-AP	0.02	0.744	−0.56	0.114	−0.49	0.219
z-PF	0.02	0.707	−0.14	0.725	−0.31	0.453
z-PB	−0.08	0.211	−0.20	0.598	−0.37	0.364
Structural arterial parameters, local and regional arterial stiffness						
z-R-CCA SD	0.10	0.123	−0.55	0.123	−0.74	**0.035**
z-R-CCA DD	0.09	0.129	−0.38	0.308	−0.59	0.120
z-R-CCA IMT	0.12	**0.060**	0.20	0.600	−0.14	0.747
z-L-CCA SD	0.10	0.100	−0.18	0.651	−0.23	0.583
z-L-CCA DD	0.09	0.136	−0.10	0.804	−0.11	0.791
z-L-CCA IMT	0.09	0.150	−0.01	0.975	−0.33	0.418
z-R-CFA SD	0.18	**0.057**	0.14	0.722	0.13	0.754
z-R-CFA DD	0.18	**0.069**	0.10	0.795	0.30	0.475
z-R-CFA IMT	0.19	0.363	0.28	0.473	−0.34	0.415
z-L-CFA SD	0.11	0.273	−0.04	0.927	−0.14	0.748
z-L-CFA DD	0.10	0.322	−0.11	0.776	0.01	0.988
z-L-CFA IMT	−0.26	0.190	−0.28	0.470	−0.52	0.184
z-R-CCA EM	0.06	0.317	0.26	0.503	−0.20	0.631
z-L-CCA EM	0.06	0.345	0.13	0.746	−0.21	0.619
z-R-CFA EM	−0.10	0.308	0.12	0.759	0.66	**0.075**
z-L-CFA EM	−0.09	0.351	−0.20	0.604	0.37	0.365
z-cfPWV	−0.03	0.621	−0.63	**0.068**	−0.35	0.390

z: z-score. BW, BH: body weight and height. BMI: body mass index. SBP, DBP, PP, MBP: systolic, diastolic, pulse and mean pressure (p: peripheral, c: central). AIx, AIx@75: augmentation index without and with heart rate adjustment. AP: augmented pressure. Pf, Pb: forward and backward pressure components. CCA, CFA: common carotid and femoral artery. EM: elastic modulus. IMT: intima-media thickness. cfPWV: carotid-femoral pulse wave velocity. DD, SD: diastolic and systolic diameter. *R*: Pearson coefficient. $p < 0.05$ (red) was considered significant. Partial correlations controlling for: [1] BW-for-BH (lenght) z-score at birth; [2] BW-for-BH z-score at birth and z-BMI at the time of CV study (18 y).

Table 9. Multiple regression analysis between CVvariables (dependent) and anthropometric and CRFsvariables (independent) in children cohort (n = 632).

Dependent	Independent Variables	βu	SE	βs	p	VIF	AdjR^2
Aortic and peripheral blood pressure, hemodynamic and wave reflection parameters							
z-pSBP	Constant	−0.069	0.097		0.477		0.071
	Current z-BMI	0.245	0.062	0.276	**<0.001**	1.00	
z-pDBP	Constant	−0.114	0.108		0.296		0.038
	Current z-BMI	0.203	0.069	0.208	**0.004**	1.00	
z-pPP	-	–	–	–	–	–	–
z-pMBP	Constant	−0.112	0.107		0.295		0.065
	Current z-BMI	0.247	0.068	0.255	**<0.001**	1.00	
z-cSBP	Constant	0.001	0.054		0.985		0.500
	z-pSBP	0.643	0.048	0.707	**<0.001**	1.00	
z-cDBP	Constant	−0.033	0.068		0.625		0.223
	z-pSBP	0.438	0.060	0.477	**<0.001**	1.00	
z-cPP	Constant	0.045	0.071		0.527		0.104
	z-pSBP	0.296	0.063	0.330	**<0.001**	1.00	
z-AIx	Constant	−0.059	0.072		0.414		0.099
	z-pSBP	−0.293	0.064	−0.323	**<0.001**	1.00	
z-AIx@75	Constant	−0.036	0.073		0.627		0.082
	z-pSBP	−0.270	0.066	−0.295	**<0.001**	1.00	
z-AP	Constant	−0.07	0.07		0.336		0.082
	z-pSBP	−0.23	0.06	−0.25	**<0.001**	1.00	
	z-BWH at birth	−0.17	0.07	−0.17	**0.018**	1.00	
z-Pf	Constant	0.069	0.073		0.343		0.149
	z-pSBP	0.361	0.065	0.386	**<0.001**	1.00	
z-Pb	Constant	−0.028	0.077		0.720		0.035
	z-pSBP	0.189	0.069	0.201	**0.007**	1.00	
Structural arterial parameters, local and regional arterial stiffness							
z-R-CCA SD	Constant	−0.222	0.127		**0.084**		0.173
	Current z-BMI	0.335	0.089	0.399	**<0.001**		
	z-pSBP	−0.205	0.091	−0.238	**0.027**		
z-R-CCA DD	Constant	−0.209	0.128		0.107		0.141
	Current z-BMI	0.325	0.090	0.385	**0.001**	1.05	
	z-pSBP	−0.200	0.092	−0.231	**0.033**	1.05	
z-R-CCA IMT	Constant	−0.147	0.146		0.317		0.117
	ΔBWH z-score (0–2y)	0.404	0.115	0.513	**0.001**	1.93	
	z-BWH at birth	0.334	0.159	0.306	**0.039**	1.93	
z-L-CCA SD	Constant	−0.121	0.096		0.207		0.100
	Current z-BMI	0.249	0.061	0.326	**<0.001**	1.00	
z-L-CCA DD	Constant	−0.071	0.086		0.414		0.099
	z-BMI	0.339	0.080	0.467	**<0.001**	1.22	
	Δz-BMI (0–6y) * current z-BMI	−0.050	0.023	−0.239	**0.032**	1.22	
z-L-CCA IMT	Constant	−0.118	0.123		0.340		0.029
	z-BMI	0.180	0.078	0.190	**0.024**	1.00	
z-R-CFA SD	Constant	−0.077	0.127		0.545		0.169
	Δz-BMI (0–6y)	0.347	0.090	0.411	**<0.001**	1.00	
z-R-CFA DD	**Constant**	−0.086	0.127		0.498		0.157
	Δz-BMI (0–6y)	0.347	0.090	0.410	**<0.001**	1.00	
z-R-CFA IMT	**Constant**	0.378	0.242		0.144		0.259
	Δz-BMI (0–6y)	−0.751	0.319	−0.562	**0.036**	1.00	

Table 9. *Cont.*

Dependent	Independent Variables	βu	SE	βs	*p*	VIF	AdjR^2
z-L-CFA SD	Constant	−0.161	0.113		0.157		0.034
	Current z-BMI	0.176	0.073	0.202	**0.018**	1.00	
z-L-CFA DD	Constant	−0.138	0.112		0.219		0.027
	Current z-BMI	0.159	0.073	0.185	**0.030**	1.00	
z-L-CFA IMT	Constant	−0.046	0.175		0.796		0.222
	z-pSBP	−0.448	0.147	−0.499	**0.005**	1.00	
z-R-CCA EM	Constant	0.028	0.108		0.794		0.07
	z-pSBP	0.264	0.100	0.29	**0.010**	1.00	
z-L-CCA EM	Constant	0.068	0.085		0.429		0.03
	z-pSBP	0.160	0.075	0.18	**0.034**	1.00	
z-R-CFA EM	-	-	-	-	-	-	-
z-L-CFA EM	-	-	-	-	-	-	-
z-cfPWV	-	-	-	-	-	-	-

βu and βs: un- and standardized coefficients. R: Pearson coefficient. Adj R^2: adjusted squared R. SE: Standard Error. VIF: variance inflation factor. z-: z-score. BMI: body mass index. SBP, DBP, PP, MBP: systolic, diastolic, pulse and mean pressure (p: peripheral, c: central). AIx, AIx@75: augmentation index without and with heart rate adjustment. AP: augmented pressure. Pf,Pb: forward and backward pressure components. CCA, CFA: common carotid and femoral artery. EM: elastic modulus. IMT: intima-media thickness. DD, SD: diastolic and systolic diameter. cfPWV: carotid-femoral pulse wave velocity. $p < 0.05$ was considered statistically significant. Variables entered in the model (forward method): z-BMI, z-BWH at birth, ΔBWH z-score 0–2y, Δ-zBMI0–6y, Sex (1: female, 0: male), z-pSBP, Hypertension (yes:1, no: 0). Interaction between growth parameters and z-BMI and z-BWH at birth were entered in the model if they showed significant association ($p < 0.005$) in the multiple linear regression. Only significant ($p < 0.05$) variables entered in the model are shown.

Explanatory variables for variations in structural parameters showed heterogeneity. At 6 y inter-individual variations in CCA SD and DD were associated with current z-BMI and z-pSBP. When considering CFA z-diameters or z-IMT levels the explanatory variables were: (a) current z-BMI (for z-left CCA IMT, CFA diameter), (b) Δz-BMI 0-6y (for z-Right CFA IMT and diameters), (c) ΔBWH z-score 0–2 y (for z-Right CCA IMT) and (d) BWH z-score at birth (for z-Right CCA IMT). Stiffness variations were not associated with anthropometric variations (Table 9). For the adolescents cohort (Table 10, Supplementary Table S14), the independent variables that remained significant in all the models ($p < 0.05$) were z-pSBP and current z-BMI (Table 10). Then, at 18 y nor BWH z-score at birth, nor the bodily changes during growth (early, intermediate, late or global), explained the CV interindividual variations (with the only exception being the interaction between current z-BMI and Δz-BMI 0-6 y for z-Right CCA IMT) (Table 10).

From the joint analysis of data from both cohorts and considering the exposure to CRFs, it can be asserted that: (1) current z-BMI was the variable mostly associated with CV characteristics; (2) the older the subject, CV properties (e.g., arterial structure) are less explained by changes in body size during the early growth phases.

Table 10. Multiple regression analysis between CVvariables (dependent) and anthropometric and CRFsvariables (independent) in adolescent cohort ($n = 340$).

Dependent Variable	Independent Variables	βu	SE	βs	*p*	VIF	Adj R^2
Aortic and peripheral blood pressure, hemodynamic and wave reflection parameters							
z-pSBP	Constant	0.259	0.08		**0.001**		0.049
	z-BMI	0.210	0.07	0.209	**0.002**	1.00	
z-pDBP	-	-	-	-	-	-	-
z-pPP	Constant	0.203	0.08		**0.011**		0.025
	z-BMI	0.164	0.07	0.160	**0.017**	1.00	
z-pMBP	Constant	0.201	0.08		**0.010**		0.027
	z-BMI	0.164	0.07	0.165	**0.014**	1.00	
z-cSBP	Constant	0.024	0.05		0.663		0.424
	z-BMI	0.587	0.05	0.653	**<0.001**	1.00	
z-cDBP	Constant	0.039	0.07		0.591		0.178
	z-pSBP	0.422	0.06	0.426	**<0.001**	1.00	
z-cPP	Constant	−0.036	0.06				0.136
	z-pSBP	0.259	0.05	0.313	**<0.001**	1.04	
	z-BMI	0.120	0.05	0.141	**0.030**	1.04	
z-Aix	Constant	0.077	0.07		0.297		0.019
	z-pSBP	−0.126	0.06	−0.138	**0.043**	1.00	
z-Aix@75	-	-	-	-	-	-	-
z-AP	Constant	0.071	0.07		0.324		0.019
	z-pSBP	−0.139	0.06	−0.154	**0.024**	1.00	
z-Pf	Constant	0.015	0.07		0.829		0.098
	z-pSBP	0.270	0.06	0.313	**<0.001**	1.00	
z-Pb	Constant	0.070	0.07		0.334		0.060
	z-pSBP	0.219	0.06	0.245	**<0.001**	1.00	
Structural arterial parameters, local and regional arterial stiffness							
z-R-CCA SD	Constant	0.080	0.08		0.309		0.097
	z-BMI	0.327	0.07	0.311	**<0.001**	1.00	
z-R-CCA DD	Constant	−0.111	0.11		0.313		0.118
	z-BMI	0.325	0.07	0.308	**<0.001**	1.02	
	Sex	0.335	0.15	0.143	**0.029**	1.02	
z-R-CCA IMT	Constant	0.086	0.084		0.308	1.00	0.035
	Δz-BMI 0–6y * current z-BMI	0.134	0.045	0.200	**0.003**		
z-L-CCA SD	Constant	0.052	0.08		0.493	1.02	0.069
	z-BMI	0.255	0.06	0.263	**<0.001**	1.02	
z-L-CCA DD	Constant	−0.113	0.10		0.267		0.101
	z-BMI	0.252	0.06	0.267	**<0.001**		
	Sex	0.298	0.14	0.139	**0.036**	1.00	
z-L-CCA IMT	Constant	0.129	0.09		0.131		0.033
	z-BMI	0.196	0.07	0.182	**0.008**	1.00	
z-R-CFA SD	Constant	0.286	0.11		**0.013**		0.239
	z-BMI	0.343	0.10	0.331	**0.001**	1.03	
	Smoking	−0.609	0.22	−0.275	**0.006**	1.02	
	z-pSBP	−0.222	0.10	−0.223	**0.025**	1.01	
z-R-CFA DD	Constant	0.249	0.12		**0.035**		0.184
	z-BMI	0.294	0.10	0.281	**0.006**	1.03	
	Smoking	−0.669	0.22	−0.299	**0.004**	1.02	
	z-pSBP	−0.201	0.10	−0.200	**0.047**	1.01	
z-R-CFA IMT	Constant	0.643	0.23		**0.011**		0.444
	z-BMI	0.594	0.18	0.559	**0.004**	1.02	
	Sex	−1.067	0.39	−0.453	**0.014**	1.02	
z-L-CFA SD	Constant	0.140	0.12		0.229		0.066
	z-BMI	0.303	0.12	0.278	**0.010**	1.00	

Table 10. *Cont.*

Dependent Variable	Independent Variables	βu	SE	βs	*p*	VIF	Adj R^2
z-L-CFA DD	Constant	0.077	0.12		0.513		0.065
	z-BMI	0.304	0.12	0.275	**0.011**	1.00	
z-L-CFA IMT	Constant	0.175	0.231		0.456		
	Hypertension	5.293	1.083	0.694	**0.000**	1.002	0.557
	Dyslipemia	2.836	1.083	0.372	**0.016**	1.002	
z-R-CCA EM	Constant	−0.061	0.07		0.377		0.099
	z-BMI	0.213	0.06	0.233	**0.001**		
	z-pSBP	0.149	0.06	0.168	**0.012**		
z-L-CCA EM	Constant	−0.267	0.12		**0.030**		0.147
	z-pSBP	0.356	0.11	0.334	**0.002**	1.00	
z-R-CFA EM	Constant	−0.267	0.12		**0.030**		0.111
	z-pSBP	0.356	0.11	0.334	**0.002**	1.00	
z-L-CFA EM	Constant	−0.403	0.11		**0.001**		0.060
	z-pSBP	0.251	0.10	0.267	**0.015**	1.00	
z-cfPWV	Constant	−0.055	0.07		0.401		0.069
	z-pSBP	0.224	0.06	0.263	**<0.001**	1.00	

βu and βs: un- and standardized coefficients. R: Pearson coefficient. Adj R^2: adjusted squaredR. SE: Standard Error. VIF: variance inflation factor. z-: z-score. BMI: body mass index. SBP, DBP, PP, MBP: systolic, diastolic, pulse and mean pressure (p: peripheral, c: central). AIx, AIx@75: augmentation index without and with heart rate adjustment. AP: augmented pressure. Pf, Pb: forward and backward pressure components. CCA, CFA: common carotid and femoral artery. EM: elastic modulus. IMT: intima-media thickness. DD, SD: diastolic and systolic diameter. cfPWV: carotid-femoral pulse wave velocity. $p < 0.05$ was considered statistically significant. Variables entered in the model (forward method): z-BMI, BWH at birth, Δ-zBMI0–6y, Sex (1: female, 0: male), z-pSBP, Hypertension (1: yes, 0: no), Dislypemia (1: yes, 0: no), Smoking (1: yes, 0: no), Sedentarism (1: yes, 0: no). Interactions between growth parameters and z-BMI or z-BWH were entered in the model if they showed significant association in multiple linear regressions. Only significant ($p < 0.05$) independent variables entered in the models are shown.

4. Discussion

To our knowledge, this is the first study to describe the association of growth-related changes in body size during early, intermediate, late, or global growth with hemodynamic (central and peripheral) and arterial (structural and functional) properties in early childhood and beginning of adulthood, adjusting for characteristics at birth, at the time of the CV study and for CRFs exposure. Associations were assessed considering three interrelated comparative analysis: (1) strength and (2) independence of the associations and (3) explanatory power of anthropometric parameters and factors associated with CV risk. Our main findings were:

- First, growth-related body size changes (0–2 and 0–6 y) were associated with interindividual variations (z-score) in CV properties at 6 y. Conversely, CV z-scores variables at 18 y were not associated with body size changes (0–6, 6–18 or 0–18 y) (Tables 2 and 3). Thus, as the subject's age increases, the association between CV properties and prior body size changes (i.e., during childhood) decreases (Table 4).
- Second, the strength of association between growth-related body changes and CV properties at 6 y was: (a) equal or greater than that observed for body size at birth and (b) lower than the obtained for current z-BMI (at 6 y). Most of the associations between ΔBWH z-score 0–2 y or Δz-BMI 0–6 y and the CV properties at 6 y were independent of the BWH z-score at birth (Tables 5 and 6). Then, in 6 y children the "hierarchical order" among explanatory variables for CV variations would be: current z-BMI > ΔBWH z-score 0–2 y or Δz-BMI 0–6 y> BWH z-score at birth (Table 2). On the contrary, only current z-BMI showed significant association with CV properties at 18 y (Table 3). In summary, while current z-BMI showed the strongest association, body size at birth showed almost no association with CV properties, regardless of subjects' age at the time of the CV study (Tables 2 and 3).
- Third, in general terms, current z-BMI was the anthropometric parameter with the greatest explanatory capacity for CV variations observed at 6 y. Though, variations in some CV parameters

were mainly explained by growth-related body changes and/or by their interaction with current z-BMI (Tables S4 and S6). Similar results were observed when the associations were analyzed considering the exposure to CRFs (e.g., hypertension, dyslipidemia) (Table 9). In turn, current z-BMI was the anthropometric variable with the greatest explanatory capacity for CV conditions and variations at 18 y.In summary, body size changes during childhood and/or adolescence contributed to explain arterial variations through the interaction with current z-BMI or BWH z-score at birth (Tables S8, S10 and S12). Among factors associated with CV risk, z-BMI and/or z-pSBP were the main explanatory variables for CV z-scores (Table 10).

The explanatory capacity of growth-related body changes was reduced or lost with, as the age at which the CV system was evaluated increased. In this regard, at least two issues must be analyzed. On the one hand, the impact (association) of anthropometric changes on the CV properties evaluated at a given age, would vary, depending on the period of "body change or gain" considered (e.g., 0–2 y vs. 0–6 y). On the other hand, the association between CV properties and the anthropometric changes observed in a given period (e.g., 0–6 y) could depend on the age at which the CV system is evaluated (e.g., 6 vs. 18 y, like in this work). Studies suggested that BW gain patterns in very early infancy (e.g., 0–6 postnatal mos.) [22–24] would be particularly important as determinants of future pBP levels, while other studies showed that BW gain during childhood would be a stronger predictor of pBP [25,26]. The exact "timing of the BW gain" associated with middle or long-term CV risk is still debated, highlighting the need for additional research to clarify and/or reconcile mixed findings. In this work, in general terms we did not find differences in the strength of association when comparing 0–2 vs. 0–6 y data, but some CV characteristics assessed at 6 y showed greater association with 0–6 y anthropometric changes. Evelein et al. (2013) reported that postnatal BW for length gain (0-3 mos.) was associated with carotid IMT (but not stiffness) in children (5 y) [21]. However, when data about growth in later infancy (3–6, 6–9 and 9–12 mos.) were considered, no associations with arterial properties were found [21]. Skilton et al. (2013) reported that BW gain, BH-adjusted-BW gain and ΔBWH z-score 0-18 mos. were positively associated with carotid IMT assessed at 8 y [27]. Unfortunately, the impact of changes in different periods was not analyzed. Linhares et al. (2015) found that the "adverse" long-term effect of accelerated growth in infancy varied depending on the time of growth acceleration. Particularly, carotid IMT at ~30 y was associated with 2–4 y BW-gain, rather than with early BW gain [7]. Additionally, Vianna et al. (2016), found that the relative BW-gain between 2 and 4 y was associated with increased aortic stiffness (evaluated by cfPWV) at ~30 y, whereas birth weight, BW-gain within the first 2 years of life (0–2 y) and linear growth (length/height gain) in childhood were not associated with cfPWV [28]. Pais et al. (2016) assessed PWV in children (8–9 y) and analyzed data considering and categorizing growth trajectories. The highest arterial stiffness levels were observed in groups with accelerated body growth during childhood, with adequate early growth pattern [29].

The dependence on the age at the time of CV study ascribed to the association between an anthropometric parameter and CV properties has been previously described, mainly for birth weight. About this, body size at birth has been associated with pBP levels, andit was reported that the relation becomes progressively stronger with increasing age, being hypothesized that the initiating process occurs in uterus and amplifies throughout life [11,30,31], satisfying theories that seek to explain the detriment of the CV system related to low birth weight and/or catch-up growth [32]. It was even postulated that interactions between increased arterial stiffness, increased pPP, stretching of vascular smooth muscles and synthesis of collagen may contribute to the amplification phenomenon through a feedback loop [33]. By contrast, Lule et al. analyzed data from studies that measured pBP at different ages and did not find an age-related increase in the strength of the association between birth weight and pBP [6]. Furthermore, the relationship between birth weight and later pBP varied depending on the age of the participants: neonates showed consistent positive association; mainly negative associations were seen in children, and studies in adolescents showed inconsistent results [6]. Then, as age increases, the positive association observed in neonates could become negative, non-existent or even positive, which is in agreement with our findings. This could be explained, at least in theory by the fact that as age increases the exposure-time to already present factors capable of impacting on the CV system also increases. As age increases, subjects could become exposed to factors (i.e., CRFs) capable of modifyingCV properties. Then, the association between anthropometricchanges and CVproperties could be modified by exposure to co-factors.

As mentioned in 6 y children the "hierarchical order" among explanatory variables for CV variations would be: current z-BMI >ΔBWH z-score 0–2 y or Δz-BMI 0–6 y> BWH z-score at birth (Table 2). Conversely, only current z-BMI showed significant association with arterial properties at 18 y (Table 3). Birth weight showed almost no association with CV properties, disregard of the subjects' age at the time of the CV study (Tables 2 and 3), and most of the associations between ΔBWH z-score 0–2 y or Δz-BMI 0–6 y and CV characteristics at 6 ywere independent of birth conditions (Tables 5 and 6). Then, the association between body-size changes during infancy or childhood and the CV system at 6 y, would not depend on having been born with low, normal or elevated BWH. When current z-BMI was considered some associations between bodily changes in childhood and CV properties at 6 y were no longer significant. In adolescents, the associations between body changes and CV variables were always dependent on z-BMI at the time of CV study (Tables 6–8).

The dependence (or independence) of the association between CV parameters and growth–related anthropometric changes on bodysize at birth and/or on current z-BMI has been previously assessed, with dissimilar findings. A positive association was observed between BW gain or adiposity accumulation during childhood and later pBP levels [23,34–37]. However, the extent to which birth size modifies the associations between postnatal growth and future pBP levels and/or arterial properties remains unclear. Belfort et al. (2007) found that infants who were thinner at birth were more susceptible to adverse effects on pBP at 3 y of accelerated BWH gain within the first 6 postnatal mos. [22]. Whether the finding is extensive to mid-childhood when BP is highly correlated with adult BP [38] is to be clarified. Leunissen et al. (2012) showed that regardless of birth-size, adiposity accumulation during childhood is a risk factor for later (~20 y) development of high BP levels [37]. Accordingly, Kelishadi's review (2014) concludes that early growth, rather than birth weight, would be important as a determinant of later BP levels [32]. Supporting a BMI-independent association between body size changes and CV properties, Thiering et al. studied children (n = 1127, age≤10 y) and reported that higher BW peak (velocity) in infancy was associated with an increase in pSBP and pDBP after confounders adjustment [39]. In contrast, it has been proposed that the association between BMI at adiposity peak and BP at 6 y would be mediated by current BMI [40]. Marinkovic et al. (2017) observed that infant peak BW velocity and BMI at adiposity peak associationwith childhood pSBP and pDBP (at 6 y), which could be explained by current BMI [12].

Our results support the proposal that the association between anthropometric parameters and pBP depends on current BMI, at the same time as they provide original information showing that unlike what was described for pBP, the association between growth-related body size changes (0–2 y) and cBP at 6 y would not depend on current z-BMI. This is further supported by the fact that reflection parameters, which are main determinants of the differences between cBPand pBP, also showed associations not explained by current BMI (Tables 5 and 6). It is to note that compared to pBP, the cBP would be of greater value in terms of association with CVchanges and risk prediction [41].

As stated above, the association between growth-related body-size changes and arterial thickness has been previously described [21,27,42]. Our results provide additional information, showing that at 6 y, the association between body size gain and thickness is independent of body size at birth and current z-BMI at 6 y, and that it is statistical significant for both carotid (elastic) and femoral (muscular) arteries. In turn, Evelein et al. (2013) described interaction between birth size and postnatal weight for length by analyzing the impact on arterial stiffness (i.e., distensibility and arterial elastic modulus). The thinner the children were at birth, the lower the distensibility (greater the elastic modulus) with increasing weight for length gain [21]. Then, the impact of birth-size and or growth-related changes would vary depending on the CV properties considered.

Finally, as mentioned, current z-BMI was the anthropometric parameter with the greatest explanatory capacity (power) for the CV variations observed at 6 and 18 y. However, interindividual variations in some hemodynamic and arterial parameters at 6 and 18 y were mainly explained by growth-related body changes and/or by their interaction with current z-BMI (Tables S4 and S6 for children; Tables S8, S10 and S12 for adolescents). Similar results were observed when the associations were analyzed taking into account the exposure to CRFs (Tables 9 and 10). In children, body change during growth, independently or by means of an interaction with current z-BMI, allowed to explain to a greater extent some CV characteristics (i.e., arterial thicknesses and diameters). In other words, disregard of birth size, exposure to CRFs and/or z-pBP, arterial wall thickness and/or diameters at 6 y could be explained by body growth between 0–2 or 0–6 y. Thus, although CV properties at 6 y would be associated with current z-BMI, knowing the history of BW gain could contribute to a better understanding of the CV characteristics of a specific child. Two children with similar z-BMI, could present CV differences associated with their "history" of body size changes (e.g., between 0–2 or 0–6y). Furthermore, for variables such as wall thickness in children, the history of weight gain would havegreater explanatory capacity than current z-BMI or factors with recognized impact on the CV system (e.g., CRFs). In adolescents, the history of BW gain would not be a primary explanatory variable for CVvariables (i.e., for IMT), but due to variables interactions it could contribute or complement data obtained from current z-BMI and/or BP.

5. Strengths and Limitations

This work has several strengths that should be considered. First, the population-based prospective cohort design, including a large number of subjects studied from early life. Repeated measures during growth-period enabled us to study the impact of growth profiles or patterns on CV properties, assessed at two specific times: early childhood (6 y) and onset of adulthood (18 y). Second, we used our own specific "reference populations" to define CV z-scores (Supplementary Tables S1 and S2). Third, many potential confounders were considered in order to isolate the effect of BW gain in the statistical models. Fourth, taking into account that the impact of body change on the CV system may depend on the period in which it occurs, we studied different periods of body gain (0–2, 0–6, 0–18, 6–18 y). Fifth, the relationship between BW gain and adult pBP is one of the most studied, based on the "fetal origin" hypothesis, but pBP is a particular variable and does not inform about central hemodynamic conditions, or about structural and/or functional arterial changes (e.g., associated with early vascular aging or atherosclerosis development). Thus, we designed an integral approach in which multiple CV parameters (e.g., pBP, cBP, arterial diametersand thicknesses, local and regional stiffness) and different arterial pathways (i.e., elastic and muscular) were evaluated. Sixth, unlike most works that analyzed the associations between body changes and the CV system considering a single age, we studied children and young adults. Up to now, most studies included premature, small for gestational age, obese and/or hypertensive subjects and data about the CVimpact of growth-related bodychanges in healthy pediatric and/or adolescent populations werescarce. In this work, healthy children and adolescents were studied.

Some limitations should be considered. First, we did not have information about blood biomarkers measured by our technicians. Therefore data about some conditions (i.e., existence of dyslipidemia) was obtained from reference physicians, registers and/or self-reports. Second, although we adjusted for several potential confounders, residual confounding factors may persist, as in any observational study. Third, in this work we chose to use change in BWH z-score or z-BMI between two time points as growth-indicators. This approach is a simple practical (clinical) method for quantifying a "change"; although more detailed growth patterns could be derived from longitudinally collected anthropometric measures in both cohorts. Fourth, we did not perform an analysis discriminating by sex; despite we are aware of data suggesting that the impact of childhood growth on the CV system may differ between boys and girls [12]. Fifth, we included subjects born at term and preterm, but as most of them belonged to the first condition (98% and 92% inchildren and adolescent cohorts, respectively) the results should be assigned to term-born subjects. Sixth, comparative analysis of the associations between anthropometric data and CV (hemodynamic and/or arterial) variables measured at 6 and 18 y was done considering two different cohorts, instead of a single cohort followed for more than 20 years. Although obtaining similar data for different cohorts could be considered as strength of the work, as a limiting factor it should be noted that for some variables data were not obtained in both cohorts and some aspects of the associations could only be evaluated in one of them. Finally, we did not analyze growth considering body composition (e.g., fat mass) and its changes as was previously done [43].

6. Conclusions

Body-size changes in infancy (0–2 y) and childhood (0–6 y) showed similar strength of association with respect to CV properties assessed at 6 y. Conversely, changes between 0–6, 6-18 or 0–18 y were not associated with CV parameters evaluated at 18 y.

The association between CV characteristics at 6 yand body-size changes during growth showed: (a) equal or greater strength than the observed for body-size at birth, and (b) lower strength with respect to that obtained when considering current z-BMI at 6 y. In 6 y children variables capable of explaining CV variations showed a "hierarchical order". Conversely, only z-BMI at 18 y showed significant associations with arterial z-scores at 18 y. Body size at birth showed almost no association with arterial characteristics at 6 or 18 y. The associations between ΔBWH z-score 0–2 y or Δz-BMI 0–6 y and CV properties at 6 y were mostly independent of body-size at birth. When current z-BMI was taken into account some associations between body changes in childhood and CV properties at 6 y were no longer significant. In adolescents, the associations between growth-related body changes and CV properties were dependent on z-BMI at the time of CVstudy.

Current z-BMI was the anthropometric parameter with the greatest capacity to explain the variations in CV properties at 6 y. However, interindividual variations in some hemodynamic and arterial parameters were mainly explained by growth-related anthropometric changes and/or by their interaction with current z-BMI. Similar findings were observed when the associations were analyzed taking into account the exposure to factors associated with CV risk. Current z-BMI at 18 y was the anthropometric variable with the greatest capacity to explain CV variations at 18 y. Body-size changes during childhood and/or adolescence contributed to explain arterial variations through the interaction with current z-BMI or BWH z-score at birth.

Supplementary Materials:
Table S1. Clinical, anthropometric hemodynamic, structural and stiffness parameters forchildren and adolescent reference subgroups; Table S2. Hemodynamic, structural and stiffness parameters z-score, forchildren and adolescent Cohorts; Table S3. Multiple linear regression analysis between CVparameters z-scores (dependent variables) and anthropometric parameters (independent variables), children cohort (n = 632); Table S4. Multiple linear regression analysis between CV parameters z-scores (dependent variables) and anthropometric parameters (independent variables), children cohort (n = 632); Table S5. Multiple linear regression analysis between CV parameters z-scores (dependent variables) and anthropometric parameters (independent variables), children cohort (n = 632); Table S6. Multiple linear regression analysis between CV parameters z-scores (dependent variables) and anthropometric parameters (independent variables), children cohort (n = 632); Table S7. Multiple linear regression analysis between CV parameters z-scores (dependent variables) and anthropometric parameters (independent variables), adolescent cohort (n = 340); Table S8. Multiple linear regression analysis between CV parameters z-scores (dependent variables) and anthropometric parameters (independent variables), adolescent cohort (n = 340); Table S9. Multiple linear regression analysis between CV parameters z-scores (dependent variables) and anthropometric parameters (independent variables), adolescent cohort (n = 340); Table S10. Multiple linear regression analysis between CV parameters z-scores (dependent variables) and anthropometric parameters (independent variables), adolescent cohort (n = 340); Table S11. Multiple linear regression analysis between CV parameters z-scores (dependent variables) and anthropometricparameters (independent variables), adolescent cohort (n = 340); Table S12. Multiple linear regression analysis between CV parameters z-scores (dependent variables) and anthropometric parameters (independent variables), adolescent cohort (n = 340); Table S13. Multiple linear regression analysis between CV parameters z-scores (dependent variables) and anthropometric parameters and CVRFs (independent variables), children cohort (n = 632) (Enter Method); Table S14. Multiple linear regression analysis between CV parameters z-scores (dependent variables) and anthropometric parameters and CVRFs (independent variables), adolescent cohort (n = 340) (Enter Method)

Author Contributions: Conceptualization, D.B. and Y.Z.; Formal analysis, J.M.C., D.B. and Y.Z.; Funding acquisition, D.B. and Y.Z.; Investigation, D.B. and Y.Z.; Methodology, J.M.C., V.G.-E., A.Z., M.M., C.S., D.B. and Y.Z.; Project administration, D.B. and Y.Z.; Visualization, J.M.C., D.B. and Y.Z.; Writing–original draft, J.M.C., D.B. and Y.Z.; Writing–review and editing, J.M.C., V.G.-E., A.Z., M.M., C.S., P.C., D.B. and Y.Z.

Acknowledgments: We thank the children, adolescents and their families for their participation in the study. The authors thank the technical staff from CUiiDARTE and IECON (Lic. Cecilia Toledo and LucíaNuñez). ELBU Study (IECON; http://fcea.edu.uy/estudio-del-bienestar-multidimensional-en-uruguay.html) is directed by Martín Leites, Gonzalo Salas and Andrea Vigorito.

Abbreviations

AIx	central (aortic) augmentation index
AIx@75	AIx adjusted to a 75 beats/min heart rate
AP	central (aortic) augmented pressure
BH	body height
BMI	body mass index
BW	body weight
BWH	body weight for body height
cBP	central (aortic) blood pressure
CCA	common carotid artery
CFA	common femoral artery
cfPWV	carotid-femoral pulse wave velocity
CRFs	cardiovascular risk factors
CV	cardiovascular
CVD	cardiovascular disease
DD	diastolic arterial diameter
EM	pressure-strain arterial elastic modulus
HBP	high blood pressure levels
HR	heart rate
IMT	intima-media thickness
LBW	low birth weight
MLR	multiple linear regression models
mos.	Months
MV	mean value
Pb	amplitude of the cBP backward component
pBP	peripheral (brachial) blood pressure
pDBP	peripheral (brachial) diastolic blood pressure
Pf	amplitude of the cBP forward component
pMBP	peripheral (brachial) mean blood pressure
pPP	peripheral (brachial) pulse pressure
pSBP	peripheral (brachial) systolic blood pressure
PWA	pulse wave analysis
SD	systolic arterial diameter
STD	standard deviation
VIF	variance inflation factor
y	years old
z	z-score

References

1. Ayer, J.G.; Harmer, J.A.; Nakhla, S.; Xuan, W.; Ng, M.K.; Raitakari, O.T.; Marks, G.B.; Celermajer, D.S. HDL-cholesterol, blood pressure, and asymmetric dimethylarginine are significantly associated with arterial wall thickness in children. *Arterioscler. Thromb. Vasc. Biol.* **2009**, *29*, 943–949. [CrossRef] [PubMed]
2. Umer, A.; Kelley, G.A.; Cottrell, L.E.; Giacobbi, P., Jr.; Innes, K.E.; Lilly, C.L. Childhood obesity and adult cardiovascular disease risk factors: A systematic review with meta-analysis. *BMC Public Health* **2017**, *17*, 683. [CrossRef] [PubMed]
3. Weihrauch-Blüher, S.; Schwarz, P.; Klusmann, J.H. Childhood obesity: Increased risk for cardiometabolic disease and cancer in adulthood. *Metabolism* **2019**, *92*, 147–152. [CrossRef] [PubMed]
4. Huxley, R.; Neil, A.; Collins, R. Unravelling the fetal origins hypothesis: Is there really an inverse association between birthweight and subsequent blood pressure? *Lancet* **2002**, *360*, 659–665. [CrossRef]
5. Leunissen, R.W.; Kerkhof, G.F.; Stijnen, T.; Hokken-Koelega, A. Timing and tempo of first-year rapid growth in relation to cardiovascular and metabolic risk profile in early adulthood. *JAMA* **2009**, *301*, 2234–2242. [CrossRef] [PubMed]
6. Lule, S.A.; Elliott, A.M.; Smeeth, L.; Webb, E.L. Is birth weight associated with blood pressure among African children and adolescents? A systematic review. *J. Dev. Orig. Health Dis.* **2018**, *9*, 270–280. [CrossRef] [PubMed]
7. da Silva Linhares, R.; Gigante, D.P.; de Barros, F.C.; Horta, B.L. Carotid intima-media thickness at age 30, birth weight, accelerated growth during infancy and breastfeeding: A birth cohort study in Southern Brazil. *PLoS ONE* **2015**, *10*, e0115166.
8. Adair, L.S.; Fall, C.H.D.; Osmond, C.; Stein, A.D.; Martorell, R.; Ramirez-Zea, M.; Sachdev, H.S.; Dahly, D.L.; Bas, I.; Norris, S.A.; et al. Associations of linear growth and relative weight gain during early life with adult health and human capital in countries of low and middle income: Findings from five birth cohort studies. *Lancet* **2013**, *382*, 525–534. [CrossRef]
9. Ong, K.K.; Ahmed, M.L.; Emmett, P.M.; Preece, M.A.; Dunger, D.B. Association between postnatal catch-up growth and obesity in childhood: Prospective cohort study. *BMJ* **2000**, *320*, 967–971. [CrossRef]
10. Jansen, M.A.C.; Uiterwaal, C.S.P.M.; van der Ent, C.K.; Grobbee, D.E.; Dalmeijer, G.W. Excess early postnatal weight gain and blood pressure in healthy young children. *J. Dev. Orig. Health Dis.* **2019**, *30*, 1–7. [CrossRef]
11. Law, C.M.; de Swiet, M.; Osmond, C.; Fayers, P.M.; Barker, D.J.; Cruddas, A.M.; Fall, C.H. Initiation of hypertension in utero and its amplification throughout life. *BMJ* **1993**, *306*, 24–27. [CrossRef] [PubMed]
12. Marinkovic, T.; Toemen, L.; Kruithof, C.J.; Reiss, I.; van Osch-Gevers, L.; Hofman, A.; Franco, O.H.; Jaddoe, V.W.V. Early infant growth velocity patterns and cardiovascular and metabolic outcomes in childhood. *J. Pediatr.* **2017**, *186*, 57–63. [CrossRef] [PubMed]
13. Garcia-Espinosa, V.; Bia, D.; Castro, J.; Zinoveev, A.; Marin, M.; Giachetto, G.; Chiesa, P.; Zócalo, Y. Peripheral and central aortic pressure, wave-derived reflection parameters, local and regional arterial stiffness and structural parameters in children and adolescents: Impact of body mass index variations. *High Blood Press. Cardiovasc. Prev.* **2018**, *25*, 267–280. [CrossRef] [PubMed]
14. Zócalo, Y.; Ungerfeld, R.; Pérez-Clariget, R.; Bia, D. Maternal nutritional restriction during gestation impacts differently on offspring muscular and elastic arteries and is associated with increased carotid resistance and ventricular afterload in maturity. *J. Dev. Orig. Health Dis.* **2019**, 1–11. [CrossRef] [PubMed]
15. Zócalo, Y.; Curcio, S.; García-Espinosa, V.; Chiesa, P.; Giachetto, G.; Bia, D. Comparative analysis of arterial parameters variations associated with inter-individual variations in peripheral and aortic blood pressure: Cross-sectional study in healthy subjects aged 2-84 years. *High Blood Press. Cardiovasc. Prev.* **2017**, *24*, 437–451. [CrossRef] [PubMed]
16. Zócalo, Y.; Castro, J.M.; Garcia-Espinosa, V.; Curcio, S.; Chiesa, P.; Giachetto, G.; Cabrera-Fischer, E.I.; Bia, D. Forward and backward aortic components and reflection indexes in children and adolescents: Determinants and role in high pressure states. *Curr. Hypertens. Rev.* **2018**, *14*, 137–153. [CrossRef] [PubMed]
17. Amarante, V.; Arim, R.; Severi, C.; Vigorito, A.; Aldabe, I.; de Melo, G.; Rodríguez, A.; Salas, G. *El Estadonutricional de los NiñOs/as y las Políticasalimentarías*; Programa Naciones Unidas para e Desarrollo (PNUD)-UNICEF: Montevideo, Uruguay, 2007.

18. Lurbe, E.; Agabiti-Rosei, E.; Cruickshank, J.K.; Dominiczak, A.; Erdine, S.; Hirth, A.; Invitti, C.; Litwin, M.; Mancia, G.; Pall, D.; et al. 2016 European Society of Hypertension guidelines for the management of high blood pressure in children and adolescents. *J. Hypertens.* **2016**, *34*, 1887–1920. [CrossRef] [PubMed]
19. García-Espinosa, V.; Curcio, S.; Marotta, M.; Castro, J.M.; Arana, M.; Peluso, G.; Chiesa, P.; Giachetto, G.; Bia, D.; Zócalo, Y. Changes in central aortic pressure levels, wave components and determinants associated with high peripheral blood pressure states in childhood: Analysis of hypertensive phenotype. *Pediatr. Cardiol.* **2016**, *37*, 1340–1350. [CrossRef] [PubMed]
20. Diedenhofen, B.; Musch, J. Cocor: A comprehensive solution for the statistical comparison of correlations. *PLoS ONE* **2015**, *10*, e0121945. [CrossRef] [PubMed]
21. Evelein, A.M.; Visseren, F.L.; van der Ent, C.K.; Grobbee, D.E.; Uiterwaal, C.S. Excess early postnatal weight gain leads to thicker and stiffer arteries in young children. *J. Clin. Endocrinol. Metab.* **2013**, *98*, 794–801. [CrossRef] [PubMed]
22. Belfort, M.B.; Rifas-Shiman, S.L.; Rich-Edwards, J.; Kleinman, K.P.; Gillman, M.W. Size at birth, infant growth, and blood pressure at three years of age. *J. Pediatr.* **2007**, *151*, 670–674. [CrossRef] [PubMed]
23. Ben-Shlomo, Y.; McCarthy, A.; Hughes, R.; Tilling, K.; Davies, D.; Smith, G.D. Immediate postnatal growth is associated with blood pressure in young adulthood: The Barry Caerphilly Growth Study. *Hypertension* **2008**, *52*, 638–644. [CrossRef] [PubMed]
24. Adair, L.S.; Martorell, R.; Stein, A.D.; Hallal, P.C.; Sachdev, H.S.; Prabhakaran, D.; Wills, A.K.; Norris, S.A.; Dahly, D.L.; Lee, N.R.; et al. Size at birth, weight gain in infancy and childhood, and adult blood pressure in 5 low- and middle-income-country cohorts: When does weight gain matter? *Am. J. Clin. Nutr.* **2009**, *89*, 1383–1392. [CrossRef] [PubMed]
25. Jones, A.; Charakida, M.; Falaschetti, E.; Hingorani, A.D.; Finer, N.; Masi, S.; Donald, A.E.; Lawlor, D.A.; Smith, G.D.; Deanfield, J.E. Adipose height growth through childhood blood pressure status in a large prospective cohort, s.t.u.d.y. *Hypertension* **2012**, *59*, 919–925. [CrossRef] [PubMed]
26. Tilling, K.; Davies, N.; Windmeijer, F.; Kramer, M.S.; Bogdanovich, N.; Matush, L.; Patel, R.; Smith, G.D.; Ben-Shlomo, Y.; Martin, R.M. Is infant weight associated with childhood blood pressure? Analysis of the promotion of breastfeeding intervention trial (probit) cohort. *Int. J. Epidemiol.* **2011**, *40*, 1227–1237. [CrossRef] [PubMed]
27. Skilton, M.R.; Marks, G.B.; Ayer, J.G.; Garden, F.L.; Garnett, S.P.; Harmer, J.A.; Leeder, S.R.; Toelle, B.G.; Webb, K.; Baur, L.A.; et al. Weight gain in infancy and vascular risk factors in later childhood. *Pediatrics* **2013**, *131*, 1821–1828. [CrossRef] [PubMed]
28. Vianna, C.A.; Horta, B.L.; Gigante, D.P.; de Barros, F.C. Pulse wave velocity at early adulthood: Breastfeeding and nutrition during pregnancy and childhood. *PLoS ONE* **2016**, *11*, e0152501. [CrossRef] [PubMed]
29. Pais, C.; Correia-Costa, L.; Moura, C.; Mota, C.; Severo, M.; Guerra, A.; Areias, J.C.; Schaefer, F.; CaldasAfonso, A.; Barros, H.; et al. Accelerated growth during childhood is associated with increased arterial stiffness in prepubertal children. *Int. J. Cardiol.* **2016**, *204*, 83–85. [CrossRef]
30. Huxley, R.R.; Shiell, A.W.; Law, C.M. The role of size at birth and postnatal catch-up growth in determining systolic blood pressure: A systematic review of the literature. *J. Hypertens.* **2000**, *18*, 815–831. [CrossRef]
31. Law, C.M.; Shiell, A.W. Is blood pressure inversely related to birth weight? The strength of evidence from a systematic review of the literature. *J. Hypertens.* **1996**, *14*, 935–941. [CrossRef]
32. Kelishadi, R.; Haghdoost, A.A.; Jamshidi, F.; Aliramezany, M.; Moosazadeh, M. Low birthweight or rapid catch-up growth: Which is more associated with cardiovascular disease and its risk factors in later life? A systematic review and cryptanalysis. *Paediatr. Int. Child Health* **2015**, *35*, 110–123. [CrossRef] [PubMed]
33. Martyn, C.N.; Greenwald, S.E. Impaired synthesis of elastin in walls of aorta and large conduit arteries during early development as an initiating event in pathogenesis of systemic hypertension. *Lancet* **1997**, *350*, 953–955. [CrossRef]
34. Uiterwaal, C.S.; Anthony, S.; Launer, L.J.; Witteman, J.C.; Trouwborst, A.M.; Hofman, A.; Grobbee, D.E. Birth weight, growth, and blood pressure: An annual follow-up study of children aged 5 through 21 years. *Hypertension* **1997**, *30*, 267–271. [CrossRef] [PubMed]
35. Adair, L.S.; Cole, T.J. Rapid child growth raises blood pressure in adolescent boys who were thin at birth. *Hypertension* **2003**, *41*, 451–456. [CrossRef] [PubMed]

36. Nishina, M.; Kikuchi, T.; Yamazaki, H.; Kameda, K.; Hiura, M.; Uchiyama, M. Relationship among systolic blood pressure, serum insulin and leptin, and visceral fat accumulation in obese children. *Hypertens. Res.* **2003**, *26*, 281–288. [CrossRef] [PubMed]
37. Leunissen, R.W.; Kerkhof, G.F.; Stijnen, T.; Hokken-Koelega, A.C. Effect of birth size and catch-up growth on adult blood pressure and carotid intima-media thickness. *Horm. Res. Paediatr.* **2012**, *77*, 394–401. [CrossRef] [PubMed]
38. Chen, X.; Wang, Y. Tracking of blood pressure from childhood to adulthood: A systematic review and meta-regression analysis. *Circulation* **2008**, *117*, 3171–3180. [CrossRef] [PubMed]
39. Thiering, E.; Bruske, I.; Kratzsch, J.; Hoffmann, B.; Herbarth, O.; von Berg, A.; Schaaf, B.; Wichmann, H.E.; Heinrich, J.; LISAplus Study Group. Peak growth velocity in infancy is positively associated with blood pressure in school-aged children. *J. Hypertens.* **2012**, *30*, 1114–1121. [CrossRef]
40. Hof, M.H.; Vrijkotte, T.G.; de Hoog, M.L.; van Eijsden, M.; Zwinderman, A.H. Association between infancy BMI peak and body composition and blood pressure at age 5–6 years. *PLoS ONE* **2013**, *8*, e80517. [CrossRef]
41. Peluso, G.; García-Espinosa, V.; Curcio, S.; Marota, M.; Castro, J.; Chiesa, P.; Giachetto, G.; Bia, D.; Zócalo, Y. High central aortic rather than brachial blood pressure is associated with carotid wall remodeling and increased arterial stiffness in childhood. *High Blood Press. Cardiovasc. Prev.* **2017**, *24*, 49–60. [CrossRef]
42. Skilton, M.R.; Sullivan, T.R.; Ayer, J.G.; Garden, F.L.; Harmer, J.A.; Leeder, S.R.; Toelle, B.G.; Webb, K.; Marks, G.B.; Celermajer, D.S. Weight gain in infancy is associated with carotid extra-medial thickness in later childhood. *Atherosclerosis* **2014**, *233*, 370–374. [CrossRef] [PubMed]
43. McCloskey, K.; Burgner, D.; Carlin, J.B.; Skilton, M.R.; Cheung, M.; Dwyer, T.; Vuillermin, P.; Ponsonby, A.L.; BIS Investigator Group. Infant adiposity at birth and early postnatal weight gain predict increased aortic intima-media thickness at 6 weeks of age: A population-derived cohort study. *Clin. Sci. (Lond.)* **2016**, *130*, 443–450. [CrossRef] [PubMed]

9

Fish, Fish Oils and Cardioprotection: Promise or Fish Tale?

Akshay Goel [1], Naga Venkata Pothineni [1], Mayank Singhal [2], Hakan Paydak [1], Tom Saldeen [1] and Jawahar L. Mehta [1,*]

1. Division of Cardiology, University of Arkansas for Medical Sciences and Central Arkansas Veterans Healthcare System, Little Rock, AR 72205, USA; AGoel@uams.edu (A.G.); NVPothineni@uams.edu (N.V.P.); HPaydak@uams.edu (H.P.); tom.saldeen@uppsalapharma.se (T.S.)
2. Cape Fear Valley Hospital, Fayetteville, NC 28304, USA; drmayanksinghal@gmail.com

* Correspondence: MehtaJL@uams.edu

Abstract: Fish and commercially available fish oil preparations are rich sources of long-chain omega-3 polyunsaturated fatty acids. Eicosapentaenoic acid (EPA) and docosahexaenoic acid (DHA) are the most important fatty acids in fish oil. Following dietary intake, these fatty acids get incorporated into the cell membrane phospholipids throughout the body, especially in the heart and brain. They play an important role in early brain development during infancy, and have also been shown to be of benefit in dementia, depression, and other neuropsychiatric disorders. Early epidemiologic studies show an inverse relationship between fish consumption and the risk of coronary heart disease. This led to the identification of the cardioprotective role of these marine-derived fatty acids. Many experimental studies and some clinical trials have documented the benefits of fish oil supplementation in decreasing the incidence and progression of atherosclerosis, myocardial infarction, heart failure, arrhythmias, and stroke. Possible mechanisms include reduction in triglycerides, alteration in membrane fluidity, modulation of cardiac ion channels, and anti-inflammatory, anti-thrombotic, and anti-arrhythmic effects. Fish oil supplements are generally safe, and the risk of toxicity with methylmercury, an environmental toxin found in fish, is minimal. Current guidelines recommend the consumption of either one to two servings of oily fish per week or daily fish oil supplements (around 1 g of omega-3 polyunsaturated fatty acids per day) in adults. However, recent large-scale studies have failed to demonstrate any benefit of fish oil supplements on cardiovascular outcomes and mortality. Here, we review the different trials that evaluated the role of fish oil in cardiovascular diseases.

Keywords: fish oil; omega-3 fatty acids; eicosapentaenoic acid (EPA); docosahexaenoic acid (DHA); cardiovascular disease

---

1. Introduction

Cardiovascular disease (CVD) is a leading cause of death in the United States [1]. However, despite extensive advances in our knowledge of nutritional options in the prevention and therapy of CVD, the benefits of dietary fish and fish oil supplementation on CVD remains debatable. Fish oil is a rich source of long-chain omega-3 (ω-3) polyunsaturated fatty acids (PUFAs)—eicosapentaenoic acid (EPA), and docosahexaenoic acid (DHA). The possible cardioprotective role of fish consumption was first identified in the early studies of Greenland's Inuit population who were found to have a low incidence of myocardial infarction (MI) compared to their Danish counterparts. The benefit was attributed to the high fish consumption by the Inuits [2,3]. This was followed by nearly four decades of research, including animal studies, epidemiological studies, randomized controlled trials (RCTs), meta-analyses of epidemiological cohort studies, and trial meta-analyses. Many of these studies demonstrated the cardioprotective effects of fish consumption and fish oil supplementation [4–10].

The rising amount of evidence led to recommendations regarding consumption of seafood/fish and/or their dietary supplementation with ω-3 PUFA from the Food and Drug Administration (FDA) [11]. In 2012, a prescription fish oil formulation was approved by the US FDA. Fish oil continues to be the most popular natural supplement in the US, used by nearly 18.8 million adults [12]. However, several recent large-scale studies have failed to demonstrate any significant benefits of fish oil supplements on cardiovascular outcomes and mortality [13–17]. In this review, we discuss the structure and metabolism of marine-derived ω-3 PUFAs, their proposed benefits and molecular mechanisms of action, and the evidence regarding their role in CVD. We conclude by providing possible reasons for the conflicting evidence and recommendations regarding the dietary intake of fish and fish oil supplements.

2. Structure and Metabolism of PUFAs

Fatty acids are long-chain hydrocarbons with a carboxylic acid group at one end (alpha terminal) and methyl group at the other end (omega terminal). They can be classified based on the number of double bonds in their side chains—saturated fatty acids (no double bond), monounsaturated fatty acids or MUFAs (single double bond), and polyunsaturated fatty acids or PUFAs (two or more double bonds). PUFAs can be classified further by the length of the carbon chain and the position of the first double bond from the methyl terminal into omega-6 (ω-6 or n-6) or omega-3 (ω-3 or n-3). For example, linoleic acid (LA) or 9,12-octadecadienoic acid ($C_{18:2}$) has 18 carbon atoms with 2 double bonds. Since the first double bond from the methyl terminal is at the sixth position, it is an ω-6 PUFA. Similarly, alpha-linolenic acid (ALA) is 9,12,15-octadecatrienoic acid ($C_{18:3}$), meaning it has 18 carbon atoms with 3 double bonds. However, in this case, the first double bond is at the third position from the methyl terminal, and hence it is an ω-3 PUFA. Both LA and ALA are considered essential fatty acids since they cannot be synthesized by humans and must be ingested via their diet.

The essential fatty acids LA and ALA are then metabolized to other fatty acids through desaturase and elongase enzymes. LA (ω-6) is metabolized to arachidonic acid (5,8,11,14-eicosatetraenoic acid, $C_{20:4}$, ω-6). Similarly, ALA (ω-3) is converted to EPA (5,8,11,14,17-eicosapentaenoic acid, $C_{20:5}$, ω-3) and DHA (4,7,10,13,16,19-docosahexaenoic acid, $C_{22:6}$, ω-3). Thus, EPA and DHA are traditionally considered non-essential since, technically speaking, they can be synthesized from ALA. However, this pathway is slow and inefficient [18]. Therefore, for all practical purposes, the dietary intake of EPA and DHA is "essential" and crucial to obtain health benefits.

After absorption from the intestine as chylomicrons, fatty acids are transported to the liver and other tissues. PUFAs are subsequently incorporated into the phospholipid bilayer of plasma membranes, and affect membrane fluidity and signaling. ω-6 and ω-3 PUFAs have opposite effects in the body. Diets rich in ω-6 are precursors of eicosanoids associated with inflammation, vasoconstriction, and platelet aggregation [19]. Acute self-limited inflammation is a protective response to infection and injury. However, excessive inappropriate inflammation has been linked to atherosclerosis and cancer. On the other hand, ω-3 PUFAs are precursors of anti-inflammatory molecules and provide benefits against chronic inflammatory conditions, like diabetes, ischemic heart disease, and cancer [20]. These molecular mechanisms are discussed in further detail in a later section of this review.

The structure and metabolism of major PUFAs is depicted in Figure 1.

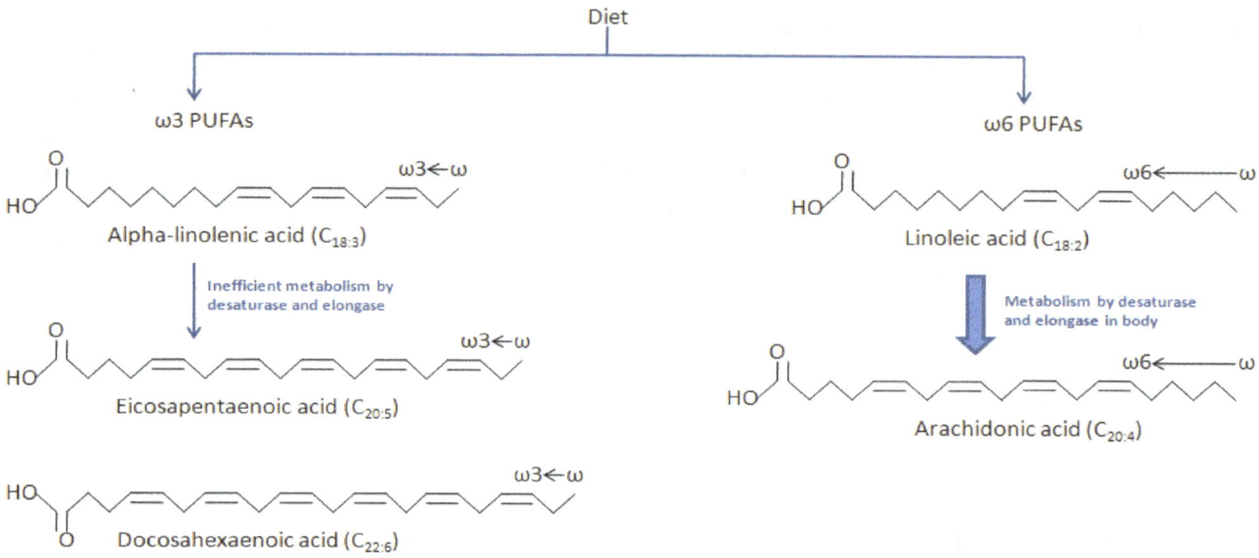

Figure 1. Structure and metabolism of major polyunsaturated fatty acids (PUFAs).

3. Dietary Sources of Major PUFAs

Most vegetable oils and crop seeds, like corn, sunflower, soybean, and canola oils, are a rich source of ω-6 LA with lesser amounts of ω-3 ALA. On the other hand, flax, walnuts, and chia seeds are a rich source of ALA, as are some green leafy vegetables.

Fatty fish and other seafood are the most important dietary sources of EPA and DHA. Wild (marine) fish feed on phyto- and zoo-planktons, and are therefore a richer source of EPA and DHA than cultivated (farmed) fish which feed on cereals and vegetable oils [20]. Cod liver and algal oil have been proposed to be non-traditional marine sources of EPA and DHA. Finally, marine-derived ω-3 fortified food products, like cereals, pastas, dairy products, eggs, meat, salad dressings, and oils are now available. They are a potential option for vegetarians and those who dislike seafood [18]. The principal dietary sources of PUFAs are shown in Table 1 [21,22].

Table 1. Dietary sources of major PUFAs.

PUFA	Dietary Source
Linoleic acid (ω-6)	Corn, safflower, soybean, sunflower oils
Alpha-linolenic acid (plant-derived ω-3)	Flaxseed oil, canola (rapeseed) oil, walnuts, seeds of chia, perilla, green leafy vegetables
Eicosapentaenoic and Docosahexaenoic acids (marine-derived ω-3)	Fish, fish oil, other seafood, beef, lamb, ω-3 fortified foods

4. Proposed Cardioprotective Benefits of ω-3 PUFAs and Their Molecular Mechanisms of Action

Fish and fish oil consumption has been shown to decrease cardiovascular events and mortality in many secondary prevention trials that included high-risk patients with recent myocardial infarction or heart failure. Several molecular mechanisms for this cardioprotective effect of ω-3 PUFAs have been proposed.

4.1. Anti-Inflammatory Effect

ω-3 PUFAs have pleiotropic anti-inflammatory effects. They readily replace arachidonic acid in cell membranes. This results in decreased production of ω-6 arachidonic acid-derived inflammatory mediators, like prostaglandin (PG) E_2, thromboxane (TX) A_2, and leukotrienes (LTs) A_4, B_4, C_4, D_4, and E_4 [23,24]. ω-3 PUFAs generate less potent inflammatory substrates, like 3-series PGs and

TXs and 5-series LTs [24]. 3-series PGs have less potent biological effects (compared to 2-series PGs) and TX A_3 lacks pro-platelet aggregatory properties. 5-series LTs are relatively less effective as pro-inflammatory molecules. EPA and DHA are metabolized to anti-inflammatory mediators, like resolvins, protectins, and the G protein-coupled receptor 120 [24,25]. Additionally, cell membranes with higher ω-3: ω-6 PUFA ratio have higher fluidity. Marine-derived ω-3 PUFAs have been shown to reduce the circulating levels of pro-inflammatory cytokines like interleukin (IL)-1, IL-6, and the tumor necrosis factor (TNF)-α [26]. ω-3 PUFAs also regulate intracellular signaling pathways to inactivate nuclear transcriptional factors. They decrease expression of inflammatory genes via the downregulation of nuclear factor (NF)-κB. The inhibition of NF-κB is mediated by the activation of peroxisome proliferator-activated receptors (PPAR) [27].

4.2. Improved Endothelial Function

Endothelial dysfunction from loss of endothelial-derived nitric oxide (NO) synthesis results in predisposition to accelerated atherosclerosis and adverse vascular events. Marine-derived ω-3 PUFAs cause translocation and activation of endothelial NO synthase (eNOS) into the cytosol, resulting in vasodilation and improved endothelial function [25,28]. Recently, EPA was shown to prevent saturated fatty acid-induced vascular endothelial dysfunction through regulation of long-chain acyl-coA synthetase expression [29]. Endothelial function is additionally improved by reduced expression of endothelial vascular cell adhesion molecules, resulting in attenuated leukocyte adhesion to endothelium [30,31].

4.3. Atherosclerotic Plaque Stabilization

EPA and DHA inhibit the proliferation and migration of smooth muscle cells (SMCs), a central step in atherosclerotic plaque formation and progression. Vasa vasorum is a network of microvessels extending up to the plaque base, which is vital for plaque progression. ω-3 PUFAs interfere with the neovascularization of vasa vasorum, thereby suppressing plaque development [25].

Apart from reducing plaque progression, ω-3 PUFAs also contribute to plaque stability. Plaque vulnerability predisposes people to plaque erosion or rupture, which causes acute coronary syndrome. High tissue levels of EPA and DHA decrease macrophage infiltration and the release of matrix metalloproteinases (MMPs), resulting in greater plaque stability [23]. The addition of EPA to statin therapy has been shown to reduce the lipid core in coronary plaques [32]. Plaques in patients receiving fish oil are more likely to be fibrous cap atheromas, with fewer macrophages and lesser inflammation, and are therefore more likely to be stable [33].

4.4. Effect on Lipid Metabolism

ω-3 PUFAs modulate the activity of genes that control lipid homeostasis. Large doses of fish oil interfere with the synthesis of very low-density lipoprotein (VLDL) via inhibition of sterol receptor element-binding protein-1c. This results in a marked lowering of serum TG levels [23]. Although ω-3 fatty acids do not affect the serum levels of total cholesterol and low-density lipoprotein (LDL), fish oil has been shown to reduce remnant lipoproteins and post-prandial lipemia after fatty meals [30,31]. Remnant lipoprotein levels and post-prandial lipemia are involved in the pathogenesis of sudden cardiac death (SCD) [23]. Marine-derived ω-3 fatty acids also cause a favorable change in high-density lipoprotein (HDL) by increasing the large, cholesterol-rich HDL2 fraction and lowering the small, TG-rich HDL3 fraction [30].

4.5. Anti-Thrombotic Effect

EPA inhibits the synthesis of platelet TXA_2 which causes platelet aggregation and vasoconstriction. Both EPA and DHA antagonize the TXA_2 and PGH_2 receptors in human platelets [34]. There are reports that ω-3 PUFA reduce fibrinogen levels and increase tissue plasminogen-activator concentrations [30,31,35].

4.6. Anti-Arrhythmic Effect

ω-3 PUFAs modulate the activity of multiple ion channels and stabilize the cardiomyocyte membrane, thereby preventing tachyarrhythmias and SCD [5]. EPA and DHA inhibit the voltage-gated sodium channels in cardiac myocytes, increase the voltage threshold for depolarization, and prolong the refractory period. They also modulate certain calcium channels, decrease free cytosolic calcium, and reduce membrane excitability further [24]. Part of the anti-arrhythmic action of these fatty acids is also due to their autonomic effects, like increased vagal tone [36]. In addition, low serum levels of EPA and DHA have been found to increase the risk of cardiogenic syncope in patients with Brugada syndrome [37].

4.7. Cardiac Remodeling

The OMEGA-REMODEL trial reported the beneficial effects of high-dose ω-3 PUFA therapy on cardiac remodeling in patients with MI. Cardiac magnetic resonance confirmed reduced ventricular remodeling and myocardial fibrosis after PUFA supplementation [38]. Similar findings of the preferential effects of ω-3 PUFAs on cardiac remodeling and heart failure were also seen in the Gruppo Italiano per lo Studio della Streptochinasi nell'Infarto Miocardico-Heart Failure (GISSI-HF) trial [10].

Cardiac myofibroblasts, activated by inflammatory signals or pressure overload, cause cardiac remodeling. Recently, a novel EPA metabolite called 18-hydroxy eicosapentaenoic acid (18-HEPE) has been identified, which prevents cardiac remodeling under pressure overload [39]. Higher dietary intake of EPA ethyl ester increases the plasma concentration of 18-HEPE, and may have beneficial long-term effects by preventing cardiac fibrosis [24].

Moreover, EPA and DHA improve cardiac mitochondrial function by increasing the efficiency of adenosine triphosphate (ATP) production [40].

4.8. Improved Exercise Tolerance

Decreased exercise capacity is a known risk factor for CVD. Recently, ω-3 PUFAs have been shown to improve exercise tolerance. This may be due to favorable effects on erythrocyte rheology and skeletal muscle function [25,41]. Improved exercise capacity may contribute to a lower risk of adverse cardiac events.

4.9. Improved Cognitive Function

Poor cognitive function is a risk factor for cardiovascular events [42]. Serum EPA levels have been shown to be independently associated with cognitive function in CVD patients [43]. Thus, improved dietary ω-3 PUFA intake might conceivably improve cognition and decrease the risk of cardiovascular events [25].

Figure 2 summarizes the various molecular mechanisms by which ω-3 PUFAs, like EPA and DHA, have been proposed to exert their cardioprotective effects.

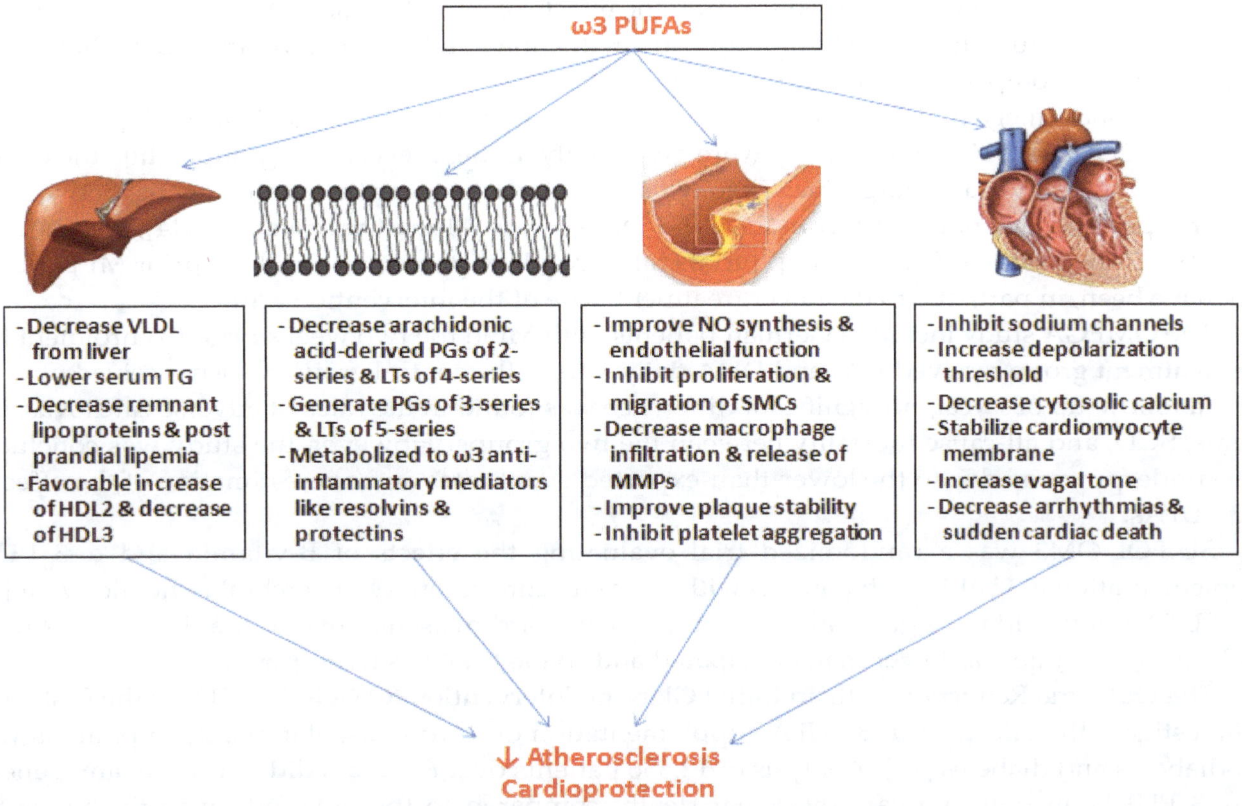

Figure 2. Pleiotropic cardioprotective effects of ω-3 PUFAs.

5. Evidence from Trials and Meta-Analyses

The Diet and Reinfarction Trial (DART) was the first RCT to assess the benefits of dietary fish and fish oil in the secondary prevention of MI [4]. A total of 2033 patients with recent MI were followed for two years. Consumption of at least two servings (200–400 g) of fish per week was associated with a reduction in all-cause mortality. Similar beneficial effects were also noticed in participants who took fish oil capsules instead of fish.

The GISSI-Prevenzione trial included 11,324 patients with previous MI (within three months) [6]. The intervention group received one fish oil capsule per day, in addition to standard care. The intervention group was noted to have a 41% reduction in all-cause mortality and 53% reduction in SCD as early as four months into the study. The difference in all-cause mortality remained significant after a follow-up of 3.5 years, and was proposed to be primarily due to the anti-arrhythmic effects of EPA and DHA.

The DART-2 was a secondary prevention study conducted in men with stable angina (and not previous MI, unlike the first DART study) [44]. Patients who were advised to consume two portions of oily fish every week or take three fish oil capsules daily had a higher risk of cardiac mortality and SCD. Subgroup analysis revealed that this difference was driven by the fish oil capsule group. The study was largely criticized for its poor design and lack of blinding.

The Japan EPA Lipid Intervention Study (JELIS), a combined primary (14,981 patients) and secondary intervention (3664 patients) trial, included a total of 18,645 patients [9]. The EPA (1.8 g daily) plus statin group showed a reduction in major coronary events compared to the statin-alone group. Subgroup analysis revealed that the significant reduction in coronary events was mainly seen in patients with a history of coronary artery disease, and there was no benefit of EPA in primary prevention. However, the results of this study may have been diluted, as the consumption of fish in the Japanese population is high at baseline.

The GISSI-HF trial was designed to study the effects of daily EPA and DHA supplementation in patients with HF [10]. The ω-3 PUFA group had a reduction in all-cause mortality and cardiovascular hospitalizations compared to the control group.

The Alpha Omega trial was a secondary prevention study using 4837 patients with prior MI [14]. Low-dose EPA and DHA in margarine were given daily to the intervention group, while the control group received only plain margarine. There was no difference in cardiovascular events between the two groups. The lack of benefit from EPA and DHA in the Alpha Omega study [14], compared to the GISSI Prevenzione [6] and JELIS [9] trials (all secondary prevention trials in prior MI patients), may have been, in part, due to the lower treatment dose of the intervention arm.

The OMEGA study included German patients with MI in the two weeks prior to enrolment [13]. The treatment group received EPA and DHA daily, versus the control group, which received olive oil. After a follow-up of 1 year, no significant difference was found in the rates of adverse cardiovascular events, SCD, and all-cause mortality between the two groups. However, the study was concluded to be underpowered due to the lower-than-expected event rates and overestimation of the effect of ω-3 PUFAs.

SU.FOL.OM3 was a randomized trial evaluating the effects of B-vitamin and ω-3 PUFA supplementation in 2501 French patients with a recent acute coronary or cerebral ischemic event [15]. ω-3 PUFA intake did not significantly affect the major cardiovascular event rate. Like the OMEGA study, the event rate was lower than anticipated and so the trial was underpowered.

The Outcome Reduction with an Initial Glargine Intervention (ORIGIN) trial was the first study to investigate the effects of ω-3 PUFA supplementation on cardiovascular events in patients with pre-diabetes and diabetes [16]. Analysis of 12,536 patients over 6.2 years did not reveal any benefits of ω-3 PUFAs in reducing cardiovascular death, compared to the olive oil given to the control group. These results were in contrast to the findings of the GISSI Prevenzione [6] and GISSI-HF [10] trials. Inter-trial differences in patient baseline characteristics and concomitant therapies could be a possible explanation.

The Risk and Prevention study investigated the efficacy of ω-3 PUFAs in Italian patients with high risk of CVD but without previous MI [17]. After a follow-up of five years, there was no difference in the primary endpoint of cardiovascular death and hospitalization between the ω-3 PUFA treatment group and olive oil control group. However, subgroup analysis revealed that the ω-3 PUFA group had fewer heart failure hospitalizations. Additionally, women in the treatment group had lower rates of primary endpoint than the control group. The results of this study may not be generalizable due to the Mediterranean dietary habits in the Italian population.

The PREDIMED trial in 7447 patients reported that a Mediterranean diet, with 50 g of extra-virgin olive oil daily, significantly reduced cardiovascular events and death at a follow-up period of 4.8 years [45]. It remains unknown whether the benefit was due to the Mediterranean diet alone, olive oil alone, or whether it was a combined effect. The OMEGA [13], ORIGIN [16], and Risk and Prevention [17] trials did not detect a significant difference between the overall outcomes in the ω-3 PUFA group and olive oil control group. However, the results of the PREDIMED trial [45] indicate that olive oil itself may have some cardioprotective benefits and is likely not an ideal control.

The Age-Related Eye Disease Study 2 (AREDS2) trial included 4203 patients at high risk of CVD and either intermediate or advanced macular degeneration [46]. Patients were randomly grouped to the ω-3 PUFA group (650 mg EPA plus 350 mg DHA), macular xanthophyll group (10 mg lutein plus 2 mg zeaxanthin), combination therapy, or matching placebos. Long-chain ω-3 PUFAs or macular xanthophylls did not reduce the risk of CVD events.

Rizos et al. performed a meta-analysis of 20 RCTs including 68,680 patients to study the role of ω-3 PUFA supplementation on major cardiovascular outcomes [47]. Overall, ω-3 PUFAs were not associated with cardiovascular benefits.

Studies have also evaluated the role of ω-3 PUFAs in the secondary prevention of atrial fibrillation [48,49]. The FORWARD trial included 586 participants with previous atrial fibrillation who were randomized to receive either ω-3 PUFA for 1 g per day, or a placebo for one year [48]. PUFA supplementation did not reduce recurrent atrial fibrillation. Mariani et al. performed a meta-analysis of 16 trials covering 4677 patients and concluded that ω-3 PUFAs have no effect in preventing recurrent or post-operative atrial fibrillation [49].

The results of the ASCEND trial were recently published [50]. It was a randomized, placebo-controlled, blinded trial in 15,480 patients followed for 7.4 years. The study aimed to assess the efficacy and safety of taking 100 mg of aspirin daily in preventing cardiovascular events and cancer in diabetic patients without known CVD. This study also investigated whether daily ω-3 PUFA supplementation decreased cardiovascular events in this population. Aspirin use was noted to prevent cardiovascular events in patients, but also caused major bleeding events. Compared to the placebo group that received olive oil capsules, 1 g of ω-3 PUFA supplementation daily failed to decrease the risk of serious vascular events in diabetics without known CVD.

The Reduction of Cardiovascular Events with EPA-Intervention Trial (REDUCE-IT) was recently concluded [51]. The study involved 8179 high-risk patients with hypertriglyceridemia on statin therapy who were randomized to receive either 4 g of ethyl EPA daily, or a placebo. After a median follow-up of 4.9 years, there was an approximately 25% reduction in the risk of major adverse cardiovascular events in the treatment group.

The Vitamin D and Omega-3 Trial (VITAL) results were recently announced [52]. The study included 25,871 participants with an objective to assess the effect of daily vitamin D_3 (2000 IU) and fish oil supplement (1 g) in the primary prevention of cancer and CVD. After a follow-up of over five years, ω-3 PUFA supplementation did not result in a lower incidence of cardiovascular events or cancer, compared to the placebo.

The STRENGTH study is an ongoing RCT that will enroll approximately 13,000 patients with hypertriglyceridemia, low HDL, and a high risk for CVD [53]. Patients are being randomized to receive either statin with corn oil or statin with prescription ω-3 carboxylic acids. The study is anticipated to be completed in 2019.

Results of various published trials and meta-analyses discussed above are presented in Table 2.

Table 2. Trials and meta-analyses of ω-3 PUFAs in cardiovascular disease (CVD).

Study	Study Design	Number of Patients	Intervention	Follow-Up	Outcome
DART [4] 1989	Secondary prevention RCT	2033	200–400 g fish per week	2 years	29% reduction in mortality
GISSI Prevenzione [6] 1999	Secondary prevention RCT	11,324	882 mg EPA and DHA daily	3.5 years	15–20% reduction in mortality and CV events
DART-2 [44] 2003	Secondary prevention RCT	3114	2 fish servings per week or 3 fish oil capsules daily	3-9 years	Higher cardiac mortality and SCD
JELIS [9] 2007	Primary and secondary prevention RCT	18,645	1.8 g EPA daily	4.6 years	19% reduction in coronary events in CAD patients, no benefit in primary prevention
GISSI-HF [10] 2008	Secondary prevention RCT	6975	840 mg EPA and DHA daily	3.9 years	9% reduction in mortality and 8% reduction in hospitalizations
Alpha Omega [14] 2010	Secondary prevention RCT	4837	226 mg EPA and 150 mg DHA daily	3.4 years	No benefit
OMEGA [13] 2010	Secondary prevention RCT	3851	460 mg EPA and 380 mg DHA daily (vs olive oil control)	1 year	No benefit
SU.FOL.OM3 [15] 2010	Secondary prevention RCT	2501	600 mg EPA and DHA daily	4.7 years	No benefit

Table 2. *Cont.*

Study	Study Design	Number of Patients	Intervention	Follow-Up	Outcome
ORIGIN [16] 2012	Secondary prevention RCT	12,536	465 mg EPA and 375 mg DHA daily (vs olive oil control)	6.2 years	No benefit
Rizos et al. [47] 2012	Meta-analysis of 20 RCTs	68,680	1000 mg EPA and DHA daily (median)	-	No benefit
Risk and Prevention [17] 2013	Primary prevention RCT	12,513	850 mg of EPA and DHA daily (vs olive oil control)	5 years	No benefit
AREDS2 [46] 2014	Primary prevention RCT	4203	650 mg EPA plus 350 mg DHA daily	4.8 years	No benefit
ASCEND [50] 2018	Primary prevention RCT	15,480	1 g ω-3 PUFA daily (vs olive oil control)	7.4 years	No benefit
REDUCE-IT [51] 2018	Primary prevention RCT	8179	4 g ethyl EPA daily	4.9 years	25% reduction in major CV events
VITAL [52] 2018	Primary prevention RCT	25,871	1 g ω-3 PUFA daily	5.3 years	No benefit

6. Available ω-3 PUFA Formulations

ω-3 PUFA ethyl esters was the first formulation approved by the FDA in the year 2004. It was marketed under the trade name Omacor® by Reliant Pharmaceuticals and approved for use in patients with serum triglyceride levels greater than 500 mg/dL. It was later renamed to Lovaza® (GlaxoSmithKline). Ethyl EPA or icosapent ethyl, marketed under the name Vascepa® by Amarin Pharmaceuticals, was approved in 2012. It differed from the earlier formulation in that it contained only ethyl esters of EPA without any DHA [54].

In 2014, ω-3 carboxylic acids, marketed under the name Epanova® by AstraZeneca, was approved for hypertriglyceridemia greater than 500 mg/dL. This formulation consists of free fatty acids instead of the prodrug, and therefore does not require pancreatic lipase for conversion to active form. Thus, it can be taken independent of meals with good bioavailability [54]. The ECLIPSE [55] and ECLIPSE II [56] studies compared the pharmacokinetics of ethyl esters and carboxylic acids. Both studies reported much higher bioavailability with the carboxylic acid formulations.

Despite newer options, ethyl esters continue to be the most commonly prescribed due to its generic options.

Differences between various ω-3 prescription products are shown in Table 3 [22].

Table 3. ω-3 PUFA formulations.

	Ethyl Esters of EPA and DHA	Ethyl Esters of EPA Only	Free Fatty Acids of EPA and DHA
Brand name	Lovaza® (GlaxoSmithKline)	Vascepa® (Amarin Pharmaceuticals)	Epanova® (AstraZeneca)
Approval date	2004	2012	2014
EPA/DHA (g per capsule)	EPA 0.465 g DHA0.375 g	EPA 1 g	EPA 0.550 g DHA 0.200 g
Dosing	2 g (2 capsules) twice daily or 4 g (4 capsules)once daily WITH MEALS	2 g (2 capsules) twice daily WITH MEALS	2 g (2 capsules)or 4 g (4 capsules) once daily WITH OR WITHOUT MEALS

7. Side-Effects and Safety Concerns

Fish oil supplements are generally well tolerated. The most common side effects are gastrointestinal, like nausea, eructation, and diarrhea. Certain large fish (like king mackerel, shark, swordfish) have a higher chance of being contaminated with methyl mercury and therefore should be avoided by pregnant/breastfeeding women and children. There have been some concerns about an increased risk of minor bleeding with ω-3 fatty acid supplementation, especially in patients taking aspirin and statins. However, no major bleeding events have been reported in trials to date.

8. Conclusions

Data from early epidemiologic and observational studies have shown there to be cardioprotective benefits from fish and fish oil consumption. However, most primary prevention trials and recent secondary prevention trials have failed to replicate similar results. Several possibilities could explain the difference in results—the high efficacy of modern-day pharmacotherapy (like statins) and revascularization that attenuates the benefit of ω-3 fatty acids, a lower dose of EPA and DHA supplementation in trials than what was needed, insufficient length of follow-up to see benefits, an improved diet with a higher consumption of fish and other seafood which may account for the decreased magnitude of benefits from fish oil capsules over time, improper study design with use of olive oil as a control (olive oil itself has cardioprotective properties making it an unideal control), and fewer-than-anticipated events leading to underpowered studies. Some trials with a large sample size and strong study design are ongoing, and may shed useful light on the subject.

Based on the current evidence, individuals are advised to consume a healthy diet with two servings of fatty fish every week. Such a food-based approach also supplies several other beneficial nutrients apart from ω-3 PUFAs. For those who cannot consume fish, fish oil supplements containing EPA and DHA have a good safety profile and may be reasonable options, especially in patients with pre-existing CVD, heart failure, and hypertriglyceridemia.

Author Contributions: All authors contributed to literature review and writing of this manuscript.

References

1. Bauer, U.E.; Briss, P.A.; Goodman, R.A.; Bowman, B.A. Prevention of chronic disease in the 21st century: Elimination of the leading preventable causes of premature death and disability in the USA. *Lancet* **2014**, *384*, 45–52. [CrossRef]
2. Bang, H.O.; Dyerberg, J.; Nielsen, A. Plasma lipid and lipoprotein pattern in Greenlandic West-coast Eskimos. *Lancet* **1971**, *297*, 1143–1146. [CrossRef]
3. Bang, H.O.; Dyerberg, J.; Sinclair, H.M. The composition of the Eskimo food in north western Greenland. *Am. J. Clin. Nutr.* **1980**, *33*, 2657–2661. [CrossRef] [PubMed]
4. Burr, M.L.; Gilbert, J.F.; Holliday, R.A.; Elwood, P.C.; Fehily, A.M.; Rogers, S.; Sweetnam, P.M.; Deadman, N.M. Effects of changes in fat, fish, and fibre intakes on death and myocardial reinfarction: Diet and reinfarction trial (DART). *Lancet* **1989** *334*, 757–761. [CrossRef]
5. Yang, B.; Saldeen, T.G.; Nichols, W.W.; Mehta, J.L. Dietary fish oil supplementation attenuates myocardial dysfunction and injury caused by global ischemia and reperfusion in isolated rat hearts. *J. Nutr.* **1993**, *123*, 2067–2074. [PubMed]
6. GISSI-Prevenzione Investigators. Dietary supplementation with n-3 polyunsaturated fatty acids and vitamin E after myocardial infarction: Results of the GISSI-Prevenzione trial. *Lancet* **1999**, *354*, 447–455. [CrossRef]
7. Whelton, S.P.; He, J.; Whelton, P.K.; Muntner, P. Meta-analysis of observational studies on fish intake and coronary heart disease. *Am. J. Cardiol.* **2004**, *93*, 1119–1123. [CrossRef] [PubMed]
8. He, K.; Song, Y.; Daviglus, M.L.; Liu, K.; Van Horn, L.; Dyer, A.R.; Greenland, P. Accumulated evidence on fish consumption and coronary heart disease mortality: A Meta-analysis of cohort studies. *Circulation* **2004**, *109*, 2705–2711. [CrossRef] [PubMed]
9. Yokoyama, M.; Origasa, H.; Matsuzaki, M.; Matsuzawa, Y.; Saito, Y.; Ishikawa, Y.; Oikawa, S.; Sasaki, J.; Hishida, H.; Itakura, H.; et al. Effects of eicosapentaenoic acid on major coronary events in hypercholesterolaemic patients (JELIS): A randomised open-label, blinded endpoint analysis. *Lancet* **2007**, *369*, 1090–1098. [CrossRef]
10. Tavazzi, L.; Maggioni, A.P.; Marchioli, R.; Barlera, S.; Franzosi, M.G.; Latini, R.; Lucci, D.; Nicolosi, G.L.; Porcu, M.; Tognoni, G. Effect of n-3 polyunsaturated fatty acids in patients with chronic heart failure (the GISSI-HF trial): A randomised, double-blind, placebo-controlled trial. *Lancet* **2008**, *372*, 1223–1230. [PubMed]

11. Kris-Etherton, P.M.; Harris, W.S.; Appel, L.J. Fish consumption, fish oil, omega-3 fatty acids, and cardiovascular disease. *Circulation* **2002**, *106*, 2747–2757. [CrossRef] [PubMed]
12. Clarke, T.C.; Black, L.I.; Stussman, B.J.; Barnes, P.M.; Nahin, R.L. *Trends in the Use of Complementary Health Approaches among Adults: United States, 2002–2012*; National Health Statistics Reports No. 79; National Center for Health Statistics: Hyattsville, MD, USA, 2015; pp. 1–16.
13. Rauch, B.; Schiele, R.; Schneider, S.; Diller, F.; Victor, N.; Gohlke, H.; Gottwik, M.; Steinbeck, G.; Del Castillo, U.; Sack, R.; et al. OMEGA, a randomized, placebo-controlled trial to test the effect of highly purified omega-3 fatty acids on top of modern guideline-adjusted therapy after myocardial infarction. *Circulation* **2010**, *122*, 2152–2159. [CrossRef] [PubMed]
14. Kromhout, D.; Giltay, E.J.; Geleijnse, J.M. n–3 Fatty acids and cardiovascular events after myocardial infarction. *N. Engl. J. Med.* **2010**, *363*, 2015–2026. [CrossRef] [PubMed]
15. Galan, P.; Kesse-Guyot, E.; Czernichow, S.; Briancon, S.; Blacher, J.; Hercberg, S. Effects of B vitamins and omega 3 fatty acids on cardiovascular diseases: A randomised placebo controlled trial. *BMJ* **2010**, *341*, c6273. [CrossRef] [PubMed]
16. ORIGIN Trial Investigators. n–3 Fatty acids and cardiovascular outcomes in patients with dysglycemia. *N. Engl. J. Med.* **2012**, *367*, 309–318. [CrossRef] [PubMed]
17. Risk and Prevention Study Collaborative Group. N–3 fatty acids in patients with multiple cardiovascular risk factors. *N. Engl. J. Med.* **2013**, *368*, 1800–1808. [CrossRef] [PubMed]
18. Bowen, K.J.; Harris, W.S.; Kris-Etherton, P.M. Omega-3 fatty acids and cardiovascular disease: Are there benefits? *Curr. Treat. Opt. Cardiovasc. Med.* **2016**, *18*, 69. [CrossRef] [PubMed]
19. Dennis, E.A.; Norris, P.C. Eicosanoid storm in infection and inflammation. *Nat. Rev. Immunol.* **2015**, *15*, 511. [CrossRef] [PubMed]
20. Saini, R.K.; Keum, Y.S. Omega-3 and omega-6 polyunsaturated fatty acids: Dietary sources, metabolism, and significance—A review. *Life Sci.* **2018**, *203*, 255–267. [CrossRef] [PubMed]
21. Dietary Guidelines Advisory Committee. *Scientific Report of the 2015 Dietary Guidelines Advisory Committee*; US Department of Health and Human Services: Washington, DC, USA, 2015.
22. Burke, M.F.; Burke, F.M.; Soffer, D.E. Review of cardiometabolic effects of prescription omega-3 fatty acids. *Curr. Atheroscler. Rep.* **2017**, *19*, 60. [CrossRef] [PubMed]
23. Kromhout, D.; Yasuda, S.; Geleijnse, J.M.; Shimokawa, H. Fish oil and omega-3 fatty acids in cardiovascular disease: Do they really work? *Eur. Heart J.* **2011**, *33*, 436–443. [CrossRef] [PubMed]
24. Endo, J.; Arita, M. Cardioprotective mechanism of omega-3 polyunsaturated fatty acids. *J. Cardiol.* **2016**, *67*, 22–27. [CrossRef] [PubMed]
25. Yagi, S.; Fukuda, D.; Aihara, K.I.; Akaike, M.; Shimabukuro, M.; Sata, M. N-3 polyunsaturated fatty acids: Promising nutrients for preventing cardiovascular disease. *J. Atheroscler. Thromb.* **2017**, *24*, 999–1010. [CrossRef] [PubMed]
26. Calder, P.C. The role of marine omega-3 (n-fatty acids in inflammatory processes, atherosclerosis and plaque stability. *Mol. Nutr. Food Res.* **2012**, *56*, 1073–1080. [CrossRef] [PubMed]
27. De Winther, M.P.; Kanters, E.; Kraal, G.; Hofker, M.H. Nuclear factor κB signaling in atherogenesis. *Arter. Thromb. Vasc. Biol.* **2005**, *25*, 904–914. [CrossRef] [PubMed]
28. Omura, M.; Kobayashi, S.; Mizukami, Y.; Mogami, K.; Todoroki-Ikeda, N.; Miyake, T.; Matsuzaki, M. Eicosapentaenoic acid (EPA) induces Ca2+-independent activation and translocation of endothelial nitric oxide synthase and endothelium-dependent vasorelaxation. *FEBS Lett.* **2001**, *487*, 361–366. [CrossRef]
29. Ishida, T.; Naoe, S.; Nakakuki, M.; Kawano, H.; Imada, K. Eicosapentaenoic acid prevents saturated fatty acid-induced vascular endothelial dysfunction: Involvement of long-chain acyl-CoA synthetase. *J. Atheroscler. Thromb.* **2015**, *22*, 1172–1185. [CrossRef] [PubMed]
30. Jain, A.P.; Aggarwal, K.K.; Zhang, P.Y. Omega-3 fatty acids and cardiovascular disease. *Eur. Rev. Med. Pharmacol. Sci.* **2015**, *19*, 441–445. [PubMed]
31. Haglund, O.; Mehta, J.L.; Saldeen, T. Effects of fish oil on some parameters of fibrinolysis and lipoprotein(a) in healthy subjects. *Am. J. Cardiol.* **1994**, *74*, 189–192. [CrossRef]
32. Niki, T.; Wakatsuki, T.; Yamaguchi, K.; Taketani, Y.; Oeduka, H.; Kusunose, K.; Ise, T.; Iwase, T.; Yamada, H.; Soeki, T.; et al. Effects of the addition of eicosapentaenoic acid to strong statin therapy on inflammatory cytokines and coronary plaque components assessed by integrated backscatter intravascular ultrasound. *Circ. J.* **2016**, *80*, 450–460. [CrossRef] [PubMed]

33. Thies, F.; Garry, J.M.; Yaqoob, P.; Rerkasem, K.; Williams, J.; Shearman, C.P.; Gallagher, P.J.; Calder, P.C.; Grimble, R.F. Association of n-3 polyunsaturated fatty acids with stability of atherosclerotic plaques: A randomised controlled trial. *Lancet* **2003**, *361*, 477–485. [CrossRef]
34. Swann, P.G.; Venton, D.L.; Le Breton, G.C. Eicosapentaenoic acid and docosahexaenoic acid are antagonists at the thromboxane A2/prostaglandin H2 receptor in human platelets. *FEBS Lett.* **1989**, *243*, 244–246. [CrossRef]
35. Atakisi, O.; Atakisi, E.; Ozcan, A.; Karapehlivan, M.; Kart, A. Protective effect of omega-3 fatty acids on diethylnitrosamine toxicity in rats. *Eur. Rev. Med. Pharmacol. Sci.* **2013**, *17*, 467–471. [PubMed]
36. Christensen, J.H.; Schmidt, E.B. Autonomic nervous system, heart rate variability and n-3 fatty acids. *J. Cardiovasc. Med.* **2007**, *8*, 19–22. [CrossRef] [PubMed]
37. Yagi, S.; Soeki, T.; Aihara, K.I.; Fukuda, D.; Ise, T.; Kadota, M.; Bando, S.; Matsuura, T.; Tobiume, T.; Yamaguchi, K.; et al. Low serum levels of eicosapentaenoic acid and docosahexaenoic acid are risk factors for cardiogenic syncope in patients with Brugada syndrome. *Int. Heart J.* **2017**, *58*, 720–723. [CrossRef] [PubMed]
38. Heydari, B.; Abdullah, S.; Pottala, J.V.; Shah, R.; Abbasi, S.; Mandry, D.; Francis, S.A.; Lumish, H.; Ghoshhajra, B.B.; Hoffmann, U.; et al. Effect of Omega-3 Acid Ethyl Esters on Left Ventricular Remodeling After Acute Myocardial Infarction Clinical Perspective: The OMEGA-REMODEL Randomized Clinical Trial. *Circulation* **2016**, *134*, 378–391. [CrossRef] [PubMed]
39. Endo, J.; Sano, M.; Isobe, Y.; Fukuda, K.; Kang, J.X.; Arai, H.; Arita, M. 18-HEPE, an n-3 fatty acid metabolite released by macrophages, prevents pressure overload–induced maladaptive cardiac remodeling. *J. Exp. Med.* **2014**, *211*, 1673–1687. [CrossRef] [PubMed]
40. Duda, M.K.; O'shea, K.M.; Stanley, W.C. ω-3 polyunsaturated fatty acid supplementation for the treatment of heart failure: Mechanisms and clinical potential. *Cardiovasc. Res.* **2009**, *84*, 33–41. [CrossRef] [PubMed]
41. Da Boit, M.; Hunter, A.M.; Gray, S.R. Fit with good fat? The role of n-3 polyunsaturated fatty acids on exercise performance. *Metabolism* **2017**, *66*, 45–54. [CrossRef] [PubMed]
42. Yagi, S.; Akaike, M.; Ise, T.; Ueda, Y.; Iwase, T.; Sata, M. Renin–angiotensin–aldosterone system has a pivotal role in cognitive impairment. *Hypertens. Res.* **2013**, *36*, 753. [CrossRef] [PubMed]
43. Yagi, S.; Hara, T.; Ueno, R.; Aihara, K.I.; Fukuda, D.; Takashima, A.; Hotchi, J.; Ise, T.; Yamaguchi, K.; Tobiume, T.; et al. Serum concentration of eicosapentaenoic acid is associated with cognitive function in patients with coronary artery disease. *Nutr. J.* **2014**, *13*, 112. [CrossRef] [PubMed]
44. Burr, M.L.; Ashfield-Watt, P.A.; Dunstan, F.D.; Fehily, A.M.; Breay, P.; Ashton, T.; Zotos, P.C.; Haboubi, N.A.; Elwood, P.C. Lack of benefit of dietary advice to men with angina: Results of a controlled trial. *Eur. J. Clin. Nutr.* **2003**, *57*, 193. [CrossRef] [PubMed]
45. Estruch, R.; Ros, E.; Salas-Salvadó, J.; Covas, M.I.; Corella, D.; Arós, F.; Gómez-Gracia, E.; Ruiz-Gutiérrez, V.; Fiol, M.; Lapetra, J.; et al. Primary prevention of cardiovascular disease with a Mediterranean diet. *N. Engl. J. Med.* **2013**, *368*, 1279–1290. [CrossRef] [PubMed]
46. Bonds, D.E.; Harrington, M.; Worrall, B.B.; Bertoni, A.G.; Eaton, C.B.; Hsia, J.; Robinson, J.; Clemons, T.E.; Fine, L.J.; Chew, E.Y. Effect of long-chain ω-3 fatty acids and lutein+ zeaxanthin supplements on cardiovascular outcomes: Results of the Age-Related Eye Disease Study 2 (AREDSrandomized clinical trial. *JAMA Intern. Med.* **2014**, *174*, 763–771. [CrossRef] [PubMed]
47. Rizos, E.C.; Ntzani, E.E.; Bika, E.; Kostapanos, M.S.; Elisaf, M.S. Association between omega-3 fatty acid supplementation and risk of major cardiovascular disease events: A systematic review and meta-analysis. *JAMA* **2012**, *308*, 1024–1033. [CrossRef] [PubMed]
48. Macchia, A.; Grancelli, H.; Varini, S.; Nul, D.; Laffaye, N.; Mariani, J.; Ferrante, D.; Badra, R.; Figal, J.; Ramos, S.; et al. Omega-3 fatty acids for the prevention of recurrent symptomatic atrial fibrillation: Results of the FORWARD (Randomized Trial to Assess Efficacy of PUFA for the Maintenance of Sinus Rhythm in Persistent Atrial Fibrillation) trial. *J. Am. Coll. Cardiol.* **2013**, *61*, 463–468. [CrossRef] [PubMed]
49. Mariani, J.; Doval, H.C.; Nul, D.; Varini, S.; Grancelli, H.; Ferrante, D.; Tognoni, G.; Macchia, A. N-3 polyunsaturated fatty acids to prevent atrial fibrillation: Updated systematic review and meta-analysis of randomized controlled trials. *J. Am. Heart Assoc.* **2013**, *2*, e005033. [CrossRef] [PubMed]
50. The ASCEND Study Collaborative Group. Effects of n-3 fatty acid supplements in diabetes mellitus. *N. Engl. J. Med.* **2018**, *379*, 1540–1550. [CrossRef] [PubMed]

51. A Study of AMR101 to Evaluate Its Ability to Reduce Cardiovascular Events in High Risk Patients with Hypertriglyceridemia and on Statin. 2016. Available online: https://clinicaltrials.gov/ct2/show/NCT01492361 (accessed on 13 October 2018).
52. Manson, J.E.; Cook, N.R.; Lee, I.M.; Christen, W.; Bassuk, S.S.; Mora, S.; Gibson, H.; Albert, C.M.; Gordon, D.; Copeland, T.; et al. Marine n− 3 fatty acids and prevention of cardiovascular disease and cancer. *N. Engl. J. Med.* **2018**. [CrossRef] [PubMed]
53. US National Institutes of Health. *Outcomes Study to Assess STatin Residual Risk Reduction With EpaNova in HiGh CV Risk PatienTs With Hypertriglyceridemia (STRENGTH)*; US National Institutes of Health: Bethesda, MD, USA, 2015.
54. Benes, L.B.; Bassi, N.S.; Kalot, M.A.; Davidson, M.H. Evolution of Omega-3 Fatty Acid Therapy and Current and Future Role in the Management of Dyslipidemia. *Cardiol. Clin.* **2018**, *36*, 277–285. [CrossRef] [PubMed]
55. Davidson, M.H.; Johnson, J.; Rooney, M.W.; Kyle, M.L.; Kling, D.F. A novel omega-3 free fatty acid formulation has dramatically improved bioavailability during a low-fat diet compared with omega-3-acid ethyl esters: The ECLIPSE (Epanova® compared to Lovaza® in a pharmacokinetic single-dose evaluation) study. *J. Clin. Lipidol.* **2012**, *6*, 573–584. [CrossRef] [PubMed]
56. Offman, E.; Marenco, T.; Ferber, S.; Johnson, J.; Kling, D.; Curcio, D.; Davidson, M. Steady-state bioavailability of prescription omega-3 on a low-fat diet is significantly improved with a free fatty acid formulation compared with an ethyl ester formulation: The ECLIPSE II study. *Vasc. Health Risk Manag.* **2013**, *9*, 563. [CrossRef] [PubMed]

10

rs2569190A>G in *CD14* is Independently Associated with Hypercholesterolemia

Ali Salami [1], Christy Costanian [2,3] and Said El Shamieh [4,*]

1 Rammal Hassan Rammal Research Laboratory, Physio-toxicity (PhyTox) Research Group, Lebanese University, Faculty of Sciences (V), Nabatieh 1700, Lebanon; a.salami@ul.edu.lb
2 Faculty of Medicine, University of Ottawa, Ottawa 61350, ON K1G 5Z3, Canada; ccostani@uottawa.ca
3 School of Medicine, Lebanese American University, Beirut 1102 2801, Lebanon
4 Department of Medical Laboratory Technology, Faculty of Health Sciences, Beirut Arab University, Beirut 115020, Lebanon
* Correspondence: s.elshamieh@bau.edu.lb

Abstract: Many studies have assessed the implication of *cluster of differentiation 14* (*CD14*) molecules and its single nucleotide polymorphism rs2569190A>G with different complex diseases, such as diabetes and cardiovascular diseases (CVDs). In this study, we investigated the association of rs2569190A>G in *CD14* with cardiovascular disease risk factors (hypercholesterolemia and hypertension) in 460 individuals from the general Lebanese population (Middle Eastern multiethnic population). Using a multiple logistic regression model adjusted for six covariates (under additive and recessive assumptions), we found that the G allele of rs2569190 in *CD14* was associated with increased levels of total cholesterol (OR = 3.10, $p = 0.009$), low-density lipoprotein cholesterol (OR = 3.87, $p = 0.003$), and decreased levels of high-density lipoprotein cholesterol (OR = 0.38, $p = 0.001$). In contrast, no significant relationship was found with hypertension. Thus, we concluded that rs2569190G in *CD14* is associated with a higher risk of developing hypercholesterolemia.

Keywords: hypercholesterolemia; *cluster of differentiation 14*; rs2569190A>G; single nucleotide polymorphisms; association analysis

1. Introduction

According to the World Health Organization, cardiovascular diseases (CVDs) represent the most significant cause of death in humans globally [1]. Around 18 million people died because of CVDs in 2016, representing 31% of all deaths worldwide, most of which occur in low- and middle-income countries [1]. In addition to modifiable risk factors such as high cholesterol and triglyceride levels, diabetes, and high blood pressure (BP) levels [2], several studies have revealed an important impact of the innate immune system on the development or the progression of many CVDs [3]. The innate immune system present in multicellular living organisms gives an immediate defense capability against foreign bodies and pathogenic organisms such as viruses, bacteria, and fungi at first exposure [4]. This system depends on the recognition of pathogens by several families of extracellular receptors, such as the cluster of differentiation 14 (*CD14*), which is responsible for triggering innate immune responses and was first identified as marker of monocytes, before being defined as a coreceptor of toll-like receptors [5].

Many studies have assessed the role of *CD14*, especially at the molecular level, and established a link between the gene product and its single nucleotide polymorphisms (SNPs) with different complex diseases such as diabetes [6] and CVDs [7]. For example, the SNP rs2569190 in the promoter region of *CD14* has been found to be implicated in coronary artery disease through changing protein levels [8,9].

Furthermore, the A allele has been reported to be functional and enhances CD14 expression, and thus the host sensitivity, for exogenous or endogenous lipopolysaccharides [10]. More importantly, soluble *CD14* levels have shown strong, independent correlations with traditional cardio-metabolic risk factors and with subclinical measures of vascular disease (carotid wall thickness, ankle-brachial index, and body mass index) [7]. Based on all of the above, we hypothesize that rs2569190 in *CD14* could be associated with CVD risk factors such as hypercholesterolemia and hypertension (HTN). Therefore, the goal of our study was to investigate the association of rs2569190 in *CD14* with CVD risk factors in individuals from the general Lebanese population.

2. Materials and Methods

2.1. Study Population

The institutional review board of the Lebanese University approved the recruitment procedure and the genetic protocols (2182/28, on 16 December 2015). This cross-sectional study involved 460 unrelated Lebanese participants who were apparently healthy (free of chronic diseases; cardiovascular or cancer) individuals.

2.2. Clinical and Biological Data Collection

All measurements, including demographic, clinical, and biochemical measurements, were assessed as described previously [11]. Nuclear DNA was extracted from whole-blood samples according to the manufacturer's recommendations (QIAamp DNA blood mini kit, Qiagen, Hilden, Germany). Very briefly, 4 μg of total DNA from 200 μL of whole human blood was extracted through lysis and continuous spinning. A KASP genotyping assay (LGC group, Berlin, Germany) was used to genotype rs2569190A>G in *CD14*. Hypercholesterolemia was defined as an elevation of total cholesterol (Tchol) and/or low-density cholesterol (LDL-C) levels. Tchol and LDL-C were considered high if their values were ≥150 and ≥100 mg/dL, respectively. High-density cholesterol (HDL-C) levels were considered low if their values were ≤50 and ≤40 mg/dL in females and males, respectively. HTN was defined as systolic blood pressure ≥130 mmHg or diastolic ≥85 mmHg.

2.3. Statistical Analyses

SPSS statistical software version 24.0 [12] was used to perform all our statistical analyses except the power analysis. GPower 3.1.9.4 software [13] was used for the power analysis. Continuous variables were presented as mean value ± standard deviation, and categorical ones were shown as numbers and percentages. A chi-squared goodness-of-fit test was performed to determine if the genotypes of rs2569190A>G in *CD14* were in Hardy–Weinberg equilibrium (HWE).

To study the association between rs2569190A>G in *CD14* and hypercholesterolemia and HTN, a multivariate logistic regression model was used while correcting for different confounding factors (age, gender, body mass index, marital status, smoking, and physical activity). This analysis was performed under the assumption of additive (AA vs. GA vs. GG) and recessive models (AA and GA vs. GG). The sample size needed to reach a statistical power of at least 0.90 in a two-sided test with $\alpha = 0.05$ and an effect size of 0.2 was 409 individuals.

3. Results

3.1. Characteristics of the Studied Participants

The demographic characteristics of the study participants are shown in Table 1. The group of participants comprised 292 females (63.5%) and 168 males (36.5%). The mean age was 40.6 years old, and approximately 70% of the participants were married (Table 1). In addition, one-fourth of participants were smokers, and only a minority practiced physical exercise once per week (Table 1).

Table 1. Demographic characteristics of the study participants.

Characteristics	Participants (n = 460)
Age	40.60 ± 14.16
Gender n (%)	
Male	168 (36.5)
Female	292 (63.5)
Smoking status n (%)	
Nonsmoker	332 (72.2)
Past smoker	6 (1.3)
Current smoker	122 (26.5)
Marital Status n (%)	
Single	121 (26.3)
Married	321 (69.8)
Divorced	18 (3.9)
Physical Activity n (%)	
<1 per week	345 (75.0)
1 per week	52 (11.3)
≥2 per week	63 (13.7)

Values are arithmetic mean ± SD for continuous variables. Categorical variables are shown as numbers (n) and percentages (%). n: sample size.

Moreover, the clinical and genetic characteristics are shown in Table 2. Approximately 75% of the participants had high total cholesterol and LDL-C levels, and around half had low HDL-C.

Table 2. Clinical and genetic characteristics of the study participants.

Characteristics	Participants (n = 460)
BMI (Kg/m^2)	25.71 ± 4.98
Total cholesterol (mg/dL)	181.41 ± 40.94
High total cholesterol levels n (%)	351 (76.3)
LDL-C (mg/dL)	117.39 ± 33.52
High LDL-C levels n (%)	347 (75.4)
HDL-C (mg/dL)	45.53 ± 14.61
Low HDL-C levels n (%)	270 (58.7)
Triglycerides (mg/dL)	145.96 ± 124.34
High triglycerides levels n (%)	174 (37.8)
SBP (mmHg)	132.07 ± 15.89
DBP (mmHg)	67.82 ± 9.12
Hypertension n (%)	255 (55.4)
MAF of rs2569190G in *CD14*	0.41
AA n (%)	158 (34.3)
GA n (%)	224 (48.7)
GG n (%)	78 (17.0)

Values are arithmetic mean ± SD for continuous variables. Categorical variables are shown as number (n) and percentages (%). n: sample size. BMI: body mass index, LDL-C: low-density lipoprotein cholesterol, HDL-C: high-density lipoprotein cholesterol, SBP: systolic blood pressure, DBP: diastolic blood pressure, MAF: minor allele frequency, *CD14*: cluster of differentiation 14.

3.2. *Association of rs2569190A>G in CD14 with Hypercholesterolemia*

Our calculations showed that the minor allele in our population was the allele G, with a frequency of 0.41 (Table 2). In addition, the allelic frequencies were consistent with HWE (p = 0.86). Interestingly, the G allele of rs2569190 in *CD14* was associated with increased levels of Tchol (OR = 3.04, p = 0.016, Table 3) and LDL-C (OR = 3.83, p = 0.006, Table 3) and decreased levels of HDL-C (OR = 0.36, p = 0.001, Table 3). Similar results were also seen with a recessive genetic model. Age was positively associated with an increase in Tchol levels (OR = 2.06 and p = 0.011, Table 3) and LDL-C levels (OR = 2.22 and p = 0.004, Table 3). Similarly, smoking was significantly associated with an increase in Tchol levels (OR = 2.18, p = 0.021, Table 3) and LDL-C (OR = 1.88, p = 0.050, Table 3) and a decrease in HDL-C (OR = 0.41, p = 0.001, Table 3). Participants that practiced physical exercise once per week had decreased Tchol (OR = 0.27 and p = 0.001, Table 3), LDL-C (OR = 0.28 and p = 0.001, Table 3), and HDL-C (OR = 0.40 and p = 0.017, Table 3) levels.

Table 3. Multiple logistic regression analysis with hyperlipidemia and hypertension.

Variables	Total Cholesterol		LDL-Cholesterol		HDL-Cholesterol		Hypertension	
	OR (95% C.I.)	p	OR (95% C.I.)	p	OR (95% C.I.)	p	OR (95% C.I.)	p
rs2569190 AA	1		1		1		1	
GA	0.97 (0.57–1.63)	0.900	0.98 (0.59–1.64)	0.939	0.89 (0.56–1.43)	0.636	0.89 (0.56–1.40)	0.607
GG	3.04 (1.23–7.48)	0.016	3.83 (1.48–9.88)	0.006	0.36 (0.19–0.67)	0.001	0.67 (0.36–1.24)	0.203
rs2569190 AA and GA	1		1		1		1	
GG	3.10 (1.33–7.23)	0.009	3.87 (1.58–9.51)	0.003	0.38 (0.22–0.67)	0.001	0.72 (0.41–1.25)	0.186
Age								
<40	1		1		1		1	
≥40	2.06 (1.18–3.59)	0.011	2.22 (1.28–3.86)	0.004	1.58 (0.99–2.51)	0.056	0.73 (0.47–1.16)	0.181
Gender								
Male	1		1		1		1	
Female	1.21 (0.69–2.12)	0.503	0.98 (0.56–1.71)	0.931	1.17 (0.72–1.90)	0.523	0.46 (0.29–0.75)	0.002
BMI								
<25	1		1		1		1	
25–29.9	0.63 (0.34–1.15)	0.132	0.51 (0.28–0.93)	0.027	2.64 (1.50–4.65)	0.001	0.74 (0.44–1.26)	0.267
≥30	1.15 (0.56–2.34)	0.704	1.19 (0.58–2.43)	0.638	1.02 (0.57–1.80)	0.956	1.40 (0.78–2.51)	0.256
Marital status								
Single	1		1		1		1	
Married	0.60 (0.31–1.15)	0.124	0.83 (0.44–1.56)	0.566	0.75 (0.43–1.30)	0.306	0.70 (0.41–1.22)	0.206
Divorced	0.76 (0.21–2.76)	0.681	1.06 (0.29–3.83)	0.935	2.06 (0.57–7.47)	0.271	0.33 (0.10–1.07)	0.065
Smoking status								
Non smoker	1		1		1		1	
Past smoker	0.71 (0.11–4.62)	0.720	0.72 (0.11–4.72)	0.735	0.63 (0.11–3.67)	0.607	0.17 (0.03–1.13)	0.067
Current smoker	2.18 (1.12–4.21)	0.021	1.88 (0.99–3.53)	0.050	0.41 (0.24–0.68)	0.001	0.74 (0.45–1.22)	0.233
Physical activity								
<1 per week	1		1		1		1	
1 per week	0.27 (0.13–0.58)	0.001	0.28 (0.13–0.60)	0.001	0.40 (0.19–0.85)	0.017	0.99 (0.48–2.04)	0.971
≥2 per week	0.69 (0.33–1.41)	0.304	1.27 (0.59–2.74)	0.536	0.57 (0.30–1.11)	0.100	0.90 (0.48–1.70)	0.752

OR: odds ratio, C.I: confidence interval, BMI: body mass index.

4. Discussion

The results of the current study indicated that rs2569190A>G in *CD14* was associated with increased levels of Tchol and LDL-C and decreased levels of HDL-C. This might point to a possible role for *CD14* in the pathophysiology of hypercholesterolemia.

Human *CD14* is located on the long arm of chromosome 5 (q23-31), which encodes the membrane (m)*CD14*, binds to lipopolysaccharides, and activates various TLRs and downstream proinflammatory pathways [14]. Additionally, *CD14* exists in a soluble form (s)*CD14* [15]. In response to interleukin-6, its expression is increased; therefore, it is regarded as an acute phase protein [16]. Of interest, Reiner et al. reported that (s)*CD14* was positively correlated with LDL-C and HTN and negatively correlated with HDL-C [7]. When combined with our results, the above suggests that the *CD14* gene and protein might be implicated in CVDs.

Increasing experimental evidence is suggesting that rs2569190A>G in the *CD14* promoter could contribute to the genetic etiology of human atherosclerosis [17,18]. This SNP was shown to be functional and increase the transcriptional activity of *CD14* [10], which leads to higher (m)*CD14* protein levels and an increased risk of myocardial infarction [17,18].

The current study is not the first to find a link between elements of the innate immune system (*CD14*) and CVD risk factors, since activated innate immune system elements and dysfunction in metabolic pathways could lead to the chronic inflammation and pathologic conditions associated with CVDs [19]. Benachour et al. reported that the expression of the antimicrobial peptide *LL-37* (a component of the immune system) was positively correlated with CVD risk factors such as systolic BP and triglyceride levels, and negatively with plasma levels of HDL-C, in a sample of 90 apparently healthy men [20]. Another component of the innate immune system that has a noteworthy association with CVD risk factors is the human formyl peptide receptor 1 (*FPR1*) [21]. We have previously identified that, in 1012 French middle-aged adults equally divided between healthy and hypertensive individuals, *FPR1* C32T (rs5030878) is associated with increased BP levels [21].

It is noteworthy to mention that a Hardy–Weinberg equilibrium for rs2569190 was found despite the participants belonging to the Middle Eastern population, where consanguinity rates are higher than in European populations. This might be explained by the fact that the majority of the studied individuals came from a northern large city (not villages), making mating less consanguineous and more random.

5. Conclusions

In conclusion, our results indicate that rs2569190A>G in *CD14* is positively associated with increased Tchol and LDL-C and negatively correlated with HDL-C. This link with hypercholesterolemia might highlight that rs2569190A>G in *CD14* could be implicated in the pathophysiology of hypercholesterolemia. Further studies are needed in order to highlight its possible role in the pathogenesis of CVDs.

Author Contributions: Conceptualization, S.E.S. and C.C.; Data curation, A.S.; Formal analysis, A.S.; Methodology, S.E.S.; Project administration, S.E.S.; Software, A.S.; Validation, A.S., C.C., and S.E.S.; Visualization, A.S. and S.E.S.; Writing—original draft, A.S. and S.E.S.; Writing—review and editing, A.S. and S.E.S.

References

1. World Health Organization. *A Report about Cardiovascular Diseases*; Avenue Appia: Geneva, Switzerland, 17 May 2017.
2. Upadhyay, R.K. Emerging risk biomarkers in cardiovascular diseases and disorders. *J. Lipids* **2015**, *2015*, 971453. [CrossRef] [PubMed]
3. Frantz, S.; Falcao-Pires, I.; Balligand, J.L.; Bauersachs, J.; Brutsaert, D.; Ciccarelli, M.; Dawson, D.; de Windt, L.J.; Giacca, M.; Hamdani, N.; et al. The innate immune system in chronic cardiomyopathy: A European Society of Cardiology (ESC) scientific statement from the Working Group on Myocardial Function of the ESC. *Eur. J. Heart Fail.* **2018**, *20*, 445–459. [CrossRef] [PubMed]
4. Turvey, S.E.; Broide, D.H. Innate immunity. *J. Allergy Clin. Immunol.* **2010**, *125*, S24–S32. [CrossRef] [PubMed]
5. Baumann, C.L.; Aspalter, I.M.; Sharif, O.; Pichlmair, A.; Bluml, S.; Grebien, F.; Bruckner, M.; Pasierbek, P.; Aumayr, K.; Planyavsky, M.; et al. CD14 is a coreceptor of Toll-like receptors 7 and 9. *J. Exp. Med.* **2010**, *207*, 2689–2701. [CrossRef] [PubMed]
6. Fernandez-Real, J.M.; Perez del Pulgar, S.; Luche, E.; Moreno-Navarrete, J.M.; Waget, A.; Serino, M.; Sorianello, E.; Sanchez-Pla, A.; Pontaque, F.C.; Vendrell, J.; et al. CD14 modulates inflammation-driven insulin resistance. *Diabetes* **2011**, *60*, 2179–2186. [CrossRef]
7. Reiner, A.P.; Lange, E.M.; Jenny, N.S.; Chaves, P.H.; Ellis, J.; Li, J.; Walston, J.; Lange, L.A.; Cushman, M.; Tracy, R.P. Soluble CD14: Genomewide association analysis and relationship to cardiovascular risk and mortality in older adults. *Arterioscler. Thromb. Vasc. Biol.* **2013**, *33*, 158–164. [CrossRef]
8. Konstantinidou, M.K.; Goutas, N.; Vlachodimitropoulos, D.; Chaidaroglou, A.; Stefanou, D.; Poumpouridou, N.; Mastorakou, R.; Gazouli, M.; Kyparissopoulos, D.; Spiliopoulou, C. TLR-4 and CD14 Genotypes and soluble cd14: Could they predispose to coronary atherosclerosis? *J. Cardiovasc. Dev. Dis.* **2016**, *3*, 9. [CrossRef]

9. Raza, S.T.; Abbas, S.; Eba, A.; Karim, F.; Wani, I.A.; Rizvi, S.; Zaidi, A.; Mahdi, F. Association of COL4A1 (rs605143, rs565470) and CD14 (rs2569190) genes polymorphism with coronary artery disease. *Mol. Cell. Biochem.* **2018**, *445*, 117–122. [CrossRef]
10. Mertens, J.; Bregadze, R.; Mansur, A.; Askar, E.; Bickeboller, H.; Ramadori, G.; Mihm, S. Functional impact of endotoxin receptor CD14 polymorphisms on transcriptional activity. *J. Mol. Med. (Berl.)* **2009**, *87*, 815–824. [CrossRef] [PubMed]
11. Assaad, S.; Costanian, C.; Jaffal, L.; Tannous, F.; Stathopoulou, M.G.; El Shamieh, S. Association of TLR4 Polymorphisms, Expression, and Vitamin D with helicobacter pylori Infection. *J. Pers. Med.* **2019**, *9*, 2. [CrossRef] [PubMed]
12. IBM Corp. *IBM SPSS Statistics for Windows, Version 24.0*; IBM Corp: Armonk, NY, USA, 2016.
13. Faul, F.; Erdfelder, E.; Lang, A.G.; Buchner, A. G*Power 3: A flexible statistical power analysis program for the social, behavioral, and biomedical sciences. *Behav. Res. Methods* **2007**, *39*, 175–191. [CrossRef] [PubMed]
14. Wright, S.D.; Ramos, R.A.; Tobias, P.S.; Ulevitch, R.J.; Mathison, J.C. CD14, a receptor for complexes of lipopolysaccharide (LPS) and LPS binding protein. *Science* **1990**, *249*, 1431–1433. [CrossRef] [PubMed]
15. Bazil, V.; Baudys, M.; Hilgert, I.; Stefanova, I.; Low, M.G.; Zbrozek, J.; Horejsi, V. Structural relationship between the soluble and membrane-bound forms of human monocyte surface glycoprotein CD14. *Mol. Immunol.* **1989**, *26*, 657–662. [CrossRef]
16. Bas, S.; Gauthier, B.R.; Spenato, U.; Stingelin, S.; Gabay, C. CD14 is an acute-phase protein. *J. Immunol.* **2004**, *172*, 4470–4479. [CrossRef] [PubMed]
17. Unkelbach, K.; Gardemann, A.; Kostrzewa, M.; Philipp, M.; Tillmanns, H.; Haberbosch, W. A new promoter polymorphism in the gene of lipopolysaccharide receptor CD14 is associated with expired myocardial infarction in patients with low atherosclerotic risk profile. *Arter. Thromb Vasc. Biol.* **1999**, *19*, 932–938. [CrossRef] [PubMed]
18. Hubacek, J.A.; Rothe, G.; Pit'ha, J.; Skodova, Z.; Stanek, V.; Poledne, R.; Schmitz, G. C(-260)–>T polymorphism in the promoter of the CD14 monocyte receptor gene as a risk factor for myocardial infarction. *Circulation* **1999**, *99*, 3218–3220. [CrossRef] [PubMed]
19. Mann, D.L. The emerging role of innate immunity in the heart and vascular system: For whom the cell tolls. *Circ. Res.* **2011**, *108*, 1133–1145. [CrossRef] [PubMed]
20. Benachour, H.; Zaiou, M.; Samara, A.; Herbeth, B.; Pfister, M.; Lambert, D.; Siest, G.; Visvikis-Siest, S. Association of human cathelicidin (hCAP-18/LL-37) gene expression with cardiovascular disease risk factors. *Nutr. Metab. Cardiovasc. Dis.* **2009**, *19*, 720–728. [CrossRef] [PubMed]
21. El Shamieh, S.; Herbeth, B.; Azimi-Nezhad, M.; Benachour, H.; Masson, C.; Visvikis-Siest, S. Human formyl peptide receptor 1 C32T SNP interacts with age and is associated with blood pressure levels. *Clin. Chim. Acta* **2012**, *413*, 34–38. [CrossRef] [PubMed]

11

Micronutrient Depletion in Heart Failure: Common, Clinically Relevant and Treatable

Natasa Cvetinovic [1], Goran Loncar [2,3], Andjelka M. Isakovic [3], Stephan von Haehling [4,5], Wolfram Doehner [6], Mitja Lainscak [7,8,*] and Jerneja Farkas [9,10,*]

1 Department of Cardiology, University Clinical Hospital Center "Dr. Dragisa Misovic—Dedinje", 11000 Belgrade, Serbia; ncvetinovic@gmail.com
2 Institute for Cardiovascular Diseases Dedinje, 11000 Belgrade, Serbia; loncar_goran@yahoo.com
3 School of Medicine, University of Belgrade, 11000 Belgrade, Serbia; andjelka.isakovic@gmail.com
4 Department of Cardiology and Pneumology, University of Goettingen Medical Center, DE-37075 Goettingen, Germany; stephan.von.haehling@med.uni-goettingen.de
5 German Center for Cardiovascular Research (DZHK), partner site Goettingen, DE-37099 Goettingen, Germany
6 Berlin Institute of Health Center for Regenerative Therapies (BCRT) and Department of Cardiology (Virchow Klinikum), German Centre for Cardiovascular Research (DZHK) partner site Berlin, Charité Universitätsmedizin Berlin, DE-13353 Berlin, Germany; wolfram.doehner@charite.de
7 Division of Cardiology, General Hospital Murska Sobota, SI-9000 Murska Sobota, Slovenia
8 Faculty of Medicine, University of Ljubljana, SI-1000 Ljubljana, Slovenia
9 Research Unit, General Hospital Murska Sobota, SI-9000 Murska Sobota, Slovenia
10 National Institute of Public Health, SI-1000 Ljubljana, Slovenia
* Correspondence: mitja.lainscak@guest.arnes.si (M.L.); jerneja.farkas@sb-ms.si (J.F.)

Abstract: Heart failure (HF) is a chronic condition with many imbalances, including nutritional issues. Next to sarcopenia and cachexia which are clinically evident, micronutrient deficiency is also present in HF. It is involved in HF pathophysiology and has prognostic implications. In general, most widely known micronutrients are depleted in HF, which is associated with symptoms and adverse outcomes. Nutritional intake is important but is not the only factor reducing the micronutrient availability for bodily processes, because absorption, distribution, and patient comorbidity may play a major role. In this context, interventional studies with parenteral micronutrient supplementation provide evidence that normalization of micronutrients is associated with improvement in physical performance and quality of life. Outcome studies are underway and should be reported in the following years.

Keywords: heart failure; micronutrients; iron; vitamins; trace elements

1. Introduction

Heart failure (HF) is a complex disease with many potential underlying causes, which affects the function of other tissues and is often followed by comorbidities [1], especially in the elderly [2]. Pathogenesis of HF has been elucidated and includes many mechanisms, such as increased hemodynamic overload, ischemic-related dysfunction, ventricular remodeling, excessive neurohormonal stimulation, abnormal cardiomyocyte calcium cycling, excessive or inadequate accumulation of extracellular matrix, accelerated apoptosis, and genetic mutations [1]. Although no single unifying pathogenetic theory can explain HF completely, there is evidence suggesting that declining bioenergy plays a major role [3]. Fatty acids and carbohydrates are the main energy source for cardiomyocytes. The conversion of these macronutrients to biological energy requires micronutrients such as coenzyme Q10, thiamine, riboflavin, etc., which are essential cofactors for energy production, energy transfer, and maintenance of the physiological heart function [4]. Moreover, patients with HF have oxidative stress, inappropriate food intake (Table 1), altered metabolism and intestinal function, and pro-inflammatory status, which leads to a deficiency of micronutrients (e.g., iron, selenium, and zinc) and consequently affects prognosis. This review aims to underline the role of micronutrients in the pathophysiology of HF, their prognostic implications, and the effects of supplementation. We reviewed micronutrients that were most represented in the literature and could potentially have the most beneficial effects when supplemented in HF patients, namely B complex vitamins (B1, B2, B6, B12), vitamin C, trace elements selenium, zinc, and iron, coenzyme Q10, with a special attention on vitamin D due to a long history of its research and supplementation, and the abundance of available data.

Table 1. Recommended micronutrient dietary allowance for the general population.

Micronutrient	RDA	Reference
Vitamin D	15–20 μg/day	[5,6]
Thiamin (B1)	1.1–1.2 mg/day	[7]
Riboflavin (B2)	0.9–1.3 mg/day	[8]
Pyridoxine (B6)	1.6–2.0 mg/day	[9]
Cobalamin (B12)	2.0–2.4 μg/day	[10]
Vitamin C	75–90 mg/day	[11]
Coenzyme Q10 *	n.a.	
Selenium	55 μg/day	[10]
Zinc	8–11 mg/day	[11]
Iron	8–18 mg/day	[11]

RDA: recommended dietary allowance. n.a.: not assessed. *: no RDA has been established.

2. Vitamin D

Although many diseases (e.g., cancer, autoimmune disorders, infertility and pregnancy complications, insulin resistance, and type 2 diabetes mellitus) are associated with vitamin D levels, its metabolism, and vitamin D-related genes [12,13], the association between vitamin D and cardiovascular disease is still controversial. Vitamin D regulates numerous processes involved in the pathogenesis of HF, such as cell proliferation and differentiation, apoptosis, oxidative stress, inflammation, endothelial function, vascular calcification, and activation of the renin-angiotensin system [14]. Observational studies have reported that subjects with lower vitamin D levels are under higher risk of developing HF [15,16]. Vitamin D deficiency (Table 2) is one of the most common types of hypovitaminosis worldwide, with a prevalence of almost 50% among the elderly [17], and is the most common vitamin deficiency in HF [18]. It is more common among patients with HF compared with healthy control individuals, independently of age [19]. While 90–99% of elderly HF patients are affected by vitamin D deficiency [17,20,21], severe deficiency is reported in 17–68% of HF patients, dependent on age, gender, functional status, HF severity, and left ventricle ejection fraction (LVEF) [17,20,22]. Pathophysiology of vitamin D deficiency includes reduced food intake and intestinal absorption of nutrients, and limited exposure to solar ultraviolet light (Table 1). Accordingly, both aging and HF predispose patients to hypovitaminosis, and they may have an additive effect on vitamin D level in elderly patients. In light of the above, it is reasonable to evaluate vitamin D status in HF patients separately according to age.

Table 2. Serum normal concentrations and definition of deficiency of micronutrients.

Micronutrient	Reference Range	Insufficiency	Deficiency	Reference
Vitamin D	>30 ng/mL >75 nmol/L	21–29 ng/mL 52.5–72.5 nmol/L	<20 ng/mL <50 nmol/L	[23]
Thiamin (B1) *	25–75 ng/mL 75–195 nmol/L			[24]
Riboflavin (B2) [a]			EGRAC ≥ 1.3	[25]
Pyridoxine (B6) [b]	5–50 ng/mL 23–223 nmol/L	20–30 nmol/L	<20 nmol/L	[26–28]
Cobalamin (B12)	180–950 pg/mL 125–701 pmol/L		<200 pg/mL <148 pmol/L	[29,30]
Vitamin C	>50 μmol/L	10–50 μmol/L	<10 μmol/L	[31]
Coenzyme Q10	0.5–1.7 μmol/L			[32]
Selenium	70–150 ng/mL 0.9–1.8 μmol/L			[33]
Zinc	0.7–1.6 μg/mL 11–25 μmol/L			[34]
Iron	45–160 μg/mL 8–23 μmol/L		<45 μg/mL <8 μmol/L	[35]

*: exact range depends on the laboratory; different cutoff values are used. [a]: expressed as erythrocyte glutathione reductase activation coefficient (EGRAC). [b]: measured as pyridoxal phosphate.

Vitamin D is associated with functional status, illness severity, and prognosis in HF [36]. Vitamin D level positively correlates with cardiopulmonary stress test performance [22] and six-minute walk test distance [37], and negatively with NYHA class [17,20]. In a study of severe HF patients, vitamin D concentration was significantly lower in hospitalized subjects requiring intravenous inotropic agents or left ventricular assist devices, compared with those treated as outpatients [22]. Vitamin D also correlates with NT-proANP [19], NT-proBNP [17,38] and left ventricle ejection fraction (LVEF) [20], which are predictors of prognosis in HF. Furthermore, vitamin D levels independently predicted all-cause mortality in an HF study with an 18-month follow-up [38] and strongly predicted mortality in a study with a longer follow-up period of 4 years [36]. Additionally, severe vitamin D deficiency was found as an independent predictor of death due to HF in a study of 3299 enrolled subjects with suspect coronary artery disease [17], and lower levels of vitamin D independently predicts mortality in end-stage HF patients [39].

Although it has been strongly confirmed that vitamin D plays an important role in the development and prognosis of HF, evidence about the effect of vitamin D supplementation in HF patients is inconsistent. It has been documented that vitamin D supplementation (800 IU/day) might protect people >60 years from HF [40]. A recent meta-analysis, which included 81 interventional studies with vitamin D supplementation in HF patients, has confirmed a positive effect on cardiovascular risk factors such as high blood pressure, dyslipidemia, and inflammation [41]. Thus, results suggest that the required dose of vitamin D for improvements in risk factors is ≥4000 IU (100 g)/day, which is above the tolerable upper intake level for adults and can be associated with toxic side effects [42,43]. Supplementation with lower doses (≤2000 IU/day) in HF patients significantly increased vitamin D levels but had no benefits on LVEF, functional capacity, or quality of life [44,45]. The EVITA, a randomized clinical trial (RCT) that compared vitamin D 4000 IU/day to a placebo in patients with advanced HF and vitamin D deficiency (vitamin D ≤ 75 nmol/L), found no difference in mortality and hospitalization rate. Furthermore, supplementation was associated with a greater need for mechanical circulatory support implant (especially in patients with initial vitamin D concentrations ≥ 30 nmol/L) and higher incidence of hypercalcemia [46]. Accordingly, vitamin D supplementation in HF can be considered but requires caution, especially in patients with no evidence of significant deficiency.

3. Other Fat-Soluble Vitamins

Although experimental data have provided evidence that vitamin A regulates the cardiac renin-angiotensin system, and that vitamin A receptors impact the development of diabetes-induced cardiac remodeling and HF in patients with diabetes mellitus [47], the association between vitamin A and HF has not been confirmed in observational studies. Only one study has evaluated vitamin A status in HF, and it found no significant difference between HF patients and sex-matched healthy controls [48]. Dietary vitamin A intake showed no association with HF mortality in the Japan Collaborative Cohort Study, which enrolled 58,696 subjects [49].

Observational studies have found no significant differences in vitamin E status between HF patients and healthy controls [48,50]. The same result was found in a rat model of HF [51]. However, in the Japan Collaborative Cohort Study, high dietary intake of vitamin E was associated with a reduced risk of HF mortality in women but not in men [49]. Although vitamin E supplementation (400 mg/day) reduces oxidative stress in HF patients [52], it has no impact on symptoms, physical functioning, or mortality [53–56]. Moreover, there are indications that vitamin E treatment may contribute to HF development [54,55].

It is known that vitamin K status is associated with reduced coronary artery calcification and cardiovascular mortality risk. Vitamin K levels, intake, and supplementation have not been evaluated in HF patients, although epidemiological studies suggest a protective role of vitamin K in cardiovascular diseases [57].

4. B Vitamins

Thiamine (vitamin B1) is a cofactor in the metabolism of carbohydrates and amino acids and is also essential for aerobic metabolism and adenosine triphosphate (ATP) production. Thiamine deficiency is associated with many cardiovascular diseases, including HF, chronic vascular inflammation, myocardial infarction, and conduction defects [58]. Furthermore, the deficiency can cause HF by depriving the heart of ATP [59]. On the other hand, HF induces thiamin deficiency by increasing urinary excretion due to therapy with loop diuretics, and poor absorption of thiamine due to cardiac cachexia and splanchnic congestion [60,61]. The addition of spironoloctone to loop diuretics has beneficial effects on thiamine levels in HF patients [62].

The prevalence of thiamine deficiency (Table 2) in HF patients is significantly higher compared with non-HF subjects and ranges from 3% in ambulatory settings to 91% in hospital settings [63]. The first observational study that evaluated the effects of thiamine supplementation in HF enrolled only six patients who were treated by intravenous thiamine (100 mg/day) for 7 days [64]. The results confirmed significant improvement in thiamine levels as assessed by LVEF and NYHA, which encouraged further research, but findings were controversial. An RCT using seven days of intravenous thiamine versus a placebo in a double-blind manner, followed by six weeks of oral thiamine (200 mg/day) in all patients, indicated significant improvement of LVEF in the thiamine group after seven days (LVEF increase was 4%), and impressive improvement of 22% in all patients at the end of treatment [65]. An RCT with oral thiamine (300 mg/day), had a small sample size (18 patients) and a short follow-up period (28 days), but confirmed LVEF improvement after supplementation [66]. However, these results were not confirmed in an RCT that enrolled 52 patients. The main difference between these two RCTs with similar designs was the use of diuretic therapy, which significantly influenced thiamine level. In the trial with no LVEF improvement, the proportion of patients who were on furosemide was low (<20%) and spironolactone was prescribed to most patients (>80%) in the thiamine group [62]. Oral supplementation may be less effective than intravenous, due to the impaired enteral absorption in HF. Limitations of all performed studies, and potential cause of inconclusive results, included small sample sizes, short follow-up periods, and subjective measures used as endpoints. Accordingly, further research is needed to elucidate the effects of thiamine supplementation on mortality, hospitalization rate, functional status, and quality of life in HF.

Riboflavin (vitamin B2) is an essential cofactor in cellular energy production, and its deficiency may contribute to the depletion of energy reserves observed in the failing heart. It is water-soluble, has limited tissue storage, and depends on intake (Table 1) and renal excretion. Prevalence of riboflavin deficiency (Table 2) is significantly higher (27%) in HF patients than in healthy controls (2.2%) [67,68]. A study on animal models of HF suggests that riboflavin supplementation significantly improves left ventricular systolic and diastolic function [69]. Further research on HF and riboflavin deficiency in humans is required.

Pyridoxine (vitamin B6) plays an important role in intermediary metabolism, as a cofactor mainly in the metabolism of amino acids, but also of carbohydrates and lipids, as well as in the biosynthesis of neurotransmitters. Pyridoxine deficiency (Table 2) prevalence is also higher in HF patients (38%) than in healthy controls [68]. There are no investigations of isolated pyridoxine supplementation in HF patients.

Cobalamin (vitamin B12) deficiency has been evaluated in the setting of HF, but results are controversial. The largest study evaluating vitamin B12 in HF, with almost 1000 patients, provided unexpected results: vitamin B12 had a weak negative correlation with LVEF and a significant positive correlation with NYHA class [70]. A possible reason for these results is the unclear selection of HF patients: a large number of patients had no systolic dysfunction (mean LVEF were 58% and 65% for men and women, respectively) and no clinical manifestations of HF (about 35% patients were NYHA class I). An observational study found that vitamin B12 deficiency (serum level <200 pg/mL) is relatively rare in HF (5%), and that vitamin B12 level is not related to prognosis [71]. However, the study was not limited to patients with reduced LVEF, and 13% of enrolled patients had LVEF >45%. Although parenteral replacement therapy should be started soon after the vitamin B12 deficiency has been established [72], an interventional study with vitamin B12 supplementation, in addition to folate and vitamin B6, in elderly HF patients (mean age 81 years) suggested no association with NT-proBNP levels [73]. In the future, vitamin B12 should be evaluated in the setting of HF with reduced ejection fraction.

5. Vitamin C

Three observational studies [48,50,74] showed significantly lower vitamin C levels among HF patients (mean 39.7 μmol/L, 61 μmol/L, 22 μmol/L, respectively) than in healthy controls, although in all of them, concentrations were above the cutoff for deficiency (Table 2) [75]. In a more recent study, patients with HF had lower vitamin C levels (43.3 μmol/L in NYHA II and 46.8 μmol/L in NYHA III/IV) than the control group had (57.2 μmol/L), but the difference was not significant [67]. Two studies, which determined vitamin C deficiency by a 3-day food diary, found a similar prevalence of the dietary deficiency (39% and 40%, respectively) among HF patients [76,77]. Furthermore, dietary deficiency predicted shorter cardiac event-free survival in both of them. Although some interventional studies have shown that vitamin C supplementation enhances the contractile response to dobutamine [78] and improves endothelial function [79] in HF, there have been no RCTs evaluating vitamin C supplementation in HF. For further research, we propose RCTs that evaluate the effects of vitamin C supplementation on biomarker status, echocardiography parameters, functional status, quality of life, and long-term outcomes in HF patients with confirmed vitamin C deficiency.

6. Coenzyme Q10

Coenzyme Q10 (CoQ10) is essential for ATP synthesis, as well as a powerful lipid-soluble antioxidant [80]. Myocardial CoQ10 deficiency has been observed in patients with HF, and it correlates with the severity of symptoms and the LVEF [81]. CoQ10 supplementation also significantly increases its concentration in the blood [82]. Lower levels of CoQ10 (Table 2) are observed in elderly patients and those with more advanced HF [83]. Since 1976, when the first interventional study with CoQ10 administration in HF suggested its therapeutic potential [84], many RCTs have been performed that confirm its benefit in the treatment of HF [85]. CoQ10 significantly improves cardiac output, cardiac index, stroke volume, and LVEF [86,87]. The administration of CoQ10 in patients with end-stage HF awaiting cardiac transplantation significantly improved functional status, clinical symptoms, and quality of life, but there were no changes in echo parameters [88]. An RCT performed 25 years ago that enrolled 641 HF patients (NYHA class III and IV) demonstrated that the addition of CoQ10 to conventional therapy (2 mg/kg daily for 1 year) significantly reduces hospitalization due to HF worsening and the incidence of serious complications [89]. The most recent Q-SYMBIO RCT (CoQ10 100 mg 3 times/day for 2 years vs. placebo) confirmed that CoQ10 as an adjunctive treatment of HF is safe, improves symptoms and functional status, and reduces major adverse cardiovascular events, such as death from HF, sudden cardiac death, and hospitalization due to HF worsening [90]. According to all of the above, we suggest that physicians should consider CoQ10 supplementation in advanced HF, especially if the deficiency is confirmed.

7. Selenium

Selenium is an essential nutrient and one of the most important antioxidants in the body. It is found within the body in various selenoproteins, such as glutathione peroxidase (GPx), thioredoxin reductase and selenoprotein P [91]. Moreover, selenium has an important role in converting thyroxin into the biologically active triiodothyronine. This may be an additional mechanism by which low concentrations of selenium compromise cardiovascular conditions [92]. The dietary intake of selenium (Table 1) differs throughout the world. In Europe, due to poor selenium content in the soil, the estimated mean intake of selenium (40 μg/day) [93] is significantly lower than the proposed dose for a normal-weighted Caucasian (75 μg/day), which is needed for optimal function of selenoprotein P [94] and cancer protection [33]. Furthermore, it is well known that selenium deficiency may be a cause of reversible HF, a condition known as Keshan Disease [95]. Also, it has been suggested that patients with HF tend to have lower circulating levels of selenium (Table 2) than individuals free from the condition [43]. A case-control-pair longitudinal study with 11,000 enrolled participants found that subjects with low selenium levels have a higher risk for myocardial infarction and cardiovascular mortality [96], but RCTs with selenium supplementation have found no evidence of cardiovascular protection [97].

The metabolism of selenium and CoQ10 are strongly associated with each other, and a deficiency of one can reduce levels or function of the other [98–100]. Accordingly, they are often used and evaluated together. An RCT of an elderly population (mean age 78) who were supplemented with 200 μg/day of organic selenium and 200 mg/day of CoQ10 versus a placebo, found that long-term supplementation reduces NT-proBNP levels and cardiovascular mortality in those with mild to moderate impaired cardiac function [101]. Although an RCT with multiple micronutrient supplementation that included selenium, suggested a beneficial effect on LVEF and quality of life in 30 HF patients (LVEF ≤ 35%, HF due to ischemic heart disease) [102], data about its effects on HF when used alone are insufficient. A recent RCT that compared selenium 200 μg/day with a placebo indicated that supplementation for 12 weeks to HF patients has beneficial effects on insulin metabolism and few markers of cardio-metabolic risk [103].

8. Zinc

Zinc, which has antioxidant properties [104], is an essential element for humans and is required for enzyme function, multiple signaling pathways and transcription factors, and is also the second most abundant trace metal in humans [105]. Although zinc is widely distributed in human tissue and has numerous functions, it has an important role in controlling cardiac contractility in cardyomyocites [106].

One of the oldest studies on zinc levels in HF patients evaluated zinc status in 20 younger HF patients (34–64 years), and indicated significantly lower levels in subjects with dilated cardiomyopathy than in healthy controls (74.5 μg/dL or 11.4 μmol/L vs. 93.1 μg/dL or 14.2 μmol/L, respectively) [107]. This finding has been supported by studies on patients with LVEF <40% and NYHA class II-IV [48,108–110], and finally confirmed by a recent meta-analysis published in 2018 [111]. Moreover, subgroup analysis found that patients with idiopathic dilated cardiomyopathy had lower zinc levels than control subjects, except for patients with ischemic cardiomyopathy. A recent study enrolled 968 hospitalized patients with decompensated HF who were divided into 3 groups based on serum zinc levels, and found the highest cardiac and all-cause mortality in the third tertile (<62 μg/dL). Serum zinc level was a predictor of cardiac and all-cause mortality, independently of age, gender, comorbidities, medications, other micronutrient levels, B-type natriuretic peptide, and LVEF [112].

Although the role of zinc in cardiovascular medicine has been well represented in molecular research and observational studies in the past few years, there have been no interventional studies or RCTs evaluating zinc supplementation in HF. Two previous studies that included zinc in multiple micronutrient supplements have suggested an association with improvement of cardiac function and quality of life [103,113].

According to the above, further research into zinc supplementation in HF is needed. We propose a study population of elderly patients with advanced HF due to non-ischemic cardiomyopathy and confirmed zinc deficiency, who could have the greatest benefit of the supplementation.

9. Iron

Iron is an essential microelement, required for transport, storage and usage of oxygen in humans. In HF, iron deficiency (Table 2) is one of the most common comorbidities, affecting 37–61% of patients [114–116]. The deficiency, even before the onset of anemia, can be severe among patients with CHF, aggravating symptoms, quality of life, functional status, and clinical outcomes, and is associated with an increased risk of mortality [114,117–120]. The 2016 European Society of Cardiology (ESC) guidelines for the diagnosis and treatment of acute and chronic HF recommend that all patients with HF should be tested for iron deficiency [121]. Moreover, intravenous iron, ferric carboxymaltose, is specifically recommended to be considered for the treatment of iron deficiency in HF, in order to alleviate symptoms and improve exercise capacity and quality of life [122,123]. Oral iron supplementation has no benefit in the setting of HF [124,125] and is not recommended by ESC guidelines. The impaired enteral absorption and other conditions characterized by immune activation are considered as causes for the ineffectiveness of oral iron administration. Findings of the IRONOUT HF RCT (oral iron therapy vs. placebo) [124] are in contrast to results from RCTs of intravenous iron repletion (FAIR-HF and CONFIRM-HF) [122,123], although patient populations were similar. Moreover, in the IRONOUT HF oral therapy produced improvement in iron stores, though the improvement was minimal and clinically not significant.

Iron deficiency is also a frequent co-morbidity in HF with preserved EF (HFpEF), which associated with reduced exercise capacity and quality of life, and its prevalence increases with increasing severity of diastolic dysfunction [126]. Beneficial effects of intravenous iron therapy in an animal model of HFpEF [127] encourage further research, which should elucidate the effects of iron therapy in HF with preserved LVEF.

10. Conclusions and Future Perspectives

Although micronutrient deficiencies are frequent among HF patients, their role in pathogenesis and treatment has not yet been completely elucidated. Besides iron supplementation, which is recommended by ESC, CoQ10 supplementation has the strongest evidence of benefit in HF. The available data suggest consideration of vitamin D supplementation in cases of confirmed deficiency in patients with HF. Some micronutrients (selenium, zinc, vitamin B2, and vitamin B6) showed improvement of various clinical parameters in HF, but were investigated only in a multiple supplementation setting, while the effects of vitamins B1 and B12 were inconsistent due to unclear selection of patients and poorly defined endpoints. The influence of vitamin C supplementation in HF is yet to be determined. Thus, interventional studies with strict selection criteria and clear endpoints for each micronutrient are still needed to gain better insight into their role in HF. Furthermore, the question remains as to whether the deficiency cutoff values drawn from the general population apply to HF patients; this should be addressed in future research. Supplementation trials should take into account reduced food intake and poor intestinal absorption of nutrients in these patients, and should investigate not only dosage with beneficial effects, but also the routes of administration (i.e., oral or intravenous). In addition, the available data on micronutrient supplementation in patients with HFpEF are scarce and should be thoroughly researched in the future.

References

1. Braunwald, E. Heart Failure. *JACC Hear. Fail.* **2013**, *1*, 1–20. [CrossRef] [PubMed]
2. Cvetinovic, N.; Loncar, G.; Farkas, J. Heart failure management in the elderly—A public health challenge. *Wien. Klin. Wochenschr.* **2016**, *128*, 466–473. [CrossRef] [PubMed]
3. Wong, A.-P.; Niedzwiecki, A.; Rath, M. Myocardial energetics and the role of micronutrients in heart failure: A critical review. *Am. J. Cardiovasc. Dis.* **2016**, *15*, 81–92.
4. Witte, K.K.; Clark, A.L. Micronutrients and their supplementation in chronic cardiac failure. An update beyond theoretical perspectives. *Heart Fail. Rev.* **2006**, *11*, 65–74. [CrossRef] [PubMed]
5. Ross, A.C.; Taylor, C.L.; Yaktine, A.L.; del Valle, H.B. *Dietary Reference Values for Vitamin D*; National Academies Press: Washington, DC, USA, 2016.
6. Ross, A.C.; Taylor, C.L.; Yaktine, A.L.; del Valle, H.B. *Dietary Reference Intakes for Calcium and Vitamin, D*; National Academies Press: Washington, DC, USA, 2011.
7. Ross, A.C.; Taylor, C.L.; Yaktine, A.L.; del Valle, H.B. *Dietary Reference Intakes for Thiamin, Riboflavin, Niacin, Vitamin B6, Folate, Vitamin B12, Pantothenic Acid, Biotin, and Choline*; National Academies Press: Washington, DC, USA, 1998.
8. Ross, A.C.; Taylor, C.L.; Yaktine, A.L.; del Valle, H.B. *Dietary Reference Intakes*; National Academies Press: Washington, DC, USA, 2003.
9. Said, H.M. Water-Soluble Vitamins. *World Rev. Nutr. Diet.* **2014**, *111*, 30–37. [PubMed]
10. Ross, A.C.; Taylor, C.L.; Yaktine, A.L.; del Valle, H.B. *Dietary Reference Intakes for Vitamin C, Vitamin E, Selenium, and Carotenoids*; National Academies Press: Washington, DC, USA, 2000.
11. Ross, A.C.; Taylor, C.L.; Yaktine, A.L.; del Valle, H.B. *Dietary Reference Intakes for Vitamin A, Vitamin K, Arsenic, Boron, Chromium, Copper, Iodine, Iron, Manganese, Molybdenum, Nickel, Silicon, Vanadium, and Zinc*; National Academies Press: Washington, DC, USA, 2001.
12. Wimalawansa, S.J.; Razzaque, M.S.; Al-Daghri, N.M. Calcium and vitamin D in human health: Hype or real? *J. Steroid Biochem. Mol. Biol.* **2018**, *180*, 4–14. [CrossRef] [PubMed]
13. Zeljic, K.; Kandolf-Sekulovic, L.; Supic, G.; Pejovic, J.; Novakovic, M.; Mijuskovic, Z. Melanoma risk is associated with vitamin D receptor gene polymorphisms. *Melanoma Res.* **2014**, *24*, 273–279. [CrossRef] [PubMed]
14. Parker, J.; Hashmi, O.; Dutton, D.; Mavrodaris, A.; Stranges, S.; Kandala, N.B.; Clarke, A.; Franco, O.H. Levels of vitamin D and cardiometabolic disorders: Systematic review and meta-analysis. *Maturitas* **2010**, *65*, 225–236. [CrossRef] [PubMed]
15. Kim, D.H.; Sabour, S.; Sagar, U.N.; Adams, S.; Whellan, D.J. Prevalence of Hypovitaminosis D in Cardiovascular Diseases (from the National Health and Nutrition Examination Survey 2001 to 2004). *Am. J. Cardiol.* **2008**, *102*, 1540–1544. [CrossRef] [PubMed]
16. Anderson, J.L.; May, H.T.; Horne, B.D.; Bair, T.L.; Hall, N.L.; Carlquist, J.F.; Lappé, D.L.; Muhlestein, J.B. Relation of vitamin D deficiency to cardiovascular risk factors, disease status, and incident events in a general healthcare population. *Am. J. Cardiol.* **2010**, *106*, 963–968. [CrossRef] [PubMed]
17. Wellnitz, B.; Seelhorst, U.; Dimai, H.P.; Dobnig, H.; Pilz, S.; Maäz, W.; Fahrleitner-Pammer, A.; Boehm, B.O. Association of vitamin D deficiency with heart failure and sudden cardiac death in a large cross-sectional study of patients referred for coronary angiography. *J. Clin. Endocrinol. Metab.* **2008**, *93*, 3927–3935.
18. Song, E.K.; Kang, S.M. Micronutrient Deficiency Independently Predicts Adverse Health Outcomes in Patients with Heart Failure. *J. Cardiovasc. Nurs.* **2017**, *32*, 47–53. [CrossRef] [PubMed]
19. Zittermann, A.; Schulze Schleithoff, S.; Tenderich, G.; Berthold, H.K.; Körfer, R.; Stehle, P. Low vitamin D status: A contributing factor in the pathogenesis of congestive heart failure? *J. Am. Coll. Cardiol.* **2003**, *41*, 105–112. [CrossRef]
20. Ameri, P.; Ronco, D.; Casu, M.; Denegri, A.; Bovio, M.; Menoni, S.; Ferone, D.; Murialdo, G. High prevalence of vitamin D deficiency and its association with left ventricular dilation: An echocardiography study in elderly patients with chronic heart failure. *Nutr. Metab. Cardiovasc. Dis.* **2010**, *20*, 633–640. [CrossRef] [PubMed]

21. Loncar, G.; Bozic, B.; Cvetinovic, N.; Dungen, H.D.; Lainscak, M.; von Haehling, S.; Doehner, W.; Radojicic, Z.; Putnikovic, B.; Trippel, T.; et al. Secondary hyperparathyroidism prevalence and prognostic role in elderly males with heart failure. *J. Endocrinol. Investig.* **2017**, *40*, 297–304. [CrossRef] [PubMed]
22. Shane, E.; Mancini, D.; Aaronson, K.; Silverberg, S.J.; Seibel, M.J.; Addesso, V.; McMahon, D.J. Bone mass, vitamin D deficiency, and hyperparathyroidism in congestive heart failure. *Am. J. Med.* **1997**, *103*, 197–207. [CrossRef]
23. Holick, M.F. The vitamin D deficiency pandemic: Approaches for diagnosis, treatment and prevention. *Rev. Endocr. Metab. Disord.* **2017**, *18*, 153–165. [CrossRef] [PubMed]
24. Whitfield, K.C.; Bourassa, M.W.; Adamolekun, B.; Bergeron, G.; Bettendorff, L.; Brown, K.H.; Cox, L.; Fattal-Valevski, A.; Fischer, P.R.; Frank, E.L.; et al. Thiamine deficiency disorders: Diagnosis, prevalence, and a roadmap for global control programs. *Ann. N. Y. Acad. Sci.* **2018**, *1430*, 3–43. [CrossRef] [PubMed]
25. Hill, M.H.E.; Bradley, A.; Mushtaq, S.; Williams, E.A.; Powers, H.J. Effects of methodological variation on assessment of riboflavin status using the erythrocyte glutathione reductase activation coefficient assay. *Br. J. Nutr.* **2009**, *102*, 273. [CrossRef] [PubMed]
26. McPherson, R.A.; Pincus, M.R. *Henry's Clinical Diagnosis and Management by Laboratory Methods*; Elsevier: Amsterdam, Switzerland, 2016.
27. Leklem, J.E. Vitamin B-6: A Status Report. *J. Nutr.* **1990**, *120*, 1503–1507. [CrossRef] [PubMed]
28. Panton, K.K.; Farup, P.G.; Sagen, E.; Sirum, U.F.; Åsberg, A. Vitamin B6 in plasma—Sample stability and the reference limits. *Scand. J. Clin. Lab. Investig.* **2013**, *73*, 476–479. [CrossRef] [PubMed]
29. Hunt, A.; Harrington, D.; Robinson, S. Vitamin B12 deficiency. *BMJ* **2014**, *349*, g5226. [CrossRef] [PubMed]
30. Klee, G.G. Cobalamin and folate evaluation: Measurement of methylmalonic acid and homocysteine vs. vitamin B(12) and folate. *Clin. Chem.* **2000**, *46*, 1277–1283. [PubMed]
31. Scientific Opinion on Dietary Reference Values for vitamin C. *EFSA J.* **2013**, *11*, 3418. [CrossRef]
32. Molyneux, S.L.; Young, J.M.; Florkowski, C.M.; Lever, M.; George, P.M. Coenzyme Q10: Is there a clinical role and a case for measurement? *Clin. Biochem. Rev.* **2008**, *29*, 71–82. [PubMed]
33. Thomson, C.D. Assessment of requirements for selenium and adequacy of selenium status: A review. *Eur. J. Clin. Nutr.* **2004**, *58*, 391–402. [CrossRef] [PubMed]
34. Livingstone, C. Zinc: Physiology, deficiency, and parenteral nutrition. *Nutr. Clin. Pract.* **2015**, *30*, 371–382. [CrossRef] [PubMed]
35. Gomella, L.G.; Haist, S.A. *Clinician's Pocket Reference*; University of Kentucky, College of Medicine, McGraw-Hill Companies, Inc: New York, NY, USA, 2007.
36. Gruson, D.; Ferracin, B.; Ahn, S.A.; Zierold, C.; Blocki, F.; Hawkins, D.M.; Bonelli, F.; Rousseau, M.F. 1,25-Dihydroxyvitamin D to PTH(1-84) ratios strongly predict cardiovascular death in heart failure. *PLoS ONE* **2015**, *10*, e0135427. [CrossRef] [PubMed]
37. Boxer, R.S.; Dauser, D.A.; Walsh, S.J.; Hager, W.D.; Kenny, A.M. The association between vitamin D and inflammation with the 6-minute walk and frailty in patients with heart failure. *J. Am. Geriatr. Soc.* **2008**, *56*, 454–461. [CrossRef] [PubMed]
38. Liu, L.C.Y.; Voors, A.A.; Van Veldhuisen, D.J.; Van Der Veer, E.; Belonje, A.M.; Szymanski, M.K.; Sillјé, H.H.; Van Gilst, W.H.; Jaarsma, T.; De Boer, R.A. Vitamin D status and outcomes in heart failure patients. *Eur. J. Heart Fail.* **2011**, *13*, 619–625. [CrossRef] [PubMed]
39. Zittermann, A.; Schleithoff, S.S.; Götting, C.; Dronow, O.; Fuchs, U.; Kühn, J.; Kleesiek, K.; Tenderich, G.; Koerfer, R. Poor outcome in end-stage heart failure patients with low circulating calcitriol levels. *Eur. J. Heart Fail.* **2008**, *10*, 321–327. [CrossRef] [PubMed]
40. Ford, J.A.; MacLennan, G.S.; Avenell, A.; Bolland, M.; Grey, A.; Witham, M. Cardiovascular disease and vitamin D supplementation: Trial analysis, systematic review, and meta-analysis. *Am. J. Clin. Nutr.* **2014**, *100*, 746–755. [CrossRef] [PubMed]
41. Mirhosseini, N.; Rainsbury, J.; Kimball, S.M. Vitamin D Supplementation, Serum 25(OH)D Concentrations and Cardiovascular Disease Risk Factors: A Systematic Review and Meta-Analysis. *Front. Cardiovasc. Med.* **2018**, *5*, 87. [CrossRef] [PubMed]
42. Ross, A.C.; Manson, J.E.; Abrams, S.A.; Aloia, J.F.; Brannon, P.M.; Clinton, S.K.; Durazo-Arvizu, R.A.; Gallagher, J.C.; Gallo, R.L.; Jones, G.; et al. The 2011 Dietary Reference Intakes for Calcium and Vitamin D: What Dietetics Practitioners Need to Know. *J. Am. Diet. Assoc.* **2011**, *111*, 524–527. [CrossRef] [PubMed]

43. McKeag, N.A.; McKinley, M.C.; Woodside, J.V.; Harbinson, M.T.; McKeown, P.P. The Role of Micronutrients in Heart Failure. *J. Acad. Nutr. Diet.* **2012**, *112*, 870–886. [CrossRef] [PubMed]
44. Schleithoff, S.S.; Zittermann, A.; Tenderich, G.; Berthold, H.K.; Stehle, P.; Koerfer, R. Vitamin D supplementation improves cytokine profiles in patients with congestive heart failure: A double-blind, randomized, placebo-controlled trial. *Am. J. Clin. Nutr.* **2006**, *83*, 754–759. [CrossRef] [PubMed]
45. Witham, M.D.; Crighton, L.J.; Gillespie, N.D.; Struthers, A.D.; McMurdo, M.E.T. The effects of vitamin D supplementation on physical function and quality of life in older patients with heart failure a randomized controlled trial. *Circ. Heart Fail.* **2010**, *3*, 195–201. [CrossRef] [PubMed]
46. Zittermann, A.; Ernst, J.B.; Prokop, S.; Fuchs, U.; Dreier, J.; Kuhn, J.; Knabbe, C.; Birschmann, I.; Schulz, U.; Berthold, H.K.; et al. Effect of Vitamin D on all-causemortality in heart failure (EVITA): A 3-year randomized clinical trial with 4000 IU Vitamin D daily. *Eur. Heart J.* **2017**, *38*, 2279–2286. [CrossRef] [PubMed]
47. Pan, J.; Guleria, R.; Zhu, S.; Baker, K. Molecular Mechanisms of Retinoid Receptors in Diabetes-Induced Cardiac Remodeling. *J. Clin. Med.* **2014**, *4*, 566–594. [CrossRef] [PubMed]
48. De Lorgeril, M.; Salen, P.; Accominotti, M.; Cadau, M.; Steghens, J.-P.; Boucher, F.; De Leiris, J. Dietary and blood ANTIOXIDANTS in patients with chronic heart failure. Insights into the potential importance of selenium in heart failure. *Eur. J. Heart Fail.* **2001**, *3*, 661–669. [CrossRef]
49. Eshak, E.S.; Iso, H.; Yamagishi, K.; Cui, R.; Tamakoshi, A. Dietary intakes of fat soluble vitamins as predictors of mortality from heart failure in a large prospective cohort study. *Nutrition* **2018**, *47*, 50–55. [CrossRef] [PubMed]
50. Keith, M.; Geranmayegan, A.; Sole, M.J.; Kurian, R.; Robinson, A.; Omran, A.S.; Jeejeebhoy, K.N. Increased oxidative stress in patients with congestive heart failure. *J. Am. Coll. Cardiol.* **1998**, *31*, 1352–1356. [CrossRef]
51. Marcocci, L.; Suzuki, Y.J. Metabolomics studies to assess biological functions of vitamin E nicotinate. *Antioxidants* **2019**, *8*, 127. [CrossRef] [PubMed]
52. Ghatak, A.; Brar, M.J.S.; Agarwal, A.; Goel, N.; Rastogi, A.K.; Vaish, A.K.; Sircar, A.R.; Chandra, M. Oxy free radical system in heart failure and therapeutic role of oral vitamin E. *Int. J. Cardiol.* **1996**, *57*, 119–127. [CrossRef]
53. Yusuf, S.; Dagenais, G.; Pogue, J.; Bosch, J.; Sleight, P. Vitamin E supplementation and cardiovascular events in high-risk patients. The Heart Outcomes Prevention Evaluation Study Investigators. *N. Engl. J. Med.* **2000**, *342*, 154–160. [PubMed]
54. Lonn, E. Effects of long-term vitamin E supplementation on cardiovascular events and cancer: A randomized controlled trial. *J. Am. Med. Assoc.* **2005**, *293*, 1338–1347.
55. Marchioli, R.; Levantesi, G.; Macchia, A.; Marfisi, R.M.; Nicolosi, G.L.; Tavazzi, L.; Tognoni, G.; Valagussa, F. Vitamin E increases the risk of developing heart failure after myocardial infarction: Results from the GISSI-Prevenzione trial. *J. Cardiovasc. Med.* **2006**, *7*, 347–350. [CrossRef] [PubMed]
56. E Keith, M.; Jeejeebhoy, K.N.; Langer, A.; Kurian, R.; Barr, A.; O'Kelly, B.; Sole, M.J. A controlled clinical trial of vitamin E supplementation in patients with congestive heart failure. *Am. J. Clin. Nutr.* **2001**, *73*, 219–224. [CrossRef] [PubMed]
57. Tsugawa, N. Cardiovascular diseases and fat soluble vitamins: Vitamin D and vitamin K. *J. Nutr. Sci. Vitam. (Tokyo)* **2015**, *61*, S170–S172. [CrossRef] [PubMed]
58. Eshak, E.S.; Arafa, A.E. Thiamine deficiency and cardiovascular disorders. *Nutr. Metab. Cardiovasc. Dis.* **2018**, *28*, 965–972. [CrossRef] [PubMed]
59. Attaluri, P.; Castillo, A.; Edriss, H.; Nugent, K. Thiamine Deficiency: An Important Consideration in Critically Ill Patients. *Am. J. Med. Sci.* **2018**, *356*, 382–390. [CrossRef] [PubMed]
60. Zenuk, C.; Healey, J.; Donnelly, J.; Vaillancourt, R.; Almalki, Y.; Smith, S. Thiamine deficiency in congestive heart failure patients receiving long term furosemide therapy. *Can J. Clin. Pharmacol.* **2003**, *10*, 184–188. [PubMed]
61. Kattoor, A.J.; Goel, A.; Mehta, J.L. Thiamine Therapy for Heart Failure: A Promise or Fiction? *Cardiovasc. Drugs Ther.* **2018**, *32*, 313–317. [CrossRef] [PubMed]
62. Rocha, R.M.; Silva, G.V.; de Albuquerque, D.C.; Tura, B.R.; Albanesi Filho, F.M. Influence of spironolactone therapy on thiamine blood levels in patients with heart failure. *Arq. Bras. Cardiol.* **2008**, *90*, 324–328. [PubMed]
63. Jain, A.; Mehta, R.; Al-Ani, M.; Hill, J.A.; Winchester, D.E. Determining the Role of Thiamine Deficiency in Systolic Heart Failure: A Meta-Analysis and Systematic Review. *J. Card. Fail.* **2015**, *21*, 1000–1007. [CrossRef] [PubMed]

64. Seligmann, H.; Halkin, H.; Rauchfleisch, S.; Kaufmann, N.; Tal, R.; Motro, M.; Vered, Z.; Ezra, D. Thiamine deficiency in patients with congestive heart failure receiving long-term furosemide therapy: A pilot study. *Am. J. Med.* **1991**, *91*, 151–155. [CrossRef]
65. Shimon, H.; Almog, S.; Vered, Z.; Seligmann, H.; Shefi, M.; Peleg, E.; Rosenthal, T.; Motro, M.; Halkin, H.; Ezra, D. Improved left ventricular function after thiamine supplementation in patients with congestive heart failure receiving long-term furosemide therapy. *Am. J. Med.* **1995**, *98*, 485–490. [CrossRef]
66. Schoenenberger, A.W.; Schoenenberger-Berzins, R.; Der Maur, C.A.; Suter, P.M.; Vergopoulos, A.; Erne, P. Thiamine supplementation in symptomatic chronic heart failure: A randomized, double-blind, placebo-controlled, cross-over pilot study. *Clin. Res. Cardiol.* **2012**, *101*, 159–164. [CrossRef] [PubMed]
67. Hughes, C.M.; Woodside, J.V.; McGartland, C.; Roberts, M.J.; Nicholls, D.P.; McKeown, P.P. Nutritional intake and oxidative stress in chronic heart failure. *Nutr. Metab. Cardiovasc. Dis.* **2012**, *22*, 376–382. [CrossRef] [PubMed]
68. Keith, M.E.; Walsh, N.A.; Darling, P.B.; Hanninen, S.A.; Thirugnanam, S.; Leong-Poi, H.; Barr, A.; Sole, M.J. B-Vitamin Deficiency in Hospitalized Patients with Heart Failure. *J. Am. Diet. Assoc.* **2009**, *109*, 1406–1410. [CrossRef] [PubMed]
69. Wang, G.; Li, W.; Lu, X.; Zhao, X. Riboflavin Alleviates Cardiac Failure in Type I Diabetic Cardiomyopathy. *Heart Int.* **2011**, *6*, e21. [CrossRef] [PubMed]
70. Herrmann, M.; Müller, S.; Kindermann, I.; Günther, L.; König, J.; Böhm, M.; Herrmann, W. Plasma B vitamins and their relation to the severity of chronic heart failure. *Am. J. Clin. Nutr.* **2007**, *85*, 117–123. [CrossRef] [PubMed]
71. Van Der Wal, H.H.; Comin-Colet, J.; Klip, I.T.; Enjuanes, C.; Beverborg, N.G.; Voors, A.A.; Banasiak, W.; van Veldhuisen, D.J.; Bruguera, J.; Ponikowski, P.; et al. Vitamin B12 and folate deficiency in chronic heart failure. *Heart* **2015**, *101*, 302–310. [CrossRef] [PubMed]
72. Briani, C.; Torre, C.D.; Citton, V.; Manara, R.; Pompanin, S.; Binotto, G.; Adami, F. Cobalamin deficiency: Clinical picture and radiological findings. *Nutrients* **2013**, *5*, 4521–4539. [CrossRef] [PubMed]
73. Andersson, S.E.; Edvinsson, M.L.; Edvinsson, L. Reduction of homocysteine in elderly with heart failure improved vascular function and blood pressure control but did not affect inflammatory activity. *Basic Clin. Pharmacol. Toxicol.* **2005**, *97*, 306–310. [CrossRef] [PubMed]
74. Demirbag, R.; Yilmaz, R.; Erel, O.; Gultekin, U.; Asci, D.E.Z. The relationship between potency of oxidative stress and severity of dilated cardiomyopathy. *Can. J. Cardiol.* **2005**, *21*, 851–855. [PubMed]
75. Jacob, R. Assessment of human vitamin C status. *J. Nutr.* **1990**, *11*, 1480–1485. [CrossRef] [PubMed]
76. Song, E.K.; Kang, S.M. Vitamin C Deficiency, High-Sensitivity C-Reactive Protein, and Cardiac Event-Free Survival in Patients with Heart Failure. *J. Cardiovasc. Nurs.* **2018**, *33*, 6–12. [CrossRef] [PubMed]
77. Wu, J.-R.; Song, E.K.; Moser, D.K.; Lennie, T.A. Dietary Vitamin C Deficiency Is Associated With Health-Related Quality of Life and Cardiac Event-free Survival in Adults With Heart Failure. *J. Cardiovasc. Nurs.* **2018**, *34*, 29–35. [CrossRef] [PubMed]
78. Shinke, T.; Shite, J.; Takaoka, H.; Hata, K.; Inoue, N.; Yoshikawa, R.; Matsumoto, H.; Masai, H.; Watanabe, S.; Ozawa, T.; et al. Vitamin C restores the contractile response to dobutamine and improves myocardial efficiency in patients with heart failure after anterior myocardial infarction. *Am. Heart J.* **2007**, *154*, e1–e8. [CrossRef] [PubMed]
79. Hornig, B.; Arakawa, N.; Kohler, C.; Drexler, H. Vitamin C improves endothelial function of conduit arteries in patients with chronic heart failure. *Circulation* **1998**, *97*, 363–368. [CrossRef] [PubMed]
80. Bentinger, M.; Brismar, K.; Dallner, G. The antioxidant role of coenzyme Q. *Mitochondrion* **2007**, *7*, S41–S50. [CrossRef] [PubMed]
81. Folkers, K.; Vadhanavikit, S.; Mortensent, S.A. Biochemical rationale and myocardial tissue data on the effective therapy of cardiomyopathy with coenzyme Q10. *Med. Sci.* **1985**, *82*, 901–904. [CrossRef] [PubMed]
82. Madmani, M.E.; Yusuf Solaiman, A.; Tamr Agha, K.; Madmani, Y.; Shahrour, Y.; Essali, A.; Kadro, W. Coenzyme Q10 for heart failure. *Cochrane Database Syst. Rev.* **2014**, *2*, CD008684. [CrossRef] [PubMed]
83. McMurray, J.J.V.; Dunselman, P.; Wedel, H.; Cleland, J.G.F.; Lindberg, M.; Hjalmarson, A.; Kjekshus, J.; Waagstein, F.; Apetrei, E.; Barrios, V.; et al. Coenzyme Q10, rosuvastatin, and clinical outcomes in heart failure: A pre-specified substudy of CORONA (Controlled Rosuvastatin Multinational Study in Heart Failure). *J. Am. Coll. Cardiol.* **2010**, *56*, 1196–1204. [CrossRef] [PubMed]

84. Ishiyama, T.; Morita, Y.; Toyama, S.; Yamagami, T.; Tsukamoto, N. A clinical study of the effect of coenzyme Q on congestive heart failure. *Jpn. Heart J.* **1976**, *17*, 32–42. [CrossRef] [PubMed]
85. Jafari, M.; Mousavi, S.M.; Asgharzadeh, A.; Yazdani, N. Coenzyme Q10 in the treatment of heart failure: A systematic review of systematic reviews. *Indian Heart J.* **2018**, *70*, S111–S117. [CrossRef] [PubMed]
86. Sander, S.; Coleman, C.I.; Patel, A.A.; Kluger, J.; Michael White, C. The Impact of Coenzyme Q10 on Systolic Function in Patients With Chronic Heart Failure. *J. Card. Fail.* **2006**, *12*, 464–472. [CrossRef] [PubMed]
87. Rosenfeldt, F.; Hilton, D.; Pepe, S.; Krum, H. Systematic review of effect of coenzyme Q10 in physical exercise, hypertension and heart failure. *Biofactors* **2003**, *18*, 91–100. [CrossRef] [PubMed]
88. Sinatra, S.T.; Berman, M. Coenzyme Q10 in patients with end-stage heart failure awaiting cardiac transplantation: A randomized, placebo-controlled study. Clin. Cardiol. 2004, 27, A26–A30. Coenzyme Q10 in patients with end-stage heart failure awaiting cardiac transplantation: A randomized, placebo-controlled study. *Clin. Cardiol.* **2004**, *27*, 295–299.
89. Morisco, C.; Trimarco, B.; Condorelli, M. Effect of coenzyme Q10therapy in patients with congestive heart failure: A long-term multicenter randomized study. *Clin. Investig.* **1993**, *71*, S134–S136. [CrossRef] [PubMed]
90. Mortensen, S.A.; Rosenfeldt, F.; Kumar, A.; Dolliner, P.; Filipiak, K.J.; Pella, D.; Alehagen, U.; Steurer, G.; Littarru, G.P. Q-SYMBIO Study Investigators. The effect of coenzyme Q10on morbidity and mortality in chronic heart failure: Results from Q-SYMBIO: A randomized double-blind trial. *JACC Hear Fail.* **2014**, *2*, 641–649. [CrossRef] [PubMed]
91. Fairweather-Tait, S.J.; Bao, Y.; Broadley, M.R.; Collings, R.; Ford, D.; Hesketh, J.E.; Hurst, R. Selenium in Human Health and Disease. *Antioxid. Redox Signal.* **2011**, *14*, 1337–1383. [CrossRef] [PubMed]
92. de Lorgeril, M.; Salen, P. Selenium and antioxidant defenses as major mediators in the development of chronic heart failure. *Heart Fail. Rev.* **2006**, *11*, 13–17. [CrossRef] [PubMed]
93. Rayman, M.P. Selenium and human health. *Lancet* **2012**, *379*, 1256–1268. [CrossRef]
94. Xia, Y.; E Hill, K.; Li, P.; Xu, J.; Zhou, D.; Motley, A.K.; Wang, L.; Byrne, D.W.; Burk, R.F. Optimization of selenoprotein P and other plasma selenium biomarkers for the assessment of the selenium nutritional requirement: A placebo-controlled, double-blind study of selenomethionine supplementation in selenium-deficient Chinese subjects. *Am. J. Clin. Nutr.* **2010**, *92*, 525–531. [CrossRef] [PubMed]
95. Ge, K.; Yang, G. The epidemiology of selenium deficiency in the etiological study of endemic diseases in China. *Am. J. Clin. Nutr.* **1993**, *57*, 259S–263S. [CrossRef] [PubMed]
96. Salonen, J.T.; Alfthan, G.; Huttunen, J.K.; Pikkarainen, J.; Puska, P. Association between cardiovascular death and myocardial infarction and serum selenium in a matched-pair longitudinal study. *Lancet* **1982**, *2*, 175–179. [CrossRef]
97. Navas-Acien, A.; Bleys, J.; Guallar, E. Selenium intake and cardiovascular risk: What is new? *Curr. Opin. Lipidol.* **2008**, *19*, 43–49. [CrossRef] [PubMed]
98. Nordman, T.; Xia, L.; Björkhem-Bergman, L.; Damdimopoulos, A.; Nalvarte, I.; Arnér, E.S.J.; Spyrou, G.; Eriksson, L.C.; Björnstedt, M.; Olsson, J.M. Regeneration of the antioxidant ubiquinol by lipoamide dehydrogenase, thioredoxin reductase and glutathione reductase. *Biofactors* **2003**, *18*, 45–50. [CrossRef] [PubMed]
99. Moosmann, B.; Behl, C. Selenoproteins, cholesterol-lowering drugs, and the consequences: Revisiting of the mevalonate pathway. *Trends Cardiovasc. Med.* **2004**, *14*, 273–281. [CrossRef] [PubMed]
100. Alehagen, U.; Aaseth, J. Selenium and coenzyme Q10 interrelationship in cardiovascular diseases-A clinician's point of view. *J. Trace Elem. Med. Biol.* **2015**, *31*, 157–162. [CrossRef] [PubMed]
101. Johansson, P.; Dahlström, Ö.; Dahlström, U.; Alehagen, U. Effect of selenium and Q10 on the cardiac biomarker NT-proBNP. *Scand Cardiovasc. J.* **2013**, *47*, 281–288. [CrossRef] [PubMed]
102. Witte, K.K.; Nikitin, N.P.; Parker, A.C.; Von Haehling, S.; Volk, H.-D.; Anker, S.D.; Clark, A.L.; Cleland, J.G. The effect of micronutrient supplementation on quality-of-life and left ventricular function in elderly patients with chronic heart failure. *Eur. Heart J.* **2005**, *26*, 2238–2244. [CrossRef] [PubMed]
103. Raygan, F.; Behnejad, M.; Ostadmohammadi, V.; Bahmani, F.; Mansournia, M.A.; Karamali, F.; Asemi, Z. Selenium supplementation lowers insulin resistance and markers of cardio-metabolic risk in patients with congestive heart failure: A randomised, double-blind, placebo-controlled trial. *Br. J. Nutr.* **2018**, *120*, 33–40. [CrossRef] [PubMed]
104. Vasto, S.; Mocchegiani, E.; Candore, G.; Listì, F.; Colonna-Romano, G.; Lio, D.; Malavolta, M.; Giacconi, R.; Cipriano, C.; Caruso, C. Inflammation, genes and zinc in ageing and age-related diseases. *Biogerontology* **2006**, *7*, 315–327. [CrossRef] [PubMed]

105. Cherasse, Y.; Urade, Y. Dietary zinc acts as a sleep modulator. *Int. J. Mol. Sci.* **2017**, *18*, 2334. [CrossRef] [PubMed]
106. Turan, B.; Tuncay, E. Impact of labile zinc on heart function: From physiology to pathophysiology. *Int. J. Mol. Sci.* **2017**, *18*, 2395. [CrossRef] [PubMed]
107. Oster, O. Trace element concentrations (Cu, Zn, Fe) in sera from patients with dilated cardiomyopathy. *Clin. Chim. Acta* **1993**, *214*, 209–218. [CrossRef]
108. Ripa, S.; Ripa, R.; Giustiniani, S. Are failured cardiomyopathies a zinc-deficit related disease? A study on Zn and Cu in patients with chronic failured dilated and hypertrophic cardiomyopathies. *Minerva Med.* **1998**, *89*, 397–403. [PubMed]
109. Topuzoglu, G.; Erbay, A.R.; Karul, A.B.; Yensel, N. Concentations of Copper, Zinc, and Magnesium in Sera from Patients with Idiopathic Dilated Cardiomyopathy. *Biol. Trace Elem. Res.* **2003**, *95*, 11–17. [CrossRef]
110. Koşar, F.; Sahin, I.; Taşkapan, C.; Küçükbay, Z.; Güllü, H.; Taşkapan, H.; Cehreli, S. Trace element status (Se, Zn, Cu) in heart failure. *Anadolu Kardiyol. Derg.* **2006**, *6*, 216–220. [PubMed]
111. Yu, X.; Huang, L.; Zhao, J.; Wang, Z.; Yao, W.; Wu, X.; Huang, J.; Bian, B. The Relationship between Serum Zinc Level and Heart Failure: A Meta-Analysis. *Biomed Res Int.* **2018**, *2018*, 1–9. [CrossRef] [PubMed]
112. Yoshihisa, A.; Abe, S.; Kiko, T.; Kimishima, Y.; Sato, Y.; Watanabe, S.; Kanno, Y.; Miyata-Tatsumi, M.; Misaka, T.; Sato, T.; et al. Association of Serum Zinc Level With Prognosis in Patients With Heart Failure. *J. Card Fail.* **2018**, *24*, 375–383. [CrossRef] [PubMed]
113. Jeejeebhoy, F.; Keith, M.; Freeman, M.; Barr, A.; McCall, M.; Kurian, R.; Mazer, D.; Errett, L. Nutritional supplementation with MyoVive repletes essential cardiac myocyte nutrients and reduces left ventricular size in patients with left ventricular dysfunction. *Am. Heart J.* **2002**, *143*, 1092–1100. [CrossRef] [PubMed]
114. Jankowska, E.A.; Rozentryt, P.; Witkowska, A.; Nowak, J.; Hartmann, O.; Ponikowska, B.; Borodulin-Nadzieja, L.; Banasiak, W.; Polonski, L.; Filippatos, G.; et al. Iron deficiency: An ominous sign in patients with systolic chronic heart failure. *Eur. Heart J.* **2010**, *31*, 1872–1880. [CrossRef] [PubMed]
115. Peyrin-Biroulet, L.; Williet, N.; Cacoub, P. Guidelines on the diagnosis and treatment of iron deficiency across indications: A systematic review. *Am. J. Clin. Nutr.* **2015**, *102*, 1585–1594. [CrossRef] [PubMed]
116. Klip, I.T.; Comín-Colet, J.; Voors, A.A.; Ponikowski, P.; Enjuanes, C.; Banasiak, W.; Lok, D.J.; Rosentryt, P.; Torrens, A.; Polonski, L.; et al. Iron deficiency in chronic heart failure: An international pooled analysis. *Am. Heart J.* **2013**, *165*, 575–582.e3. [CrossRef] [PubMed]
117. Jankowska, E.A.; Von Haehling, S.; Anker, S.D.; MacDougall, I.C.; Ponikowski, P. Iron deficiency and heart failure: Diagnostic dilemmas and therapeutic perspectives. *Eur. Heart J.* **2013**, *34*, 816–829. [CrossRef] [PubMed]
118. Anker, S.D.; Kirwan, B.A.; van Veldhuisen, D.J.; Filippatos, G.; Comin-Colet, J.; Ruschitzka, F.; Lüscher, T.F.; Arutyunov, G.P.; Motr, M.; Mori, C.; et al. Effects of ferric carboxymaltose on hospitalisations and mortality rates in iron-deficient heart failure patients: An individual patient data meta-analysis. *Eur. J. Heart Fail.* **2018**, *20*, 125–133. [CrossRef] [PubMed]
119. Enjuanes, C.; Bruguera, J.; Grau, M.; Cladellas, M.; Gonzalez, G.; Meroño, O.; Moliner-Borja, P.; Verdú, J.M.; Farré, N.; Comín-Colet, J. Iron Status in Chronic Heart Failure: Impact on Symptoms, Functional Class and Submaximal Exercise Capacity. *Rev. Esp. Cardiol. (Engl. Ed)* **2016**, *69*, 247–255. [CrossRef] [PubMed]
120. Lam, C.S.P.; Doehner, W.; Comin-Colet, J.; Lam, C.S. Iron deficiency in chronic heart failure: Case-based practical guidance. *ESC Heart Fail.* **2018**, *5*, 764–771. [CrossRef] [PubMed]
121. Ponikowski, P.; Voors, A.A.; Anker, S.D.; Bueno, H.; Cleland, J.G.F.; Coats, A.J.S.; Falk, V.; González-Juanatey, J.R.; Harjola, V.-P.; Jankowska, E.A.; et al. 2016 ESC Guidelines for the diagnosis and treatment of acute and chronic heart failure. *Eur. Heart J.* **2016**, *37*, 2129–2200. [CrossRef] [PubMed]
122. Anker, S.D.; Colet, J.C.; Filippatos, G.; Willenheimer, R.; Dickstein, K.; Drexler, H.; Lüscher, T.F.; Bart, B.; Banasiak, W.; Niegowska, J.; et al. Ferric Carboxymaltose in Patients with Heart Failure and Iron Deficiency. *N. Engl. J. Med.* **2009**, *361*, 2436–2448. [CrossRef] [PubMed]
123. Ponikowski, P.; Van Veldhuisen, D.J.; Comin-Colet, J.; Ertl, G.; Komajda, M.; Mareev, V.; McDonagh, T.; Parkhomenko, A.; Tavazzi, L.; Levesque, V.; et al. Beneficial effects of long-term intravenous iron therapy with ferric carboxymaltose in patients with symptomatic heart failure and iron deficiency. *Eur. Heart J.* **2015**, *36*, 657–668. [CrossRef] [PubMed]

124. Lewis, G.D.; Malhotra, R.; Hernandez, A.F.; McNulty, S.E.; Smith, A.; Felker, G.M.; Tang, W.H.W.; LaRue, S.J.; Redfield, M.M.; Semigran, M.J.; et al. Effect of oral iron repletion on exercise capacity in patients with heart failure with reduced ejection fraction and iron deficiency the IRONOUT HF randomized clinical trial. *JAMA* **2017**, *317*, 1958–1966. [CrossRef] [PubMed]
125. Beck-Da-Silva, L.; Piardi, D.; Söder, S.; Rohde, L.E.; Pereira-Barretto, A.C.; De Albuquerque, D.; Bocchi, E.; Vilas-Boas, F.; Moura, L.Z.; Montera, M.W.; et al. IRON-HF study: A randomized trial to assess the effects of iron in heart failure patients with anemia. *Int. J. Cardiol.* **2013**, *168*, 3439–3442. [CrossRef] [PubMed]
126. Bekfani, T.; Pellicori, P.; Morris, D.; Ebner, N.; Valentova, M.; Sandek, A.; Doehner, W.; Cleland, J.G.; Lainscak, M.; Schulze, P.C.; et al. Iron deficiency in patients with heart failure with preserved ejection fraction and its association with reduced exercise capacity, muscle strength and quality of life. *Clin. Res. Cardiol.* **2019**, *108*, 203–211. [CrossRef] [PubMed]
127. Paterek, A.; Kępska, M.; Sochanowicz, B.; Chajduk, E.; Kołodziejczyk, J.; Polkowska-Motrenko, H.; Kruszewski, M.; Leszek, P.; Mackiewicz, U.; Mączewski, M. Beneficial effects of intravenous iron therapy in a rat model of heart failure with preserved systemic iron status but depleted intracellular cardiac stores. *Sci. Rep.* **2018**, *8*, 15758. Available online: http://www.nature.com/articles/s41598-018-33277-2 (accessed on 4 November 2018). [CrossRef] [PubMed]

12

Nutrition and Cardiovascular Health

Rosa Casas [1,2], Sara Castro-Barquero [1], Ramon Estruch [1,2] and Emilio Sacanella [1,2,*]

1. Department of Internal Medicine, Hospital Clinic, Institut d'Investigació Biomèdica August Pi i Sunyer (IDIBAPS), University of Barcelona, Villarroel, 170, 08036 Barcelona, Spain; rcasas1@clinic.cat (R.C.); sacastro@clinic.cat (S.C.-B.); restruch@clinic.cat (R.E.)
2. CIBER 06/03: Fisiopatología de la Obesidad y la Nutrición, Instituto de Salud Carlos III, 28029 Madrid, Spain

* Correspondence: esacane@clinic.ub.es

Abstract: Cardiovascular disease (CVD) is the leading cause of death in Western countries, representing almost 30% of all deaths worldwide. Evidence shows the effectiveness of healthy dietary patterns and lifestyles for the prevention of CVD. Furthermore, the rising incidence of CVD over the last 25 years has become a public health priority, especially the prevention of CVD (or cardiovascular events) through lifestyle interventions. Current scientific evidence shows that Western dietary patterns compared to healthier dietary patterns, such as the 'Mediterranean diet' (MeDiet), leads to an excessive production of proinflammatory cytokines associated with a reduced synthesis of anti-inflammatory cytokines. In fact, dietary intervention allows better combination of multiple foods and nutrients. Therefore, a healthy dietary pattern shows a greater magnitude of beneficial effects than the potential effects of a single nutrient supplementation. This review aims to identify potential targets (food patterns, single foods, or individual nutrients) for preventing CVD and quantifies the magnitude of the beneficial effects observed. On the other hand, we analyze the possible mechanisms implicated in this cardioprotective effect.

Keywords: Mediterranean diet; cardiovascular disease; inflammation; nutrients; polyphenols; MUFA; PUFA; bioactive compounds; phytosterols; dietary pattern

---

1. Introduction

Data obtained in 2013 showed that the leading global cause of death in Western countries is cardiovascular disease (CVD), accounting for 17.3 million of all deaths worldwide per year (or 31.5% of all global deaths), despite steadily decreasing during the past 10 years [1,2]. One in three deaths in the United States and one in four deaths in Europe are caused by CVD [3]. So, in 2035, 45.1% (>130 million adults) of the US population are projected to have clinical expression of CVD [1,4]. CVD describes a range of disorders that affect the heart and blood vessels, such as hypertension, stroke, atherosclerosis, peripheral artery disease, and vein diseases [4]. The probability of developing CVD is associated with unhealthy dietary patterns (i.e., excessive intake of sodium and processed foods; added sugars; unhealthy fats; low intake of fruit and vegetables, whole grains, fiber, legumes, fish, and nuts), together with a lack of exercise, overweight and obesity, stress, alcohol consumption, or a smoking habit (Figure 1) [5–7]. Additionally, CVD often coincides with multiple co-morbidities, such as obesity, diabetes, hypertension, or dyslipidemia, which represent four of the 10 greatest risk factors for all-cause mortality worldwide [8]. Furthermore, the rising incidence of CVD over the last 25 years has become a public health priority, especially the prevention of CVD (or cardiovascular events) through lifestyle interventions [9]. On the one hand, a large body of scientific evidence has reported that nutrition might be the most preventive factor of CVD death [10], and could even reverse heart disease [8]. On the other hand, diet seems to play an important role in the management of other risk factors, such as excess weight, hypertension, diabetes, or dyslipidemia [8]. In this sense, the identification and classification of nutrients, foods, or dietary patterns that can enhance CVD prevention is a priority.

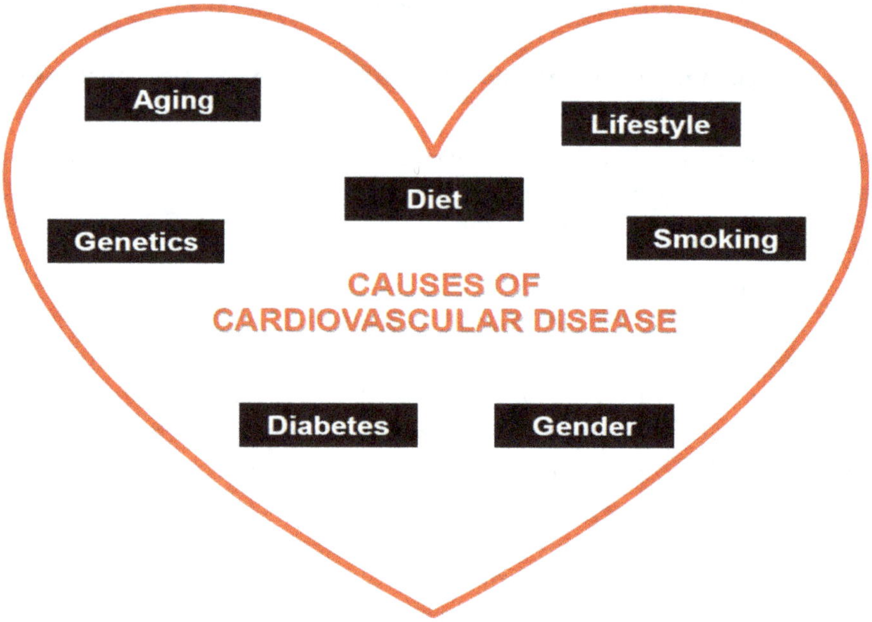

Figure 1. Unhealthy dietary patterns, together with a lack of exercise, overweight and obesity, aging, gender, genetics, or a smoking habit, among others, might lead to the development of cardiovascular disease (CVD).

Atherosclerosis is an inflammatory disease that contributes to major incidence and mortality of CVD. Oxidative stress and systemic inflammation are modifiable by nutrition [10–13], with an excess energy intake and physical inactivity as contributors of pro-inflammatory cytokines' secretion [14]. Inflammatory processes involve the sub-endothelial area of the arterial wall, accumulating lipids and lipid-laden macrophages among other cell types [15,16]. Current scientific evidence shows that chronic inflammation plays a key role in the pathogenesis of coronary artery disease (CAD), including the initiation and progression of atheroma plaque and rupture, and post-angioplasty and restenosis [17]. The main mediators of CAD development are C-reactive protein (CRP), interleukin (IL)-1, IL-6, IL-8, IL-1β, IL-18, monocyte chemoattractant protein (MCP)-1, and tumor necrosis factor (TNF)-α, among others. Moreover, those mediators are considered potential inflammation biomarkers and their expression may correlate with CAD severity [17–19].

As such, current evidence indicates that Western dietary patterns compared to healthier dietary patterns, such as the "Mediterranean diet" (MeDiet), leading to an excessive production of proinflammatory cytokines associated with a reduction of the synthesis of anti-inflammatory cytokines [20–23]. Therefore, the intake of fruits, vegetables, whole grains, nuts, seeds, and legumes is associated with lower inflammation [24–28], whereas red meat intake has been correlated with a higher inflammatory level [24,29–31]. Consequently, increased adherence to healthier dietary patterns, characterized by higher intake of fruits, vegetables, legumes, nuts, and whole grains, may mitigate low grade inflammation, preventing CVD [32–35].

In addition, microbiota has been linked to intestinal health, the immune, system and bioactivation and metabolism of nutrients, such as vitamins B and K and bioactive compounds. Recent clinical studies suggest a correlation between elevated plasma trimethylamine N-oxide (TMAO), which is produced by gut bacteria metabolism of dietary components, such as L-carnitine, betaine, and choline, and a higher risk of diabetes, hypertension, and atherosclerosis [36–38]. Therefore, it has been well studied that diet affects the composition and activity of gut microbiota and situations of gut microbiota dysbiosis may be involved in the development of CVD.

This review aims to identify potential targets (food patterns, single foods, or individual nutrients) for CVD prevention, quantify the magnitude of the beneficial effects observed, and analyze the mechanisms implicated in these cardioprotective effects. Besides, studies were limited to humans with no time restriction. Relevant studies, systematic reviews, and meta-analyses were searched to obtain the reference lists. The Medical Subject Headings search terms included: Inflammation, oxidative stress, inflammatory markers, IL, CRP, TNF-α, IL-6, dietary pattern, Mediterranean diet, Dietary Approach to Stop Hypertension (DASH diet), atherosclerosis, fruits and vegetables, olive oil, nuts, wine, fiber, micronutrients, vitamins, minerals, omega-3 fatty acids, lycopene, phytosterols, and polyphenols.

2. Atherosclerosis

Early stages of atherosclerosis are involved the internalization of lipids in the intima, mainly low-density lipoproteins (LDL), which is translated to endothelial dysfunction [39]. The disruption of the endothelial function promotes the inflammatory response, thrombus formation, and multiple pathological consequences, such as calcifications, stenosis, rupture, or hemorrhage [15,40].

The inflammatory response is enhanced by the infiltration of low-density lipoproteins (LDL) particles in the extracellular matrix (EM) while circulating monocytes are attached to the endothelium and transformed into macrophages infiltrating into the sub-endothelial area. The retention of LDL in EM is mediated by proteoglycans, which facilitate retention in the intima [41]. The LDL particles attached in the intima are susceptible to oxidative modifications by reactive oxygen species (ROS) and enzymatic modification released from inflammatory cells. Macrophages are converted into foam cells after oxidized LDL (oxLDL) particles are absorbed by them. Additionally, endothelial dysfunction enhances platelets' adhesion, which secretes chemotactic substances and growth factors, promoting plaque progression [42]. Vascular smooth muscle cells (VSMC) are also involved in plaque progression. Foam cells' growth factors and cytokines' secretion enhance VSMC migration to the intima where they contribute to the formation of the fibrous cap [43]. If the progression of lipid accumulation persists, foam cells and macrophages' apoptosis is induced jointly with pro-thrombotic molecules' secretion [44,45]. Atherosclerotic plaque progression and plaque disruption, promoted by pro-thrombotic agents, initiate platelet activation and aggregation, which leads to the coagulation cascade and, consequently, thrombus formation [46]. The clinical manifestations of advanced atherosclerosis are coronary heart disease, ischemic stroke, peripheral artery disease, heart failure, or sudden death [47].

3. Oxidative Stress and Inflammation

Oxidative stress has been related to the pathogenesis of atherosclerosis [48]. ROS and reactive nitrogen species (RNS) are mainly produced through mitochondrial activity and other pathways, such as nitric oxide (NO) synthase, and oxidase enzymes, such as Nicotinamide adenine dinucleotide phosphate (NADPH) oxidases (Nox), xanthine oxidase (XO), lipoxygenase, myeloperoxidase, uncoupled endothelial nitric oxide synthase (eNOS), and the mitochondrial respiratory chain via a one-electron reduction of molecular oxygen. Note the role of Nox in oxidative stress, as upregulated and overactive Nox enzymes contribute to oxidative stress and CVD. Several signaling pathways regulate inactivation and degradation of ROS and RNS, including catalase, glutathione peroxidase, and superoxide dismutase among others. An excess of ROS and RNS leads to oxidative stress, promoting cell proliferation, migration, autophagy, necrosis, DNA damage, endoplasmic reticulum stress, endothelial dysfunction, and higher levels of oxLDL [49,50]. Moreover, ROS activate the inflammatory response that directly affects plaque progression and endothelial function, increasing the levels of inflammatory cytokines, such as interleukins (IL-6, IL-8), TNF-α, and MCP-1, and adhesion molecules, such as intercellular adhesion molecule 1 (sICAM-1) and vascular cell adhesion molecule (sVCAM-1) [51]. Simultaneously, transcription factors activation, mainly nuclear factor kappa B

(NF-κβ) and nuclear factor (erythroid-derived 2)-like 2 (Nrf2), and signal transduction cascades result in a high production of inflammatory cytokines and inducible nitric oxide synthase [52]. NO has important anti-inflammatory, antihypertensive, and antithrombotic actions due to its strong vasodilator activity and anti-platelet aggregation. Additionally, anti-inflammatory effects are enhanced by the ability of NO to inhibit NF-κβ expression and the subsequent adhesion molecules [53]. Oxidative stress contributes to endothelial eNOS dysfunction [54,55]. Dysfunctional eNOS generates superoxide anions instead of NO, which is translated to a higher ROS production and contributes to atherogenesis [56]. In the case of inducible NOS (iNOS), which is expressed in cells after cytokines or bacterial lipopolysaccharide stimulation, an excessive and sustained production of NO has been linked with inflammatory diseases and septic shock [57]. Therefore, a decrease of NO production by eNOS leads to endothelial dysfunction while an excessive NO production by iNOS may induce pro-inflammatory and pro-atherogenic factors.

The causes and risk factor of atherosclerosis and oxidative stress are not well defined. However, certain health conditions and habits may contribute to atherosclerosis development, such as high total cholesterol and low-high-density lipoprotein cholesterol (HDL-c) levels, hypertension, type 2 diabetes mellitus (T2DM), obesity, and physical inactivity. Additionally, healthy dietary patterns and lifestyle modifications are potential strategies for atherosclerosis and oxidative stress prevention.

4. Dietary Patterns

Several studies correlate healthy dietary patterns with lower plasmatic concentrations of pro-inflammatory markers [58], whilst a Western-type diet (meat-based dietary pattern) is associated with higher levels of low-grade inflammation [31]. For that reason, CVD guidelines recommend a healthy diet. Dietary intervention allows a better combination of multiple foods and nutrients. Therefore, healthy dietary patterns support a greater magnitude of beneficial effects than the potential effects of a single nutrient supplementation, because of the synergistic health effects among them. The current body of evidence shows that healthy dietary patterns share similarities, such as a high intake of fiber, antioxidants, vitamins, minerals, polyphenols, monounsaturated, and polyunsaturated fatty acids (MUFA and PUFA, respectively); low intake of salt, refined sugar, saturated, and trans fats; and carbohydrates of low glycemic load [59]. This translates to a high intake of fruits, vegetables, legumes, fish and seafood, nuts, seeds, whole grains, vegetable oils (mainly, extra virgin olive oil [EVOO]), and dairy foods together with a low intake of pastries, soft drinks, and red and processed meat [59,60].

Mediterranean and DASH dietary interventions are well studied for CV outcomes. Both dietary patterns may reduce the incidence CVD through the down-regulation of low-grade inflammation and better control of body weight, which also improve other risk factors, and are correlated with lower numbers of clinical events [59,60]. Thus, this will be the focus of this research.

4.1. Mediterranean Diet

Until now, the main benefits of the Mediterranean diet (MeDiet) against CVD (Figure 2) have been associated with a better control of risk factors to improve blood pressure (BP), lipid profile, glucose metabolism, arrhythmic risk, or gut microbiome [59]. Also, some authors have suggested that MeDiet may exert an anti-inflammatory effect (Table 1) in the vascular wall as a possible mechanism to explain the link between MeDiet and low CVD prevalence [61]. Interestingly, MeDiet seems to modulate the expression of pro-atherogenic genes as cyclooxygenase-2 (COX-2), MCP-1, and low-density lipoprotein receptor-related protein (LRP1) [62], reducing plasmatic levels of plaque stability and rupture related molecules as MMP-9, IL-10, IL-13, or IL-18 [63,64].

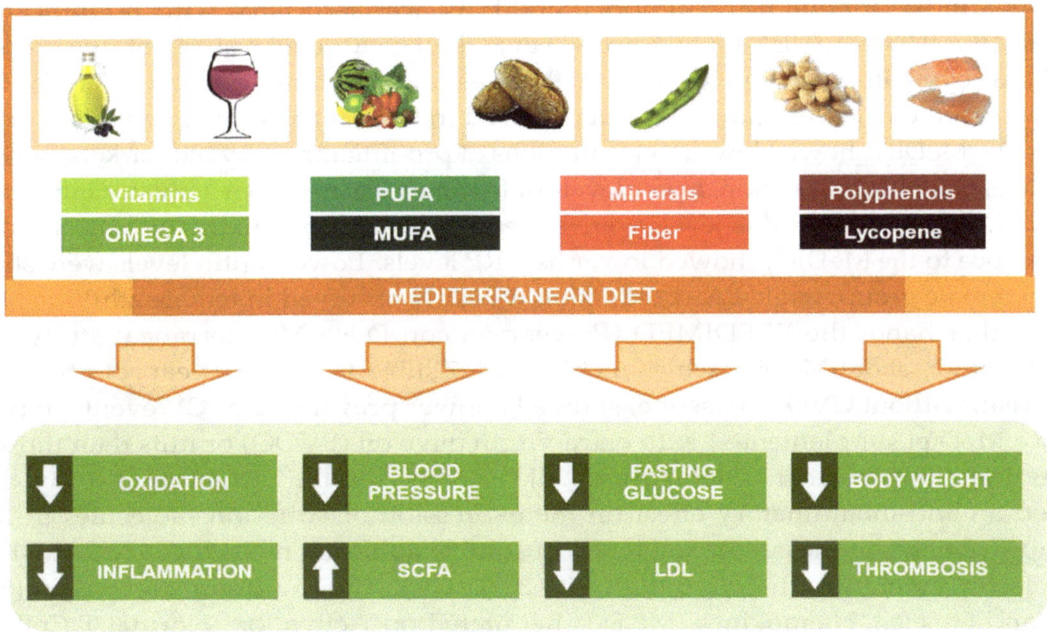

Figure 2. Main protection mechanisms of the Mediterranean diet against cardiovascular disease.

Table 1. Potential inflammatory effects of Mediterranean and DASH diet on CVD.

	Pro- and Anti-Inflammatory Markers and Genes	Leukocyte Expression	Oxidative Stress Markers
MeDiet	sVCAM-1, sICAM-1, RANTES, MIP-1β, TNF-α, TNFR-60, IL-1β, IL-6, IL-7, IL-10, IL-12p70, IL-13, IL-18, MMP-9, VEGF, CRP, TCF7L2, APOA2, CETP, COX-2, MCP-1, LRP1	Lymphocytes: CD11a, CD49d, CD40 Monocytes: CD11a, CD11b, CD49d, CD40	MDA, oxLDL
DASH diet	sICAM-1, IL-6, CRP, PAI-1	-	-

APOA2: Apolipoprotein A2; CETP: Cholesteryl ester transfer protein plasma; COX-2: Cyclooxygenase-2; CRP: C-reactive protein; IL: Interleukin; LRP1: Low-density lipoprotein receptor-related protein; MCP-1: Monocyte chemoattractant protein; MDA: Malondialdehyde; MMP-9: Metallopeptidase-9; oxLDL: Oxidized LDL; PAI-1: Plasminogen activator inhibitor 1; sICAM-1: Soluble intercellular adhesion molecule 1; sVCAM-1: Soluble vascular cell adhesion molecule; TNF-α: Tumor necrosis factor; TNFR: Tumor necrosis factor receptor; TCF7L2: Transcription factor 7-like 2; VEGF: Vascular endothelial growth factor.

The observational study, ATTICA, evaluated the link between MeDiet and the incidence of metabolic syndrome (MetS) in 1514 men and 1528 women (>18 y) without clinical evidence of CVD or any other chronic disease [65] during 10 years. Authors found that an increase of 10% in the MeDiet adherence score was associated with a 15% lower odds for CVD incidence. Nevertheless, the inflammatory factors studied (adiposity, CRP, IL-6), whose components are associated with a higher likelihood of CVD, showed a higher incidence (29%) in those subjects away from the MD [65]. Also, the Multi-Ethnic Study of Atherosclerosis (MESA) investigated if a dietary quality score based in a MeDiet pattern was related with regional adiposity [66]. Authors studied 5079 individuals free of CVD (61 ± 10 years) and found that a high quality dietary pattern was associated with less regional adiposity and a lower body mass index (BMI), CRP, and insulin resistance. Thus, Lahoz et al. [67] conducted a cross-sectional analysis of 1411 subjects of the Screening PRE-diabetes and type 2 DIAbetes (SPREDIA-2) study (mean age 61 years, 43.0% males) to assess whether the 14-point Mediterranean Diet Adherence Screener (MEDAS) was associated with serum CRP levels. After adjusting for confounders, the authors showed an inverse correlation between the adherence to MeDiet and CRP levels ($p = 0.041$). Also, a substudy of the MOLI-SANI cohort (6879 women and 6892 men) found that men with a higher adherence to a healthy high-antioxidant diet (HAC), vitamins, and phytochemicals enriched diet, inside a MeDiet pattern, were more protected against hypertension and inflammation than those with a healthy low-antioxidant diet [68]. Authors found HAC was associated with a significant decrease in CRP levels ($\beta = 0.03$, $p = 0.03$). Finally, Sureda et al. [69] conducted a study of two cross-sectional nutritional surveys with men and women (219 males and 379 females) aged among 12–65 years old, who lived on the Balearic Islands. Results showed that the male adult population with a higher adherence to the MeDiet showed lower concentrations of pro-inflammatory biomarkers, such as TNF-α and hs-CRP. Also, in this population, lower levels of leptin or plasminogen activator inhibitor 1 (PAI-1) were observed, while adiponectine levels were increased. Moreover, females (young and old), with a higher adherence to the MeDiet, showed lower hs-CRP levels. Lower leptin levels were showed only in the young female group, while PAI-1 reduction was only observed in female adults.

On the other hand, the PREDIMED (Prevención con Dieta Mediterránea) study, the largest interventional study about MeDiet, which included 7447 subjects (55 to 80 years of age, 57% women) at high CV risk, without CVD at baseline, showed a lower prevalence of CV events in participants assigned to a MeDiet supplemented with extra-virgin olive oil (EVOO) or nuts than those assigned to a low-fat diet after five years intervention [70]. Focusing on the PREDIMED study, the MeDiet has reported an anti-inflammatory effect on the expression of adhesion molecules in leukocytes, but also improvements in the circulating levels of soluble adhesion molecules (sVCAM-1, sICAM-1, E- and P-selectin, cytokines (IL-1, IL-6, IL-8, IL-12p70, CRP, TNF-α, tumor necrosis factor receptor (TNFR)-60 and 80, etc.), chemokines (MCP-1, Regulated on Activation, Normal T Cell Expressed and Secreted [RANTES], macrophage inflammatory proteins [MIP-1β], etc.) and molecules related with vulnerability atheroma plaque (IL-10, IL-13, IL-18, or Matrix metallopeptidase-9 [MMP-9]) after three months, one, three, and five years intervention in those participants that followed a MeDiet supplemented with EVOO or nuts [63,64,71–74]. On the one hand, the results obtained support that MeDiet exerts an important immunomodulatory effect, reducing proinflammatory biomarkers, especially those related to atheroma stability plaque. On the other hand, these anti-inflammatory effects seem to appear in the short and medium-term (three months, one year) and later is maintained in the long-term (three and five years). In a Swedish randomized crossover study [75], the adherence to a Medierranean-style diet and its correlation with inflammatory biomarkers (CRP, IL-6), vasoregulation, vascular endothelial growth factor (VEGF), and serum phospholipid fatty acid composition was investigated. The 22 subjects free of CVD (10 women) received a Mediterranean-type diet or Swedish diet for four weeks. No changes were observed for CRP or IL-6 although the MeDiet group showed significant reductions in leukocytes and platelets levels (by 10% and 15%, respectively) and in VEGF levels (15%). Esposito and et al. [76] assessed the effects of a Mediterranean dietary pattern on endothelial function and vascular inflammatory markers in patients with the MetS during two years (90 patients/intervention group). Compared with controls, the MeDiet group showed lower serum concentrations of high-sensitivity ((hs)-CRP, IL-6, IL-7, and IL-18 ($p \leq 0.04$; all)) and improved the endothelial function score ($p < 0.001$), defined as a measure of BP and platelet aggregation response to l-arginine. These results are in agreement with Azzini et al. [77], who also reported improvements in the CV risk profile and modulation of inflammatory levels (IL-10 and TNF-α), and a reduction in oxidative stress (malondialdehyde [MDA]).

The influence of polyphenols' content of a MeDiet pattern was also studied in the PREDIMED study [78]. Total polyphenol excretion (TPE) in urine was analyzed in 1139 participants homogenously and randomly in one of the three groups. Authors observed that MeDiet (supplemented with EVOO or nuts) significantly increased their TPE after one year of dietary intervention, decreasing inflammatory biomarkers compared with baseline (sVCAM-1, sICAM-1, IL-6 MCP-1, TNF-α).

Epigenetic studies have also reported similar results. Thus, Arpón et al. [79,80] conducted a substudy on 36 participants of the PREDIMED cohort after five years of intervention, where the main results were that a MeDiet supplemented with EVOO or nuts may influence the methylation status of peripheral white blood cell (PWBCs) genes. These changes were mainly observed in genes related to intermediate metabolism, diabetes, inflammation, and signal transduction. However, interactions among MeDiet and COX-2, IL-6, apolipoprotein A2 (APOA2), cholesteryl ester transfer protein plasma (CETP), and transcription factor 7-like 2 (TCF7L2) gene polymorphisms have been demonstrated [81–84].

4.2. DASH Diet

A large body of evidence supports that adherence to a DASH dietary pattern is linked to improvements in BP [85], body weight [86], glucose-insulin homeostasis [87], blood lipids and lipoproteins [88], inflammation grade [89,90], endothelial function [91,92], the gut microbiome [93,94], CVD risk [95,96], and total mortality [97,98]. The DASH diet is characterized by a high intake of fruits and vegetables, legumes, low fat dairy, whole grain products, nuts, fish, and poultry; a reduced intake of saturated fat, red meat and processed meats, and sweet beverages; and a low intake of sodium and refined grains [89,99].

Focusing on inflammatory markers and oxidative stress, several studies have shown the protective effect of the DASH diet on CVD (Table 1). A recent systematic review and meta-analysis of randomized trials [89], which included six randomized control trials (RCT) with 451 participants who were followed for 3–24 weeks, studied the effect of the DASH diet on inflammatory biomarkers. Results showed that the DASH diet significantly reduced high hs-CRP concentrations (mean difference (MD) = −1.01, 95% confidence interval (CI): −1.64, −0.38; I-squared (I2) = 67.7%) compared to other diets. When the follow up of participants was longer, the reduction of hs-CRP serum levels was greater. However, when the DASH diet effect was compared to other healthy diets, no significant changes were observed. Besides, a meta-analysis conducted by Neale et al. [100] about 17 RCTs observed that following a healthy diet (MeDiet, Nordic diet, Tibetan diet, and DASH diet) was associated with a significant reduction of CRP levels (−0.75, 95% confidence interval (CI): −1.16, −0.35; $p = 0.003$). No changes were found for the other biomarkers (TNF-α, total adiponectin, high-molecular-weight adiponectin, adiponectin:leptin ratio, resistin, or retinol binding protein 4). Eichelmann et al. [101] studied the link between plant-based diets (Nordic diet, MeDiet, vegetarian diet, plant-based diet, Paleolithic diet, and DASH) and obesity-related pro-inflammatory markers (CRP, IL-6, TNF-α, sICAM-1, leptin, adiponectin, and resistin) on 29 interventional trials with a total of 2689 participants. Results showed improvements in obesity-related inflammatory profiles after following plant-based diets: CRP (−0.55 mg/L), IL-6 (−0.25 ng/L), and sICAM-1 (−25.07 ng/mL). No significant changes were observed for TNF-α, resistin, adiponectin, and leptin.

In a cross-sectional analysis of 1493 men and women (aged 50–69 years), potential associations between dietary quality (through the DASH dietary quality score), adiposity, and biomarkers of glucose metabolism, lipid profile, and inflammation were assessed [102]. Results showed that a higher adherence to the DASH dietary pattern was associated with improvements in adiposity measures (BMI, $p < 0.05$, waist circumference, $p < 0.001$), and lower concentrations of TNF-α, IL-6, CRP, WBC, and PAI-1 ($p < 0.05$; all), such as pro-inflammatory, pro-thrombotic, and pro-atherogenic markers. Improvements in lipoprotein profile parameters (LDL-c, HDL-c, and lower large very low density lipoprotein [VLDL] particles, $p < 0.001$ all) and glucose homeostasis biomarkers (HOMA, insulin and glucose, $p < 0.05$ all) were also shown.

With respect to interventional studies, the DASH diet has reported improvements on insulin resistance, inflammation, and oxidative stress in women with gestational diabetes [103]. The RCT was performed with 32 pregnant women diagnosed with gestational diabetes (GD) at 24- to 28-week gestation. All of them were randomly assigned to a DASH diet group or a control group (16 participants/group) and were followed up for four weeks. The DASH diet compared with the control showed significant reductions in serum insulin levels (−2.62 μIU/mL, $p = 0.03$), fasting plasma glucose (FPG) (−7.62 mg/dL, $p = 0.02$), and the homeostasis model of assessment-insulin resistance (HOMA-IR) score (−0.8, $p = 0.03$). Furthermore, Kawamura et al. [104] also reported significant reductions in the BMI, BP, FPG, and fasting insulin level ($p \leq 0.003$; all) after analyzing 58 Japanese participants with untreated high-normal BP or stage 1 hypertension (30 men and 28 women; mean age 54.1 ± 8.1 years), who followed a modified DASH diet (salt 8.0 g/day) during two months. Finally, the DASH diet also increased the plasma total antioxidant capacity (45.2 mmol/L, $p < 0.0001$) and total glutathione levels (108.1 μmol/L, $p < 0.0001$). Neither group showed changes in serum hs-CRP levels. Saneei et al. [105] conducted a cross-over study, which examined the effects of the DASH diet on markers of systemic inflammation in 60 post-pubescent girls with MetS (aged 11–18 years and weight mean was 69 kg). Participants were randomized into two groups: The DASH diet or usual dietary advice (control group) and were followed for six weeks. Results did not show significant changes on TNF-α, IL-2, IL-6, and adiponectin levels, whereas hs-CRP levels were significantly lower (−0.09 mg/L, $p = 0.002$) in those participants with higher adherence to a DASH diet compared to the control group.

5. Foods

5.1. Fruits and Vegetables

The European Society of Cardiology (ESC) and American Heart Association Nutrition Committee strongly endorse the daily consumption of multiple servings of both fruits and vegetables in order to reduce CVD risk [106,107]. These recommendations are based upon epidemiological studies and meta-analysis, mainly [106–113]. A recent meta-analysis [108] with 83 studies (71 clinical trials and 12 observational studies) showed that a higher intake of fruit or vegetable was significantly inversely associated with CRP and TNF-α levels ($p < 0.05$; both) and directly associated with an increased proliferation of γδ-T cell populations ($p < 0.05$). Also, Corley et al. [111] studied, in 792 participants aged 70 years from the Lothian Birth Cohort 1936, the association between biomarkers of systemic inflammation (such as CRP and fibrinogen) and specific single foods (fruits and vegetables). The dietary intake was measured using a 168-item Food Frequency Questionnaire (FFQ). Authors described that a higher fresh fruit intake was associated with lower CRP levels (≤3 mg/L) (β = 0.100, 95% CI 0.82, 0.99). No significant association was found between vegetables and CRP. Similar results ($p < 0.05$) were found between fibrinogen levels and fruit intake (β = 0.083) or combined fruits and vegetables intake (β = 0.084).

Also, in the cross-sectional study conducted by Holt et al. [112], in 285 healthy adolescent boys and girls aged 13 to 17 years, it was found that serum CRP levels were inversely associated with fruit intake (r = −0.19; $p = 0.004$), while IL-6 was inversely associated with fruit and vegetable intake and TNF-α only with vegetable consumption ($p < 0.05$; both). The HELENA Cross-Sectional Study [113], which aimed to demonstrate that a healthy diet might reduce adiposity and systemic inflammation, found that fruits and nuts were negatively linked with IL-4 (all subjects, $p < 0.05$; both) and TNF-α (only girls, $p = 0.036$). Contrastingly, vegetables showed only significant inverse correlations with sE-selectin (all subjects, $p \leq 0.0012$; both). This study was carried out in 464 adolescents (13–17 years) of the European HELENA cohort. In a cross-sectional analysis [114], in 1005 Chinese women aged 40 to 70 years, the association between vegetable intake and inflammatory and oxidative stress markers was studied. Results showed that a higher intake of cruciferous vegetables was associated with lower concentrations of TNF-α (p trend = 0.001), IL-1β (p trend = 0.004), and IL-6 (p trend = 0.02). Additionally, the mean difference of concentrations among the highest and the lowest quintiles of cruciferous vegetables intake were 12.66% for TNF-α, 18.18% for IL-1β, and 24.68% for IL-6. Any association was observed between the consumption of cruciferous vegetable and oxidative stress markers (F2-isoprostanes and 2,3-dinor-5,6-dihydro-15-F2t-IsoP).

Finally, in a sub-study from the PREDIMED study, Urpí-Sardà et al. [77] found that the participants who increased more than 62.7 g/day of their consumption of vegetables after one year decreased their plasma concentration of TNFR60 from 1.7 μg/L to 1.5 μg/L ($p < 0.05$), as shown in Table 2.

Table 2. Potential inflammatory effects of different foods on CVD.

	Pro- and Anti-Inflammatory Markers and Genes	Leukocyte Expression	Oxidative Stress Markers
Fruits & vegetables	TNF-α, TNFR-60, IL-1β, IL-4, IL-6, γδ-T cell, fibrinogen, sE-selectin	-	F2-isoprostanes, 2,3-dinor-5,6-dihydro-15-F2t-IsoP
Olive oil	sVCAM-1, sICAM-1, RANTES, MIP-1β, TNF-α, TNFR-60, IL-1β, IL-6, IL-7, IL-10, IL-12p70, IL-13, IL-18, MMP-9, CRP, MCP-1, NT-proBNP, NF-κβ	-	plasma antioxidant capacity, antioxidant enzymes-catalase, and glutathione peroxidase
Nuts	CRP, IL-6, TNF-α, TNF-β, TNF-R2, sICAM-1, fibrinogen, PF4, resistin	-	oxLDL
Wine and beer	IL-1α, IL-5, IL-6, IL-6r, IL-8, IL-10, IL-15, IL-18, CRP, MDC, sVCAM-1, sICAM-1, E-selectin, fibrinogen, CD40 ligand, MCP-1, factor VII, PAI-1, IFN-γ, RANTES, TNF-β	Lymphocytes: LFA-1 Monocytes: LFA-1, MAC-1, VLA-4, CCR2, CD36, CD15	SOD, MDA

CCR2: C-C chemokine receptor type 2; CD15: Sialil-Lewis X; CRP: C-reactive protein; IL: Interleukin; LFA: Lymphocyte function-associated antigen 1; MAC-1: T-lymphocytes and macrophage-1 receptor; MCP-1: Monocyte chemoattractant protein; MDA: Malondialdehyde; MDC: Macrophage-derived chemokine; MMP-9: Metallopeptidase-9; NT-proBNP: Pro-brain natriuretic peptide; oxLDL: Oxidized LDL; PAI-1: Plasminogen activator inhibitor 1; PF4: Platelet factor 4; sICAM-1: Soluble intercellular adhesion molecule 1; SOD: Superoxide dismutase; sVCAM-1: Soluble vascular cell adhesion molecule; TNF: Tumor necrosis factor; TNFR: Tumor necrosis factor receptor; IFN-γ: Interferon gamma.

5.2. Olive Oil

Several studies and meta-analyses have demonstrated the anti-inflammatory effects of olive oil (OO) rich diets [115–117]. Bioactive components of EVOO, the main key food of the MeDiet, have demonstrated improvements in inflammatory status, oxidative stress, and endothelial dysfunction [115]. A recent meta-analysis conducted by Schwingshackl et al. [118] in 30 RCT (3106 participants and daily consumption of 1 mg and 50 mg OO) found a significant decrease in CRP (−0.64 mg/L, $p < 0.0001$, n = 15 trials) and IL-6 (−0.29 mg/L, $p < 0.04$, n = 7 trials) compared to controls. Also, the flow-mediated dilatation (FMD) value was significantly increased in subjects with highest OO intake (0.6%, $p < 0.002$).

Several studies from the PREDIMED study and others related to the MeDiet have reported that a MeDiet supplemented with EVOO leads to decreased levels of N-terminal pro-brain natriuretic peptide (NT-proBNP) [119], the progression of intima media thickness (IMT) in those with elevated baseline IMT [120,121], improved systolic and diastolic BP in both hypertensive and non-hypertensive patients [122–124], and decreased expression and concentration of circulating inflammatory biomarkers related to atherosclerosis [63,64,71–74]. Urpí-Sardà et al. [72] reported that those participants with a higher adherence to a MeDiet + EVOO and whose intake of VOO was higher than 24 g/day showed lower plasma concentrations of TNFR60 after one year of intervention. Moreover, Camargo et al. [125] observed that, after isolation of peripheral blood mononuclear cells (PBMCs), the MeDiet exerted an inhibitory effect on the expression of genes related to plaque progression, such as MMP-9, NF-κβ or MCP-1, by increasing IκB kinase (IκBα) expression after the intake of a MeDiet + EVOO compared with two other diets ($p < 0.05$; all). IκBα stabilizes the NF-κβ molecule in the cytoplasm, maintaining it in an "unactivated" state. Widmer et al. [126] observed that daily consumption of 30 mL of OO or 30 mL of OO supplemented with epigallocatechin 3-gallate (EGCG) in 82 subjects (≥18-y) with early atherosclerosis showed improvements of endothelial dysfunction, independently of EGCG supplementation, after four months of intervention. However, the OO + EGCG group showed significant reductions in inflammatory parameters, such as sICAM-1 ($p \leq 0.001$), white blood cells ($p < 0.05$), monocytes, and lymphocytes ($p < 0.05$; both). Additionally, Oliveras-López et al. [127] showed an increase in plasma antioxidant capacity, antioxidant enzymes-catalase, and glutathione peroxidase, as well as an improvement in the superoxide dismutase (SOD) expression after analyzing

45 healthy adults (age: 21–45 years old, mean BMI: 21.4 $\pm$ 0.5 kg/m^2) who ingested 50 mL of EVOO for 30 days. Along with the other studies, the intake of EVOO seems to have positive effects on endothelial function. Finally, in the VOLOS (Virgin Olive Oil Study), participants with mild dyslipemia were randomized in two groups of intervention (daily 40 mL of EVOO with 166 mg/L of hydroxytyrosol vs. refined OO with 2 mg/L of hydroxytyrosol) during seven weeks. Results showed significant reduction of thromboxane B2 (TXB2) levels of 20% in the EVOO groups [128], as shown in Table 2.

5.3. *Nuts*

Nuts, specifically peanuts and walnuts, have been demonstrated to reduce the CVD morbidity and mortality in numerous large prospective cohort studies [129,130]. Mente et al. [131] predicted that nut intake might offer a preventative risk reduction on heart disease (RR = 0.67 [95% CI: 0.57–0.77]). Also, nut intake is associated with weight loss improvements [132], lower LDL-c levels [71,133,134], hypertension risk [133,135], and T2DM, improving hyperglycemia and insulin resistance [136], and inflammatory and oxidants mediators [134,137–139].

In a recent extensive meta-analysis, 23 RCTs were evaluated [139] to investigate the effects of nut intake over some inflammatory biomarkers (CRP, sICAM-1, sVCAM-1, IL-6, E-selectin, TNF-α). Authors found significant reductions of sICAM-1 (-0.17 ng/mL, p = 0.01) after nut intake. No changes were observed among the others inflammatory markers. Similar results were found in the meta-analysis conducted by Neale et al. [138]. No significant differences were shown after analyzing a wide number of inflammatory biomarkers, such as CRP, adiponectin, IL-6, sICAM-1, sVCAM-1, and FMD, in a total of 32 RCT studies. A significant improvement in FMD after nut intake was observed.

On the one hand, Yu et al. [137] conducted a cross-sectional study to investigate if nut intake was correlated to inflammatory biomarkers levels (CRP, IL-6, and tumor necrosis factor receptor 2 (TNFR2)) from 5013 participants in the Nurses' Health Study (NHS) and Health Professionals Follow-Up Study (HPFS) who were non-diabetic. Results showed that a higher nut intake showed lower inflammatory biomarkers levels (CRP: RR = 0.80 [95% CI: 0.69, 0.90, p-trend = 0.0003]; and IL-6: RR = 0.86 [95% CI: 0.77, 0.97, p-trend = 0.006]).

However, a randomized, parallel-group study on 50 patients with MetS and supplemented with 30 g/day of raw nuts (15 g walnuts, 7.5 g almonds, and 7.5 g hazelnuts) showed significant reductions of plasma concentrations of IL-6 (-1.1 ng/L; p = 0.035) compared with a control diet [140]. These results are according with the data showed by Hernández-Alonso et al. [141], who reported, in a randomized cross-over study in 54 participants, significant reductions of fibrinogen, oxLDL, and platelet factor 4 levels in the pistachio-supplemented group compared with control group ($p < 0.05$; all) after four months of intervention. Additionally, the pistachio-supplemented group showed lower IL-6 (-9%) and resistin gene expression (-6%) ($p < 0.05$; both). Similar results (-10.3% for IL-6 and CRP, -15.7% for TNF-α) were showed in a randomized, crossover study for 12-weeks carried out by Liu et al. [142] in 20 Chinese subjects with T2DM with mild hyperlipidemia (nine men and 11 women, mean age of 58 years, and BMI of 26 kg/m^2). See Table 2.

5.4. *Wine and Other Fermented Alcoholic Beverages*

Nowadays, there is enough evidence from both epidemiologic studies and RCTs to conclude that regular moderate consumption of fermented alcoholic beverages, mainly red wine and beer, has cardioprotective effects and can exert a positive effect on CV risk factors [143–145].

5.4.1. Wine

Wine or wine-derived phenolic compounds that exert effects through mechanisms on atherosclerosis are clearly identified. On the one hand, wine and their phenolic compounds decrease oxidation of LDL-c and oxidation stress, and increase in NO, improving endothelial function. Also, ethanol increases HDL-c levels and inhibits platelet aggregation, promotes fibrinolysis, and reduces systemic inflammation [144,146].

Janssen et al. [147] investigated the relationship of wine consumption and CV risk markers (CRP, fibrinogen, factor VII, and PAI-1) in a multi-ethnic sample of 2900 healthy women of middle-age, who were followed up for seven years. Authors concluded that moderate wine consumption may protect against CVD, after observing lower concentrations of CRP ($p < 0.001$), fibrinogen ($p < 0.001$), factor VII ($p < 0.01$), and PAI-1 ($p < 0.05$) compared to abstainers or women that drink little wine.

On the other side, Estruch et al. [148] reported that both red wine and gin have anti-inflammatory properties in the atherosclerotic process through the reduction of fibrinogen levels (−9%) and IL-1α (−21%), as well as lower plasma hs-CRP (−21%), sVCAM-1 (−17%), and sICAM-1 (−9%) levels. Moreover, monocyte expression was significantly reduced by 27–32% (LFA-1, MAC-1, VLA-4). In another randomized, crossover consumption trial in 67 males at high risk of CVD, Chiva-Blanch et al. [149] investigated the effects of ethanol and phenolic compounds of 30 g alcohol/day of red wine, and the equivalent amount of dealcoholized red wine and gin (30 g alcohol/d) for four weeks on the expression of inflammatory biomarkers related to atherosclerosis. Thirty g/day of alcohol of red wine showed an increase in plasma concentrations of IL-10 and decreased macrophage-derived chemokine (MDC). On the other hand, sICAM-1, E-selectin, and IL-6 were reduced by phenolic compounds of red wine. Phenolic compounds also inhibited the expression of LFA-1 in T-lymphocytes and MAC-1, and CCR2 expressions in monocytes. Concentrations of CD40 antigen, CD40 ligand IL-16, MCP-1, and sVCAM-1 were downregulated in both groups: Ethanol and phenolic compounds of red wine. A current study conducted by Roth et al. [150] found that aged white wine presents a greater ability to repair and maintain endothelial integrity than gin. In this randomized, controlled, crossover study, 38 high-risk male volunteers (55–80 years), who received 30 g ethanol/day as aged white wine or gin for three weeks, were evaluated. After intervention, T-lymphocytes' expression of CD31 and CD40 and monocytes expression of CCR2 and CD36 were lower after consumption of aged white wine. Additionally, for aged white wine, a significant reduction was observed in plasma concentrations of IL-8 and IL-18, sICAM-1 and sVCAM-1. Both beverages showed significant reductions in LFA-1, MAC-1, VLA4, CD40, and CD31 expression, as well as lower concentrations of interferon gamma (IFN-γ). Finally, Estruch et al. [151], in a new study, where wine and gin were compared again, found that wine intake significantly decreased plasma SOD activity [8.1 U/gHb (95% CI: 138, 25; $p = 0.009$)] and MDA levels [11.9 nmol/L (95% CI: 21.4, 2.5; $p = 0.020$)] compared to the gin group, as shown in Table 2.

5.4.2. Beer

Among fermented beverages, beer has a moderate polyphenol content that confers grater cardioprotective effects than spirits and distilled beverages [145]. So, De Gaetano et al. [152] described in a consensus document the effects of moderate beer consumption on health and disease, where they concluded that epidemiological studies showed that low-moderate doses of beer intake protect against CV risk and its effect is comparable to that reported for moderate red wine consumption.

In 1999, Wannamethee et al. [153] studied 7735 British men during 17 years and found that regular beer intake was associated with lower total mortality (HR = 0.84 (CI: 0.71–10.01)).

Finally, Chiva-Blanch et al. [154] performed a randomized, crossover controlled clinical trial with 33 subjects to evaluate the effects of three beverages types: A non-phenolic alcoholic beverage, such as gin; beer, which is a moderate phenolic alcoholic beverage; and a non-alcoholic beer, with the same amount of phenolic compounds. Beer and gin showed improvements in the HDL cholesterol levels (around 5%) and adiponectin (around 7%) compared to the non-alcoholic beer intervention. Related to circulating inflammatory biomarkers, IL-1α levels increased (around 24%) and IL-5 levels decreased around 14% after beer and gin intervention. However, non-alcoholic beer showed significant improvements in homocysteine concentration (decreased by around 6%) and improved folic acid levels around 9%. Related to inflammatory biomarkers, non-alcoholic beer intervention showed significant decreases of IL-6r, IL-15, RANTES, and TNF-β levels, as shown in Table 2.

6. Nutrients

It is important to focus on the possible benefits of the intake of specific nutrients to avoid possible deficiencies of these nutrients, which can lead to the development of atherosclerotic disease. We have only included information about fiber, some vitamins, and minerals, but no other nutrients—such as carbohydrates, fats, or proteins—which have also been demonstrated to have a certain effect on the risk of developing atherosclerosis.

6.1. Fiber

A wide number of studies and scientific publications have reported the health benefits of dietary fiber intake decreasing cholesterol concentrations and BP, while a deficiency of fiber intake is associated with CVD development [155].

On the one hand, several meta-analyses have displayed that a higher dietary fiber intake is linked with a lower relative risk of total all-cause mortality among 16–23% [156–158]. On the other hand, several clinical trials have studied the link between diet and inflammation, and more specifically, the impact of dietary fiber. Although, to date, the implicated mechanisms are still unknown, the proposed mechanisms are that dietary fiber decreases the glucose absorption, and down-regulates the expression of oxidative stress related cytokines or the inflammatory response mediated by gut microbiota exposed to fiber [159].

In an observational study of 1958 postmenopausal women (age 50–79 years), dietary fiber consumption was associated with higher levels of inflammatory markers (CRP and IL-6) [160]. Also, in the Women's Health Initiative Observational Study (13,745 US men and women), a higher fiber intake (24.7 g/day) was associated with lower plasma concentrations of IL-6 and TNFR2 compared with the lowest fiber intake group (7.7 g/day) [161]. Similar results were expressed by Qi et al. [162], who observed that concentrations of CRP and TNFR2 were among 8% to 18% lower in the highest quintile of cereal fiber intake compared to the lowest quintile. Similar results were obtained by Estruch et al. [163] for CRP levels and other inflammatory cytokines (IL-6, sICAM-1, sVCAM-1), whose decrease was inversely related with dietary fiber intake, but not significantly. Additionally, cross-sectional data (1088 participants without T2DM at baseline and aged 40 y–60 y) from the Insulin Resistance Atherosclerosis Study [164] showed that whole grain products' intake was inversely related to PAI-1 ($\beta = -0.102$; SEM = 0.038; $p = 0.0077$) and CRP plasma concentrations ($\beta = -0.102$; SEM = 0.048; $p = 0.0340$).

In interventional studies, North et al. [165] studied, in 554 subjects (192 men, 362 women), the associations between dietary fiber and CRP levels, showing significantly lower CRP concentrations (−25–54%) with higher fiber intakes ($\geq$3.3 g/MJ). An interventional cross-over study [166] with a total of 60 participants (50% patients with newly diagnosed T2DM, 50% nondiabetic subjects) received three isoenergetic meals separated by one week intervals: A high-fiber (16.8 g) meal; a high-fat meal; and a low-fiber (4.5 g) meal. Results showed that a high fiber intake showed lower plasma IL-18 concentrations and greater stimulation of adiponectin plasmatic levels. Finally, significant reductions of TNF-α (−3.7 pg/mL; $p < 0.001$), were observed after whole grain product intake in a randomized parallel arm feeding trial in 49 subjects who were overweight or obese, and low fruits, vegetables, and whole grain products' intake [167]. See Table 3.

Table 3. Potential inflammatory effects of different nutrients on CVD.

	Pro- and Anti-Inflammatory Markers and Genes
Fiber	sVCAM-1, sICAM-1, TNF-α, TNFR2, IL-6, IL-18, CRP, PAI-1
Micronutrients	IL-6, CRP, TNF-α, leptin, tHcy

CRP: C-reactive protein; IL: Interleukin; PAI-1: Plasminogen activator inhibitor 1; sICAM-1: Soluble intercellular adhesion molecule 1; sVCAM-1: Soluble vascular cell adhesion molecule; tHcy: Total homocysteine; TNF-α: Tumor necrosis factor; TNFR: Tumor necrosis factor receptor.

6.2. Micronutrients

Nowadays, there are great experimental, epidemiological, and clinical evidence showing how micronutrients' ingestion may protect against CVD [168–170]. Micronutrients exert their protective effect through three possible ways: 1. Reducing endothelial cells damage; 2. improving the production of NO; and 3. inhibiting oxidation of LDL-c [168–170]. Both in adolescence and in adulthood, pro-inflammatory biomarkers have been associated with dietary antioxidants, such as Zn, Se, and vitamin C and E, whose deficiency leads to a higher CVD risk [171–175]. Also, a meta-analysis [176] suggested that Mg supplementation might significantly reduce serum CRP levels (−1.33 mg/L, 95% CI: −2.63, −0.02) after analyzing eight RCTs. Similar results were showed in another meta-analysis [177], where after stratifying by the baseline plasma CRP values of ≤3 and >3 mg/L, found significant reductions of CRP levels (1.12 mg/L, 95% CI: −2.05, −0.18, $p = 0.019$) for the last subgroup. Finally, a recent meta-analysis [178] of seven studies (all RCTs) showed that vitamin D-supplemented groups had lower levels of TNF-α ($p = 0.04$) compared with control groups. No differences between vitamin D and control groups were observed for CRP, IL-10, or IL-6. Relative to vitamin E, a recent meta-analysis [179] suggested that supplementation with vitamin E might reduce serum CRP levels (−0.62 mg/L, 95% CI = −0.92, −0.31; $p < 0.001$) after analyzing 12 trials with 246 participants in the intervention arms and 249 participants in control arms.

De Oliveira Otto et al. [180] investigated the association between dietary micronutrients (heme iron, nonheme iron, zinc (Zn), magnesium (Mg), β-carotene, vitamin C, and vitamin E) with inflammatory markers (CRP, IL-6, total homocysteine (tHcy), fibrinogen, coronary artery calcium, and common and internal carotid artery-IMT) and subclinical atherosclerosis in 5181 participants free of diabetes and CVD from the Multi-Ethnic Study of Atherosclerosis (aged 45 y–84 y). Authors found that Mg and nonheme iron were inversely associated with tHcy concentrations, whilst vitamin C was positively associated with tHcy concentrations. Besides, CRP levels were positively associated with Zn and heme iron, whereas Mg concentrations showed an inverse association with CCA-IMT. Finally, no significant association was observed between dietary intake of carotene or vitamin E and inflammatory markers. Wang et al. [181] also reported that serum vitamin D levels were negatively associated with IL-6 ($r = -0.244$, $p = 0.002$) and hs-CRP ($r = -0.231$, $p = 0.004$) levels after studying 152 acute stroke patients. Furthermore, for vitamin D, several observational studies have reported that reduced vitamin D levels are linked with endothelial dysfunction and higher arterial stiffness [182,183], and this deficiency might be related to foam cell formation and decreased expression of adhesion molecules in endothelial cells [184].

Recently, Tabesh et al. [185] examined the effects of co-supplementation of vitamin D and calcium on inflammatory biomarkers and adipokines in 118 diabetic participants with insufficient vitamin D levels. The placebo-controlled clinical trial after eight weeks with four intervention groups ((1) vitamin D + calcium placebo; (2) calcium + vitamin D placebo; (3) vitamin D + calcium; or (4) vitamin D placebo + calcium placebo) showed that supplementation with calcium and vitamin D decreased leptin (−9 ± 18 ng/mL), IL-6 (−4 ± 1 pg/mL, $p < 0.001$), and TNF-α (−3.4 ± 1.3, $p < 0.05$) concentrations compared with the placebo. Also, Shargorodsky et al. [186] studied the effect of vitamin C (500 mg), vitamin E (200 IU), coenzyme Q10 (60 mg), and selenium (120 μg) on inflammatory markers in the long-term (six months) in participants at high CVD risk. No significant changes were observed for homocysteine, endothelin, aldosterone, and renin in participants who received antioxidant supplementation, while there was a significant decrease in HbA1C and a significant increase in HDL-c. Large and small artery elasticity was also significantly increased after antioxidant supplementation intake. In addition, an RCT conducted by Ellulu et al. [187] in 64 obese patients, who were hypertensive and/or diabetic, reported the potential anti-inflammatory effect of 500 mg of vitamin C, twice daily. Vitamin C might decline hs-CRP ($p = 0.01$), IL-6 ($p = 0.001$), and fasting blood glucose ($p < 0.01$) after eight weeks of treatment. Christen et al. [188] also conducted a randomized, double-blind, placebo-controlled sub-study from the Women's Antioxidant and Folic Acid Cardiovascular Study. They tested a daily combination of folic acid (2.5 mg), vitamin B6 (50 mg), vitamin B_{12} (1 mg), or placebo on 300 participants (half for each group). After 7.3 years, the supplemented group showed significant reductions in homocysteine concentrations (−18%), whereas no changes were observed in CRP, IL-6, sICAM-1, and fibrinogen levels, as shown in Table 3.

7. Bioactive Compounds

Multiple bioactive compounds (omega-3 fatty acids, lycopene, or polyphenols) present in the diet have been associated with beneficial effects on atherosclerosis development. All of them act to reduce levels of LDL-c, improving inflammatory and oxidative stress biomarkers. Next, we analyze those cited above.

7.1. Omega-3 Fatty Acids

PUFAs, as Omega-3 fatty acid (Ω-3 PUFA), α-linolenic acid (ALA), eicosapentaenoic acid (EPA), and docosahexaenoic acid (DHA), have been reported as potential anti-atherogenic agents for the atherosclerotic process [189]. Mechanisms, through which they might reduce CV risk, include improvements in the lipid and lipoprotein profile, oxidation, thrombosis, endothelial function, BP, plaque stability, CV mortality, platelet aggregation, modulating concentration or expression of pro-inflammatory markers (adhesion molecules, cytokines, etc.), and immune cells [190–192].

In a meta-analysis conducted by Wang et al. [193] of 16 randomized placebo-controlled trials in 901 participants, it was reported that Ω-3 PUFA intake (0.45–4.5 g/day, for 56 days) increased FMD by 2.30% (95% CI: 0.89, 3.72%, $p = 0.001$) compared with the placebo group. Additionally, a meta-analysis of 38 RCTs [194] reported reductions by 20–30% in serum triglycerides levels in healthy participants after daily consumption of ≥4 g of EPA and DHA through either supplementation or consumption of enriched foods.

In an observational study [195], 102 Japanese individuals with acute coronary syndrome were analyzed and were stratified in three groups: ≤50, 51–74, and ≥75 years. It was found that low serum DHA concentrations leads to CVD, with DHA useful as a predictive marker of endothelial dysfunction. Similar results were reported by Kelley et al. [196].

On the one hand, Cawood et al. [197] showed that patients in the Ω-3 PUFA group (1.8 g EPA + DHA/day), followed up for 21 days, had a lower number of foam cells ($p = 0.0390$) and T-lymphocytes ($p = 0.0097$), less inflammation ($p = 0.0108$), and improved stability of atheroma plaque ($p = 0.0209$) after analyzing data obtained from a randomized placebo-controlled trial. On the other hand, patients who received Ω-3 PUFAs showed lower expression of mRNA for MMP-7 ($p = 0.0055$), -9 ($p = 0.0048$), -12 ($p = 0.0044$), and for IL-6 ($p = 0.0395$) and sICAM-1 ($p = 0.0142$). Similar results were reported by Thies et al. [198], where after administering dietary fish oil supplements (1.4 g EPA + DHA/day) in patients with advanced atherosclerotic plaque, less inflammation, inhibition of macrophages and lymphocytes infiltration and an increase in plaque stability was observed. Besides, several RCTs have pointed out that Ω-3 PUFAs might modulate the expression of cell adhesion molecules (sICAM-1, sVCAM-1, or sP-selectin) as well as CRP, IL-1β, IL-6, serum amyloid A (SAA), TNF-receptor concentrations, TNF-α, or PAI-1 levels among others [195,199], as shown in Table 4.

Table 4. Potential inflammatory effects of different bioactive compounds on CVD.

	Pro- and Anti-Inflammatory Markers and Genes	Leukocyte Expression
Ω-3 PUFA	sVCAM-1, sICAM-1, sP-selectin, TNF-α, TNFR, IL-1β, IL-6, MMP-7, MMP-9, CRP, PAI-1, SAA	T-lymphocytes
Lycopene	sVCAM-1, IL-6, IL-10, IL-18, MCP-1, tHcy, PAI-1	T-lymphocytes: LFA
Phytosterols	IL-1β, IL-6, CRP	-

CRP: C-reactive protein; IL: Interleukin; LFA: Lymphocyte function-associated antigen 1; MCP-1: Monocyte chemoattractant protein; MMP: Metallopeptidase; PAI-1: Plasminogen activator inhibitor 1; SAA: Serum amyloid A; sICAM-1: Soluble intercellular adhesion molecule 1; sVCAM-1: Soluble vascular cell adhesion molecule; tHcy: Total homocysteine; TNF-α: Tumor necrosis factor; TNFR: Tumor necrosis factor receptor.

7.2. Lycopene

Lycopene is a lipophilic and an unsaturated carotenoid, present in red-colored fruits and vegetables, such as tomatoes, papaya, or watermelons among others. Epidemiological observational and interventional studies [200,201] suggest that lycopene might reduce atherosclerotic risk, particularly in early stages of atherosclerosis, preventing endothelial dysfunction (NO bioavailability and blood flow) and LDL oxidation. Others mechanisms through which lycopene might exert effects is improvement of the metabolic profile (by impairing cholesterol synthesis) and BP, through reductions in arterial stiffness, and modulation of the expression of pro-inflammatory markers and platelet aggregation [202]. Furthermore, dietary lycopene confers CV benefits and significant reduction in CV mortality and major CV events in postmenopausal women free of CVD or cancer [202]. Focusing on the risk of develops atherosclerosis, several studies have pointed out lycopene's antioxidant power as a possible mechanism to explain its health benefits [203].

Additionally, in a recent meta-analysis [204], dietary interventions supplemented with tomatoes significantly decreased LDL-c (−0.22 mmol/L; $p = 0.006$), IL-6 (−0.25; $p = 0.03$) and improved FMD by 2.53% ($p = 0.01$), while lycopene supplementation reduced SBP (−5.66 mmHg; $p = 0.002$). In another study with 40 participants with heart failure [205] (lycopene intervention, 29.4 mg/day of lycopene vs. control group), CRP levels decreased significantly in the intervention group, but only in women ($p = 0.04$).

Dietary data collected from the National Health and Nutrition Examination Survey (NANHES) 2003–2006 [206] showed significant inverse associations with tHcy and CRP for dietary lycopene intake ($p < 0.05$).

Therefore, Valderas-Martinez et al. [201] investigated the postprandial effects of a single dose of raw tomatoes (RT), tomato sauce (TS), and tomato sauce with refined olive oil (TSOO) on CVD. In this randomized, cross-over, controlled feeding trial in 40 subjects free of CVD, authors found that tomato intake significantly decreased some inflammatory biomarkers levels, such as LFA-1, IL-6, IL-18, MCP-1, and VCAM-1, and increased plasma IL-10 levels. In another interventional study [207], with 80 subjects, 40 early atherosclerosis cases, and 40 control subjects, the authors pointed out that serum carotenoids concentrations are linked with the risk of atherosclerosis development. They observed that serum lutein was negatively associated with IL-6 ($p < 0.001$) and directly associated with IFN-γ ($p = 0.002$). Moreover, zeaxanthin was inversely associated with VCAM-1 ($p = 0.001$) and apolipoprotein E ($p = 0.022$) levels, while lycopene was inversely associated with sVCAM-1 ($p = 0.011$) and LDL ($p = 0.046$). However, in a single-blind, randomized controlled intervention trial [208] with healthy volunteers (94 men and 131 women, aged 40 y–65 y), no changes were observed for inflammatory markers (oxLDL, sICAM-1, and IL-6), insulin resistance, and sensitivity markers after 12 weeks of dietary intervention, as shown in Table 4.

7.3. Phytosterols

A large body of scientific evidence has concluded that a daily dose of 2–3 g of plant sterols or phytosterols is associated with an LDL-c reduction of around 6–15% of the total concentration [209,210]. These reductions were also observed in a meta-analysis conducted by Demonty et al. [211], where after administering a daily dose of 2.15 g of phytosterols, LDL-c was reduced by 8.8%. In fact, plant sterols have been proposed as a complement of statins treatment in order to decrease the risk of CVD. However, available data is inconsistent, so more research is needed. In this other meta-analysis [212] of 20 RCTs with 1308 participants, the effect of phytosterols intake on pro-inflammatory markers was evaluated. Significant reductions of CRP levels (−0.10 mg/dL) were observed after plan sterols' intake.

In addition, clinical studies have evaluated the association between phytosterols' consumption and inflammatory markers, such as CRP and cytokines. Although the results showed by Ras et al. [213] are in aggregement with the data reported by Demonty, no changes in CRP levels were observed. In a new study conducted by Ras et al. [209], in 240 hypercholesterolaemic voluntaries who consumed a low-fat spread with added phytosterols (3 g/day) for 12 weeks, no changes in any of the markers evaluated (CRP, SAA, IL-6, IL-8, TNF-α, and sICAM-1) were observed. Devaraj et al. [214] described significant reductions of IL-6 and IL1β levels after the intake of an orange juice-based beverage fortified with sterols (2 g sterols/day). In addition, results of a double-blinded, randomized, crossover trial [215] with 58 hypercholesterolemic participants during 12 weeks of intervention with margarine supplemented with phytosterols (3 g/day) did not show changes in CRP, IL-6, or TNF-α levels, as shown in Table 4.

8. Polyphenols

Polyphenols are the most abundant dietary antioxidants present in most plant origin foods and beverages, which possess a wide range of health effects in the prevention of CVD [216]. The most relevant food sources are fruit and vegetables, red wine, black and green tea, coffee, EVOO, and chocolate, as well as nuts, seeds, herbs, and spices [217].

Numerous scientific reports accumulated in the last years suggest that polyphenols might exert their positive effects by delaying progression of atherosclerosis through several mechanisms: Regulation of signaling and transcription pathways, such as NF-κβ; antioxidant systems; prevention of leukocyte migration and later infiltration inside plaque; reduction of adhesion molecules levels; inhibition of the encoding of pro-inflammatory cytokines; reduction of BP because of the enhanced NO production; and improvements of lipid metabolism, coagulation activity, and endothelial function, among others [218,219].

Several epidemiological studies have reported a negative association between consumption of polyphenols or polyphenols-rich foods and CVD [220–222]. A meta-analysis [223], including 14 prospective cohort studies with 1,279,804 participants and 36,352 CVD cases, showed that moderate consumption of coffee (three to five cups/day) was associated with a lower CVD risk compared with non-consumers. Similar results were found in the meta-analysis conducted by Larsson et al. [224]. Additionally, in another meta-analysis (14 prospective studies, with 513,804 participants and a median of follow-up of 11.5 years), it was found that a daily intake of ≥3 cups of tea was associated with a lower risk of stroke (−13%) and ischemic stroke (−24%) [225].

Focusing on the action of polyphenols on endothelial function, a large number of studies that have tested red wine, grape juice, black tea, soy, or dark cocoa showed an increase in FMD [226]. Besides, a daily consumption of dark chocolate (50 g) was associated with an improvement of FMD by 3.99% in acute and 1.45% in chronic intake and reduced systolic (−5.88 mm Hg) and diastolic BP (−3.30 mm Hg) [227]. Additionally, and contrary to the expected, acute consumption of black tea was associated with an increase of SBP (5.69 mm Hg) and DBP (2.56 mm Hg) while FMD was increased by 3.40%. Contrary to black tea, green tea led to a significant reduction in LDL-c (−0.23 mmol/L) [227]. Furthermore, alcohol and red wine moderate consumption were associated with an increase of FMD after analyzing 801 individual foods with food frequency questionnaires (FFQs) from the 2000 Hoorn Study (women = 399; age 68.5 ± 7.2 years) [228].

So, several meta-analyses of RCTs [229,230] have reported significant reductions of LDL-c, SBP, fasting glucose, BMI, hemoglobin A1c, or TNF-α levels, and significant increments of HDL-c.

Additionally, hs-CRP, IL-1β, and sP-selectin levels were significantly decreased after anthocyanin extract interventions. A larger cross-sectional study (BELSTRESS) with observational data from 1031 healthy men (49 years on average) found that drinking tea might reduce the inflammatory processes underlying CVD, as tea intake leads to lower levels of CRP ($p = 0.004$), SAA ($p = 0.001$), and haptoglobin ($p = 0.02$) [231].

Anti-inflammatory and immune-modulating effects of polyphenols have also been suggested as a potential pathway for polyphenols' health benefits. Several RCTs showed the relationship between cocoa polyphenols and inflammatory biomarkers related to atherosclerosis disease progression. In this sense, Vazquez-Agell et al. [232] suggested that the acute consumption of 40 g of cocoa with water might inhibit the NF-κβ transcription and down-regulate adhesion molecules' production (sICAM-1 and sE-selectin). Moreover, Monagas et al. [233], in a cross-interventional trial, showed that cocoa powder intake led to a reduced expression of adhesion molecules on monocyte surfaces (VLA-4, CD40, and CD36, $p \leq 0.028$; all) and lower serum levels of soluble adhesion molecules (sP-selectin and sICAM-1; both $p = 0.007$) in 42 subjects (mean age 69.7 years) at high risk of CVD and after four weeks of intervention. Additionally, Basu et al. [234] found that green tea consumption, as a beverage or extract, did not alter inflammatory biomarkers (adiponectin, CRP, IL-6, IL-1β, sVCAM-1, sICAM-1, leptin, or leptin:adiponectin ratio) related to MetS after eight weeks of intervention. Only SAA was significantly decreased after green tea beverage and extracts' intake ($p < 0.005$). Also, Zhang et al. [235] reported a significant decrease of CXCL7 by 12.32%, CXCL5 by 9.95%, CXCL8 by 6.07%, CXCL12 by 8.11%, and CCL2 levels by 11.63% after 320 mg intake of purified anthocyanins during 24 weeks. Similar results were observed after administering 320 mg of purified anthocyanins in 150 hypercholesterolemic patients during 24 weeks [236]. In this case, significant reductions of β-thromboglobulin, sP-selectin, and RANTES (regulated on activation, normal T cell expressed and secreted) were observed. Anthocyanins have also been correlated with lower levels of oxidative stress biomarkers. In an interventional study with 42 overweight and smoker participants, significant reductions in oxLDL and 8-iso-prostaglandin F2α were observed after the supplementation with an extract of maqui berry (162 mg anthocyanins) for 40 days [237]. Isoflavones and stilbens (mainly resveratrol) have also shown anti-inflammatory and immunomodulatory effects. Isoflavones improved CRP concentrations of 117 healthy European postmenopausal women after 50 mg/day of isoflavones intake [238]. Other RCT on postmenopausal American women who received daily 25 g of soy protein supplementation, showed reductions of subclinical atherosclerosis progression by 16% as well as reductions of carotid thickness progression by a mean of 68% [239]. Relative to stilbens, Tomé-Carneiro et al. [240] found significant reductions of oxLDL, apolipoprotein B (ApoB), and LDL-c after analyzing the effect of the intake of a grape supplement containing 8 mg resveratrol for six months. Also, a significant reduction of inflammatory markers levels (IL-18, sICAM-1, and sVCAM-1; $p \leq 0.037$; all) related with atheroma plaque development was observed in 44 healthy participants who ingested the resveratrol extract during four weeks [241]. Additionally, a randomized, double-blind, placebo-controlled clinical trial conducted by Seyyedebrahimi et al. [242] with 48 diabetics type 2 participants and supplemented with 800 mg/day of resveratrol for eight weeks showed a reduction in plasmatic levels of protein carbonyl content and ROS in PBMCs. Furthermore, after resveratrol supplement intake, an increase in the expression of Nrf2 and SOD was observed, as shown in Table 5.

Table 5. Potential inflammatory effects of polyphenols on CVD.

	Pro- and Anti-Inflammatory Markers and Genes	**Leukocyte Expression**	**Oxidative Stress Markers**
Polyphenols	NF-κβ, sICAM-1, sE- and sP-selectin, IL-1β, IL-18, CRP, SAA, CXCL5, CXCL7, CXCL8, CXCL12, CCL2, TNF-α, β-thromboglobulin, RANTES, ApoB	Monocytes: VLA-4, CD40, CD36	oxLDL, 8-iso-prostaglandin F2α, ROS, SOD, Nrf2

ApoB: Apolipoprotein B; CRP: C-reactive protein; CXCL: Chemokine (C-X-C motif) ligand; IL: Interleukin; NF-κβ: Nuclear factor kappa B; Nrf2: Nuclear factor (erythroid-derived 2)-like 2; oxLDL: Oxidized LDL; RANTES: Regulated on activation, normal T cell expressed and secreted; ROS: Reactive oxygen species; SAA: Serum amyloid A; sICAM-1: Soluble intercellular adhesion molecule 1; SOD: Superoxide dismutase; TNF-α: Tumor necrosis factor.

9. Conclusions

We have shown the intimate relationship between nutrition and CVD. Thus, the challenge is in promoting healthy dietary habits as well as an active lifestyle as early as possible in children and young adults. The evidence favors consumption of healthy dietary patterns, such as the Mediterranean diet or DASH diet, against other unhealthy dietary patterns, such as the Western diet, based on a high consumption of salt, added sugars, and saturated and trans-fats. Despite the fact that strong evidence shows the potential health benefits of a great amount of foods, nutrients, bioactive compounds, and dietary antioxidants, such as polyphenols, may exert on CV risk factors or directly on CVD development, it is necessary to conduct more interventional studies with a higher number of cases and longer follow up. To date, a lot of results obtained have produced few conclusions and sometimes, even contradictions. Therefore, due to a lack of information about possible mechanisms implicated in the cardioprotective effect of diet, foods, nutrients, or bioactive compounds, this needs to be more investigated.

Author Contributions: Conceptualization, R.C. and E.S.; Methodology, R.C. and R.E.; Investigation, R.C. and S.C.-B.; Writing—Original Draft Preparation, R.C. and S.C.-B.; Writing—Review & Editing, R.C. and R.E.; Visualization, E.S.; Supervision, E.S.; project administration, E.S.; funding acquisition, R.E.

Acknowledgments: This research was funded by the Instituto de Salud Carlos III, Spain. CIBER OBN is an initiative of the Instituto de Salud Carlos III, Spain.

References

1. Benjamin, E.J.; Blaha, M.J.; Chiuve, S.E.; Cushman, M.; Das, S.R.; Deo, R.; de Ferranti, S.D.; Floyd, J.; Fornage, M.; Gillespie, C.; et al. Heart Disease and Stroke Statistics-2017 Update: A Report from the American Heart Association. *Circulation* **2017**, *35*, e146–e603. [CrossRef] [PubMed]
2. Ravera, A.; Carubelli, V.; Sciatti, E.; Bonadei, I.; Gorga, E.; Cani, D.; Vizzardi, E.; Metra, M.; Lombardi, C. Nutrition and cardiovascular disease: Finding the perfect recipe for cardiovascular health. *Nutrients* **2016**, *8*, 363. [CrossRef] [PubMed]
3. Mozaffarian, D.; Benjamin, E.J.; Go, A.S.; Arnett, D.K.; Blaha, M.J.; Cushman, M.; Das, S.R.; de Ferranti, S.; Despres, J.P.; Fullerton, H.J.; et al. Heart disease and stroke statistics-2016 update: A report from the American Heart Association. *Circulation* **2016**, *133*, e38–e360. [CrossRef] [PubMed]
4. Benjamin, E.J.; Virani, S.S.; Callaway, C.W.; Chamberlain, A.M.; Chang, A.R.; Cheng, S.; Chiuve, S.E.; Cushman, M.; Delling, F.N.; Deo, R.; et al. Heart Disease and Stroke Statistics-2018 Update: A report from the American heart association. *Circulation* **2018**, *137*, e67–e492. [CrossRef] [PubMed]
5. Artinian, N.T.; Fletcher, G.F.; Mozaffarian, D.; Kris-Etherton, P.; Van Horn, L.; Lichtenstein, A.H.; Kumanyika, S.; Kraus, W.E.; Fleg, J.L.; Redeker, N.S. Interventions to promote physical activity and dietary lifestyle changes for cardiovascular risk factor reduction in adults: A scientific statement from the American Heart Association. *Circulation* **2010**, *122*, 406–441. [CrossRef] [PubMed]
6. GBD 2013 Mortality and Causes of Death Collaborators. Global, regional, and national age-sex specific all-cause and cause-specific mortality for 240 causes of death, 1990–2013: A systematic analysis for the global burden of disease study 2013. *Lancet* **2015**, *385*, 117–171. [CrossRef]
7. Anand, S.S.; Hawkes, C.; de Souza, R.J.; Mente, A.; Dehghan, M.; Nugent, R.; Zulyniak, M.A.; Weis, T.; Bernstein, A.M.; Krauss, R.M. Food consumption and its impact on cardiovascular disease: Importance of solutions focusedon the globalized food system: A report from the workshop convened by the world heart federation. *J. Am. Coll. Cardiol.* **2015**, *66*, 1590–1614. [CrossRef]
8. Lacroix, S.; Cantin, J.; Nigam, A. Contemporary issues regarding nutrition in cardiovascular rehabilitation. *Ann. Phys. Rehabil. Med.* **2017**, *60*, 36–42. [CrossRef]
9. O'Rourke, K.; Vander Zanden, A.; Shepard, D.; Leach-Kemon, K. For the Institute for Health Metrics and Evaluation. Cardiovascular disease worldwide, 1990–2013. *JAMA* **2015**, *314*, 1905. [CrossRef]
10. Mozaffarian, D.; Ludwig, D.S. Dietary guidelines in the 21st century: A time for food. *JAMA* **2010**, *304*, 681–682. [CrossRef]
11. Libby, P. Interleukin-1 beta as a target for atherosclerosis therapy: Biological basis of CANTOS and beyond. *J. Am. Coll. Cardiol.* **2017**, *70*, 2278–2289. [CrossRef] [PubMed]
12. Libby, P.; Hansson, G.K. Taming immune and inflammatory responses to treat atherosclerosis. *J. Am. Coll. Cardiol.* **2018**, *71*, 173–176. [CrossRef] [PubMed]
13. Micha, R.; Peñalvo, J.L.; Cudhea, F.; Imamura, F.; Rehm, C.D.; Mozaffarian, D. Association between dietary factors and mortality from heart disease, stroke, and type 2 diabetes in the United States. *JAMA* **2017**, *317*, 912–924. [CrossRef] [PubMed]
14. Cardoso Lde, O.; Carvalho, M.S.; Cruz, O.G.; Melere, C.; Luft, V.C.; Molina, M.C.; Faria, C.P.; Benseñor, I.M.; Matos, S.M.; Fonseca, M.D.; et al. Eating patterns in the Brazilian Longitudinal Study of Adult Health (ELSA-Brasil): An exploratory analysis. *Cad. Saude Publica* **2016**, *32*, e00066215. [CrossRef] [PubMed]
15. Lu, H.; Daugherty, A. Recent Highlights of ATVB Atherosclerosis. *Arterioescler. Thromb. Vasc. Biol.* **2015**, *35*, 485–491. [CrossRef] [PubMed]

16. Arbab-Zadeh, A.; Fuster, V. The Myth of the "Vulnerable Plaque": Transitioning from a Focus on Individual Lesions to Atherosclerotic Disease Burden for Coronary Artery Disease Risk Assessment. *J. Am. Coll. Cardiol.* **2015**, *65*, 846–855. [CrossRef] [PubMed]
17. Jolliffe, I.T.; Cadima, J. Principal component analysis: A review and recent developments. *Philos. Trans. A Math. Phys. Eng. Sci.* **2016**, *374*, 20150202. [CrossRef]
18. Ozawa, M.; Shipley, M.; Kivimaki, M.; Singh-Manoux, A.; Brunner, E.J. Dietary pattern, inflammation and cognitive decline: The Whitehall II prospective cohort study. *Clin. Nutr.* **2017**, *36*, 506–512. [CrossRef]
19. Atkins, J.L.; Whincup, P.H.; Morris, R.W.; Lennon, L.T.; Papacosta, O.; Wannamethee, S.G. Dietary patterns and the risk of CVD and all-cause mortality in older British men. *Br. J. Nutr.* **2016**, *116*, 1246–1255. [CrossRef]
20. Viscogliosi, G.; Cipriani, E.; Liguori, M.L.; Marigliano, B.; Saliola, M.; Ettorre, E.; Andreozzi, P. Mediterranean dietary pattern adherence: Associations with prediabetes, metabolic syndrome, and related microinflammation. *Metab. Syndr. Relat. Disord.* **2013**, *11*, 210–216. [CrossRef]
21. Denova-Gutiérrez, E.; Tucker, K.L.; Flores, M.; Barquera, S.; Salmerón, J. Dietary patterns are associated with predicted cardiovascular disease risk in an urban mexican adult population. *J. Nutr.* **2016**, *146*, 90–97. [CrossRef] [PubMed]
22. Okada, E.; Takahashi, K.; Takimoto, H.; Takabayashi, S.; Kishi, T.; Kobayashi, T.; Nakamura, K.; Ukawa, S.; Nakamura, M.; Sasaki, S.; et al. Dietary patterns among Japanese adults: Findings from the National Health and Nutrition Survey, 2012. *Asia Pac. J. Clin. Nutr.* **2018**, *27*, 1120–1130. [CrossRef] [PubMed]
23. Hu, F.B. Dietary patterns analysis: a new direction in nutritional epidemiology. *Curr. Opin. Lipidol.* **2002**, *13*, 3–9. [CrossRef] [PubMed]
24. Wood, A.D.; Strachan, A.A.; Thies, F.; Aucott, L.S.; Reid, D.M.; Hardcastle, A.C.; Mavroeidi, A.; Simpson, W.G.; Duthie, G.G.; Macdonald, H.M. Patterns of dietary intake and serum carotenoid and tocopherol status are associated with biomarkers of chronic low-grade systemic inflammation and cardiovascular risk. *Br. J. Nutr.* **2014**, *112*, 1341–1352. [CrossRef] [PubMed]
25. Sijtsma, F.P.; Meyer, K.A.; Steffen, L.M.; Van Horn, L.; Shikany, J.M.; Odegaard, A.O.; Gross, M.D.; Kromhout, D.; Jacobs, D.R., Jr. Diet quality and markers of endothelial function: The CARDIA study. *Nutr. Metab. Cardiovasc. Dis.* **2014**, *24*, 632–638. [CrossRef] [PubMed]
26. Piccand, E.; Vollenweider, P.; Guessous, I.; Marques-Vidal, P. Association between dietary intake and inflammatory markers: Results from the CoLaus study. *Public Health Nutr.* **2018**, *18*, 1–8. [CrossRef] [PubMed]
27. Slavin, J.L.; Lloyd, B. Health benefits of fruits and vegetables. *Adv. Nutr.* **2012**, *3*, 506–516. [CrossRef]
28. Noad, R.L.; Rooney, C.; McCall, D.; Young, I.S.; McCance, D.; McKinley, M.C.; Woodside, J.V.; McKeown, P.P. Beneficial effect of a polyphenol-rich diet on cardiovascular risk: A randomised control trial. *Heart* **2016**, *102*, 1371–1379. [CrossRef]
29. Quintana Pacheco, D.A.; Sookthai, D.; Wittenbecher, C.; Graf, M.E.; Schübel, R.; Johnson, T.; Katzke, V.; Jakszyn, P.; Kaaks, R.; Kühn, T. Red meat consumption and risk of cardiovascular diseases-is increased iron load a possible link? *Am. J. Clin. Nutr.* **2018**, *107*, 113–119. [CrossRef]
30. Oude Griep, L.M.; Wang, H.; Chan, Q. Empirically-derived dietary patterns, diet quality scores, and markers of inflammation and endothelial dysfunction. *Curr. Nutr. Rep.* **2013**, *2*, 97–104. [CrossRef]
31. Barbaresko, J.; Koch, M.; Schulze, M.B.; Nöthlings, U. Dietary pattern analysis and biomarkers of low-grade inflammation: A systematic literature review. *Nutr. Rev.* **2013**, *71*, 511–527. [CrossRef] [PubMed]
32. Badimon, L.; Chagas, P.; Chiva-Blanch, G. Diet and Cardiovascular Disease: Effects of Foods and Nutrients in Classical and Emerging Cardiovascular Risk Factors. *Curr. Med. Chem.* **2017**. [CrossRef] [PubMed]
33. Ros, E.; Martínez-González, M.A.; Estruch, R.; Salas-Salvadó, J.; Fitó, M.; Martínez, J.A.; Corella, D. Mediterranean diet and cardiovascular health: Teachings of the PREDIMED study. *Adv. Nutr.* **2014**, *5*, 330S–336S. [CrossRef] [PubMed]
34. Ahluwalia, N.; Andreeva, V.A.; Kesse-Guyot, E.; Hercberg, S. Dietary patterns, inflammation and the metabolic syndrome. *Diabetes Metab.* **2013**, *39*, 99–110. [CrossRef] [PubMed]
35. Tapsell, L.C.; Neale, E.P.; Satija, A.; Hu, F.B. Foods, nutrients, and dietary patterns: Interconnections and implications for dietary guidelines. *Adv. Nutr.* **2016**, *7*, 445–454. [CrossRef] [PubMed]
36. Húc, T.; Nowinski, A.; Drapala, A.; Konopelski, P.; Ufnal, M. Indole and indoxyl sulfate, gut bacteria metabolites of tryptophan change arterial blood pressure via peripheral and central mechanisms in rats. *Pharmacol. Res.* **2018**, *130*, 172–179. [CrossRef] [PubMed]

37. Koeth, R.A.; Wang, Z.; Levison, B.S.; Buffa, J.A.; Org, E.; Sheehy, B.T.; Britt, E.B.; Fu, X.; Wu, Y.; Li, L.; et al. Intestinal microbiota metabolism of L-carnitine, a nutrient in red meat, promotes atherosclerosis. *Nat. Med.* **2013**, *19*, 576–585. [CrossRef]
38. Nowinski, A.; Ufnal, M. Trimethylamine N-oxide: A harmful, protective or diagnostic marker in lifestyle diseases? *Nutrition* **2018**, *46*, 7–12. [CrossRef] [PubMed]
39. Mehta, D.; Malik, A.B. Signaling mechanisms regulating endothelial permeability. *Physiol. Rev.* **2016**, *86*, 279–367. [CrossRef] [PubMed]
40. Virmani, R.; Joner, M.; Sakakura, K. Recent highlights of ATVB: Calcification. *Arterioscler. Thromb. Vasc. Biol.* **2014**, *34*, 1329–1332. [CrossRef] [PubMed]
41. Kwon, G.P.; Schroeder, J.L.; Amar, M.J.; Remaley, A.T.; Balaban, R.S. Contribution of macromolecular structure to the retention of low-density lipoprotein at arterial branch points. *Circulation* **2008**, *117*, 2658–2664. [CrossRef] [PubMed]
42. Jennings, L.K. Mechanisms of platelet activation: Need for new strategies to protect against platelet-mediated atherothrombosis. *Thromb. Haemost.* **2009**, *102*, 248–257. [CrossRef] [PubMed]
43. Chistiakov, D.A.; Melnichenko, A.A.; Myasoedova, V.A.; Grenchko, A.V.; Orekhov, A.N. Mechanisms of foam cell formation in atherosclerosis. *J. Mol. Med.* **2017**, *95*, 1153–1165. [CrossRef] [PubMed]
44. Salvayre, R.; Auge, N.; Benoist, H.; Negre-Salvayre, A. Oxidized low-density lipoprotein-induced apoptosis. *Biochim. Biophys. Acta* **2002**, *1585*, 213–221. [CrossRef]
45. Ghosh, S.; Zhao, B.; Bie, J.; Song, J. Macrophage cholesteryl ester mobilization and atherosclerosis. *Vasc. Pharmacol.* **2010**, *52*, 1–10. [CrossRef] [PubMed]
46. Legein, B.; Temmerman, L.; Biessen, E.A.; Lutgens, E. Inflammation and immune system interactions in atherosclerosis. *Cell. Mol. Life Sci.* **2013**, *70*, 3847–3869. [CrossRef]
47. Low Wang, C.C.; Hess, C.N.; Hiatt, W.R.; Goldfine, A.B. Atherosclerotic cardiovascular disease and hearth failure in type 2 diabetes-mechanisms, management, and clinical considerations. *Circulation* **2016**, *133*, 2459–2502. [CrossRef]
48. Harrison, D.; Griendling, K.K.; Landmesser, U.; Hornig, B.; Drexler, H. Role of oxidative stress in atherosclerosis. *Am. J. Cardiol.* **2003**, *91*, 7A–11A. [CrossRef]
49. Brown, D.I.; Griendling, K.K. Regulation of signaling transduction by reactive oxygen species in the cardiovascular system. *Circ. Res.* **2015**, *116*, 531–549. [CrossRef]
50. Littlewood, T.D.; Bennett, M.R. Apoptotic cell death in atherosclerosis. *Curr. Opin. Lipodol.* **2003**, *14*, 469–475. [CrossRef]
51. Li, H.; Horke, S.; Förstermann, U. Vascular oxidative stress, nitric oxide and atherosclerosis. *Atherosclerosis* **2014**, *237*, 208–219. [CrossRef] [PubMed]
52. Reuter, S.; Gupta, S.C.; Chaturvedi, M.M.; Aggarwal, B.B. Oxidative stress, inflammation, and cancer: How are they linked? *Free Radic. Biol. Med.* **2010**, *49*, 1603–1616. [CrossRef] [PubMed]
53. Torres, N.; Guevara-Cruz, M.; Velázquez-Villegas, L.A.; Tovar, A.R. Nutrition and atherosclerosis. *Arch. Med. Res.* **2015**, *46*, 408–426. [CrossRef] [PubMed]
54. Li, H.; Forstermann, U. Uncoupling of endothelial NO synthase in atherosclerosis and vascular disease. *Curr. Opin. Pharmacol.* **2013**, *13*, 161–167. [CrossRef] [PubMed]
55. Badimon, L.; Vilahur, G.; Padro, T. Lipoproteins, platelets and atherothrombosis. *Rev. Esp. Cardiol.* **2009**, *62*, 1161–1178. [CrossRef]
56. Kattoor, A.J.; Pothineni, N.V.K.; Palagiri, D. Oxidative strees in atherosclerosis. *Curr. Atheroscler. Rep.* **2017**, *19*, 42. [CrossRef] [PubMed]
57. Guzik, T.J.; Korbut, R.; Adamek-Guzik, T. Nitric oxide and superoxide in inflammation and immune regulation. *J. Physiol. Pharmacol.* **2003**, *54*, 469–487. [PubMed]
58. Centritto, F.; Iacoviello, L.; di Giuseppe, R.; De Curtis, A.; Costanzo, S.; Zito, F.; Grioni, S.; Sieri, S.; Donati, M.B.; de Gaetano, G.; et al. Dietary patterns, cardiovascular risk factors and C-reactive protein in a healthy Italian population. *Nutr. Metab. Cardiovasc. Dis.* **2009**, *19*, 697–706. [CrossRef]
59. Mozaffarian, D. Dietary and policy priorities for cardiovascular disease, diabetes, and obesity: A comprehensive review. *Circulation* **2016**, *133*, 187–225. [CrossRef]
60. Silveira, B.K.S.; Oliveira, T.M.S.; Andrade, P.A.; Hermsdorff, H.H.M.; Rosa, C.O.B.; Franceschini, S.D.C.C. Dietary pattern and macronutrients profile on the variation of inflammatory biomarkers: Scientific Update. *Cardiol. Res. Pract.* **2018**, *2018*, 4762575. [CrossRef]

61. Esposito, K.; Ciotola, M.; Giugliano, D. Mediterranean diet, endothelial function and vascular inflammatory markers. *Public Health Nutr.* **2006**, *9*, 1073–1076. [CrossRef] [PubMed]
62. Llorente-Cortés, V.; Estruch, R.; Mena, M.P.; Ros, E.; González, M.A.; Fitó, M.; Lamuela-Raventós, R.M.; Badimon, L. Effect of Mediterranean diet on the expression of pro-atherogenic genes in a population at high cardiovascular risk. *Atherosclerosis* **2010**, *208*, 442–450. [CrossRef] [PubMed]
63. Casas, R.; Sacanella, E.; Urpí-Sardà, M.; Chiva-Blanch, G.; Ros, E.; Martínez-González, M.A.; Covas, M.I.; Lamuela-Raventos, R.M.; Salas-Salvadó, J.; Fiol, M.; et al. The effects of the mediterranean diet on biomarkers of vascular wall inflammation and plaque vulnerability in subjects with high risk for cardiovascular disease. A randomized trial. *PLoS ONE* **2014**, *9*, e100084. [CrossRef] [PubMed]
64. Casas, R.; Urpi-Sardà, M.; Sacanella, E.; Arranz, S.; Corella, D.; Castañer, O.; Lamuela-Raventós, R.M.; Salas-Salvadó, J.; Lapetra, J.; Portillo, M.P.; et al. Anti-Inflammatory Effects of the Mediterranean Diet in the Early and Late Stages of Atheroma Plaque Development. *Mediat. Inflamm.* **2017**, *2017*, 3674390. [CrossRef] [PubMed]
65. Kastorini, C.M.; Panagiotakos, D.B.; Chrysohoou, C.; Georgousopoulou, E.; Pitaraki, E.; Puddu, P.E.; Tousoulis, D.; Stefanadis, C.; Pitsavos, C.; ATTICA Study Group. Metabolic syndrome, adherence to the Mediterranean diet and 10-year cardiovascular disease incidence: The ATTICA study. *Atherosclerosis* **2016**, *246*, 87–93. [CrossRef] [PubMed]
66. Cainzos-Achirica, M.; Miedema, M.D.; McEvoy, J.W.; Cushman, M.; Dardari, Z.; Greenland, P.; Nasir, K.; Budoff, M.J.; Al-Mallah, M.H.; Yeboah, J.; et al. The prognostic value of high sensitivity C-reactive protein in a multi-ethnic population after >10 years of follow-up: The Multi-Ethnic Study of Atherosclerosis (MESA). *Int. J. Cardiol.* **2018**, *264*, 158–164. [CrossRef] [PubMed]
67. Lahoz, C.; Castillo, E.; Mostaza, J.M.; de Dios, O.; Salinero-Fort, M.A.; González-Alegre, T.; García-Iglesias, F.; Estirado, E.; Laguna, F.; Sanchez, V.; et al. Relationship of the Adherence to a Mediterranean Diet and Its Main Components with CRP Levels in the Spanish Population. *Nutrients* **2018**, *10*, 379. [CrossRef] [PubMed]
68. Pounis, G.; Costanzo, S.; di Giuseppe, R.; de Lucia, F.; Santimone, I.; Sciarretta, A.; Barisciano, P.; Persichillo, M.; de Curtis, A.; Zito, F.; et al. Consumption of healthy foods at different content of antioxidant vitamins and phytochemicals and metabolic risk factors for cardiovascular disease in men and women of the Moli-sani study. *Eur. J. Clin. Nutr.* **2013**, *67*, 207–213. [CrossRef]
69. Sureda, A.; Bibiloni, M.D.M.; Julibert, A.; Bouzas, C.; Argelich, E.; Llompart, I.; Pons, A.; Tur, J.A. Adherence to the Mediterranean Diet and Inflammatory Markers. *Nutrients* **2018**, *10*, 62. [CrossRef]
70. Estruch, R.; Ros, E.; Salas-Salvadó, J.; Covas, M.I.; Corella, D.; Arós, F.; Gómez-Gracia, E.; Ruiz-Gutiérrez, V.; Fiol, M.; Lapetra, J.; et al. Primary Prevention of Cardiovascular Disease with a Mediterranean Diet Supplemented with Extra-Virgin Olive Oil or Nuts. *N. Engl. J. Med.* **2018**, *378*, e34. [CrossRef]
71. Estruch, R.; Martínez-González, M.A.; Corella, D.; Salas-Salvadó, J.; Ruiz-Gutiérrez, V.; Covas, M.I.; Fiol, M.; Gómez-Gracia, E.; López-Sabater, M.C.; Vinyoles, E.; et al. Effects of a Mediterraneanstyle diet on cardiovascular risk factors: A randomized trial. *Ann. Intern. Med.* **2006**, *145*, 1–11. [CrossRef] [PubMed]
72. Urpi-Sarda, M.; Casas, R.; Chiva-Blanch, G.; Romero-Mamani, E.S.; Valderas-Martínez, P.; Salas-Salvadó, J.; Covas, M.I.; Toledo, E.; Andres-Lacueva, C.; Llorach, R.; et al. The Mediterranean diet pattern and its main components are associated with lower plasma concentrations of tumor necrosis factor receptor 60 in patients at high risk for cardiovascular disease. *J. Nutr.* **2012**, *142*, 1019–1025. [CrossRef] [PubMed]
73. Mena, M.P.; Sacanella, E.; Vazquez-Agell, M.; Morales, M.; Fitó, M.; Escoda, R.; Serrano-Martínez, M.; Salas-Salvadó, J.; Benages, N.; Casas, R.; et al. Inhibition of circulating immune cell activation: A molecular antiinflammatory effect of the Mediterranean diet. *Am. J. Clin. Nutr.* **2009**, *89*, 248–256. [CrossRef] [PubMed]
74. Casas, R.; Sacanella, E.; Urpí-Sardà, M.; Corella, D.; Castañer, O.; Lamuela-Raventos, R.M.; Salas-Salvadó, J.; Martínez-González, M.A.; Ros, E.; Estruch, R. Long-Term Immunomodulatory Effects of a Mediterranean Diet in Adults at High Risk of Cardiovascular Disease in the PREvención con DIeta MEDiterránea (PREDIMED) Randomized Controlled Trial. *J. Nutr.* **2016**, *146*, 1684–1693. [CrossRef] [PubMed]
75. Ambring, A.; Johansson, M.; Axelsen, M.; Gan, L.; Strandvik, B.; Friberg, P. Mediterranean-inspired diet lowers the ratio of serum phospholipid n-6 to n-3 fatty acids, the number of leukocytes and platelets, and vascular endothelial growth factor in healthy subjects. *Am. J. Clin. Nutr.* **2006**, *83*, 575–581. [CrossRef] [PubMed]
76. Esposito, K.; Marfella, R.; Ciotola, M.; Di Palo, C.; Giugliano, F.; Giugliano, G.; D'Armiento, M.; D'Andrea, F.; Giugliano, D. Effect of a Mediterranean-Style Diet on Endothelial Dysfunction and Markers of Vascular Inflammation in the Metabolic Syndrome: A Randomized Trial. *JAMA* **2004**, *292*, 1440. [CrossRef] [PubMed]

77. Azzini, E.; Polito, A.; Fumagalli, A.; Intorre, F.; Venneria, E.; Durazzo, A.; Zaccaria, M.; Ciarapica, D.; Foddai, M.S.; Mauro, B.; et al. Mediterranean diet effect: An Italian picture. *Nutr. J.* **2011**, *10*, 125. [CrossRef] [PubMed]
78. Medina-Remón, A.; Casas, R.; Tressserra-Rimbau, A.; Ros, E.; Martínez-González, M.A.; Fitó, M.; Corella, D.; Salas-Salvadó, J.; Lamuela-Raventos, R.M.; Estruch, R.; et al. Polyphenol intake from a Mediterranean diet decreases inflammatory biomarkers related to atherosclerosis: A substudy of the PREDIMED trial. *Br. J. Clin. Pharmacol.* **2017**, *83*, 114–128. [CrossRef]
79. Arpón, A.; Milagro, F.I.; Razquin, C.; Corella, D.; Estruch, R.; Fitó, M.; Marti, A.; Martínez-González, M.A.; Ros, E.; Salas-Salvadó, J.; et al. Impact of consuming extra-virgin olive oil or nuts within a Mediterranean diet on DNA methylation in peripheral white blood cells within the PREDIMED-Navarra randomized controlled trial: A role for dietary lipids. *Nutrients* **2017**, *10*, 15. [CrossRef]
80. Arpón, A.; Riezu-Boj, J.I.; Milagro, F.I.; Marti, A.; Razquin, C.; Martínez-González, M.A.; Corella, D.; Estruch, R.; Casas, R.; Fitó, M.; et al. Adherence to Mediterranean diet is associated with methylation changes in inflammation-related genes in peripheral blood cells. *J. Physiol. Biochem.* **2016**, *73*, 445–455. [CrossRef]
81. Corella, D.; González, J.I.; Bulló, M.; Carrasco, P.; Portolés, O.; Díez-Espino, J.; Covas, M.I.; Ruíz-Gutierrez, V.; Gómez-Gracia, E.; Arós, F.; et al. Polymorphisms cyclooxygenase-2-765G>C and interleukin-6-174G>C are associated with serum inflammation markers in a high cardiovascular risk population and do not modify the response to a Mediterranean diet supplemented with virgin olive oil or nuts. *J. Nutr.* **2009**, *139*, 128–134. [CrossRef] [PubMed]
82. Corella, D.; Tai, E.S.; Sorlí, J.V.; Chew, S.K.; Coltell, O.; Sotos-Prieto, M.; García-Rios, A.; Estruch, R.; Ordovas, J.M. Association between the APOA2 promoter polymorphism and body weight in Mediterranean and Asian populations: Replication of a gene-saturated fat interaction. *Int. J. Obes.* **2011**, *35*, 666–675. [CrossRef] [PubMed]
83. Corella, D.; Carrasco, P.; Fitó, M.; Martínez-González, M.A.; Salas-Salvadó, J.; Arós, F.; Lapetra, J.; Guillén, M.; Ortega-Azorín, C.; Warnberg, J.; et al. Gene-environment interactions of CETP gene variation in a high cardiovascular risk Mediterranean population. *J. Lipid Res.* **2010**, *51*, 2798–2807. [CrossRef] [PubMed]
84. Corella, D.; Carrasco, P.; Sorlí, J.V.; Estruch, R.; Rico-Sanz, J.; Martínez-González, M.Á.; Salas-Salvadó, J.; Covas, M.I.; Coltell, O.; Arós, F.; et al. Mediterranean diet reduces the adverse effect of the TCF7L2-rs7903146 polymorphism on cardiovascular risk factors and stroke incidence: A randomized controlled trial in a high-cardiovascular-risk population. *Diabetes Care* **2013**, *36*, 3803–3811. [CrossRef] [PubMed]
85. Saneei, P.; Salehi-Abargouei, A.; Esmaillzadeh, A.; Azadbakht, L. Influence of dietary approaches to stop hypertension (DASH) diet on blood pressure: A systematic review and meta-analysis on randomized controlled trials. *Nutr. Metab. Cardiovasc. Dis.* **2014**, *24*, 1253–1261. [CrossRef] [PubMed]
86. Soltani, S.; Shirani, F.; Chitsazi, M.J.; Salehi-Abargouei, A. The effect of dietary approaches to stop hypertension (DASH) diet on weight and body composition in adults: A systematic review and meta-analysis of randomized controlled clinical trials. *Obes. Rev.* **2016**, *17*, 442–454. [CrossRef]
87. Shirani, F.; Salehi-Abargouei, A.; Azadbakht, L. Effects of dietary approaches to stop hypertension (DASH) diet on some risk for developing type 2 diabetes: A systematic review and meta-analysis on controlled clinical trials. *Nutrition* **2013**, *29*, 939–947. [CrossRef]
88. Millen, B.E.; Abrams, S.; Adams-Campbell, L.; Anderson, C.A.; Brenna, J.T.; Campbell, W.W.; Clinton, S.; Hu, F.; Nelson, M.; Neuhouser, M.L.; et al. The 2015 Dietary Guidelines Advisory Committee Scientific Report: Development and Major Conclusions. *Adv. Nutr.* **2016**, *7*, 438–444. [CrossRef]
89. Soltani, S.; Chitsazi, M.J.; Salehi-Abargouei, A. The effect of dietary approaches to stop hypertension (DASH) on serum inflammatory markers: A systematic review and meta-analysis of randomized trials. *Clin. Nutr.* **2018**, *37*, 542–550. [CrossRef]
90. Woo, J.; Yu, B.W.M.; Chan, R.S.M.; Leung, J. Influence of Dietary Patterns and Inflammatory Markers on Atherosclerosis Using Ankle Brachial Index as a Surrogate. *J. Nutr. Health Aging* **2018**, *22*, 619–626. [CrossRef]
91. Rifai, L.; Pisano, C.; Hayden, J.; Sulo, S.; Silver, M.A. Impact of the DASH diet on endothelial function, exercise capacity, and quality of life in patientswith heart failure. *Bayl. Univ. Med. Cent. Proc.* **2015**, *28*, 151–156. [CrossRef]
92. d'El-Rei, J.; Cunha, A.R.; Trindade, M.; Neves, M.F. Beneficial Effects of Dietary Nitrate on Endothelial Function and Blood Pressure Levels. *Int. J. Hypertens.* **2016**, *2016*, 6791519. [CrossRef]

93. Marques, F.Z.; Mackay, C.R.; Kaye, D.M. Beyond gut feelings: How the gut microbiota regulates blood pressure. *Nat. Rev. Cardiol.* **2018**, *15*, 20–32. [CrossRef] [PubMed]
94. Derkach, A.; Sampson, J.; Joseph, J.; Playdon, M.C.; Stolzenberg-Solomon, R.Z. Effects of dietary sodium on metabolites: The Dietary Approaches to Stop Hypertension (DASH)-Sodium Feeding Study. *Am. J. Clin. Nutr.* **2017**, *106*, 1131–1141. [CrossRef] [PubMed]
95. Mertens, E.; Markey, O.; Geleijnse, J.M.; Lovegrove, J.A.; Givens, D.I. Adherence to a healthy diet in relation to cardiovascular incidence and risk markers: Evidence from the Caerphilly Prospective Study. *Eur. J. Nutr.* **2018**, *57*, 1245–1258. [CrossRef] [PubMed]
96. Jones, N.R.V.; Forouhi, N.G.; Khaw, K.T.; Wareham, N.J.; Monsivais, P. Accordance to the Dietary Approaches to Stop Hypertension diet pattern and cardiovascular disease in a British, population-based cohort. *Eur. J. Epidemiol.* **2018**, *33*, 235–244. [CrossRef]
97. Saglimbene, V.M.; Wong, G.; Craig, J.C.; Ruospo, M.; Palmer, S.C.; Campbell, K.; Garcia-Larsen, V.; Natale, P.; Teixeira-Pinto, A.; Carrero, J.J.; et al. The Association of Mediterranean and DASH Diets with Mortality in Adults on Hemodialysis: The DIET-HD Multinational Cohort Study. *J. Am. Soc. Nephrol.* **2018**, *29*, 1741–1751. [CrossRef]
98. Neelakantan, N.; Koh, W.P.; Yuan, J.M.; van Dam, R.M. Diet-quality indexes are associated with a lower risk of cardiovascular, respiratory, and all-cause mortality among Chinese adults. *J. Nutr.* **2018**, *148*, 1323–1332. [CrossRef]
99. Rai, S.K.; Fung, T.T.; Lu, N.; Keller, S.F.; Curhan, G.C.; Choi, H.K. The Dietary Approaches to Stop Hypertension (DASH) diet, Western diet, and risk of gout in men: Prospective cohort study. *BMJ* **2017**, *357*, j1794. [CrossRef]
100. Neale, E.P.; Batterham, M.J.; Tapsell, L.C. Consumption of a healthy dietary pattern results in significant reductions in C-reactive protein levels in adults: A meta-analysis. *Nutr. Res.* **2016**, *36*, 391–401. [CrossRef]
101. Eichelmann, F.; Schwingshackl, L.; Fedirko, V.; Aleksandrova, K. Effect of plantbased diets on obesity-related inflammatory profiles: A systematic review and meta-analysis of intervention trials. *Obes. Rev.* **2016**, *17*, 1067–1079. [CrossRef] [PubMed]
102. Phillips, C.M.; Harrington, J.M.; Perry, I.J. Relationship between dietary quality, determined by DASH score, and cardiometabolic health biomarkers: A cross-sectional analysis in adults. *Clin. Nutr.* **2018**, *S0261–S5614*, in press. [CrossRef] [PubMed]
103. Asemi, Z.; Samimi, M.; Tabassi, Z.; Sabihi, S.S.; Esmaillzadeh, A. A randomized controlled clinical trial investigating the effect of DASH diet on insulin resistance, inflammation, and oxidative stress in gestational diabetes. *Nutrition* **2013**, *29*, 619–624. [CrossRef] [PubMed]
104. Kawamura, A.; Kajiya, K.; Kishi, H.; Inagaki, J.; Mitarai, M.; Oda, H.; Umemoto, S.; Kobayashi, S. Effects of the DASH-JUMP dietary intervention in Japanese participants with high-normal blood pressure and stage 1 hypertension: An open-label single-arm trial. *Hypertens. Res.* **2016**, *39*, 777–785. [CrossRef] [PubMed]
105. Saneei, P.; Hashemipour, M.; Kelishadi, R.; Esmaillzadeh, A. The Dietary Approaches to Stop Hypertension (DASH) diet affects inflammation in childhood metabolic syndrome: A randomized cross-over clinical trial. *Ann. Nutr. Metab.* **2014**, *64*, 20–27. [CrossRef] [PubMed]
106. Dauchet, L.; Amouyel, P.; Hercberg, S.; Dallongeville, J. Fruit and vegetable consumption and risk of coronary heart disease: A metaanalysis of cohort studies. *J. Nutr.* **2006**, *136*, 2588–2593. [CrossRef]
107. Dauchet, L.; Amouyel, P.; Dallongeville, J. Fruits, vegetables and coronary heart disease. *Nat. Rev. Cardiol.* **2009**, *6*, 599–608. [CrossRef] [PubMed]
108. Hosseini, B.; Berthon, B.S.; Saedisomeolia, A.; Starkey, M.R.; Collison, A.; Wark, P.A.B.; Wood, L.G. Effects of fruit and vegetable consumption on inflammatory biomarkers and immune cell populations: A systematic literature review and meta-analysis. *Am. J. Clin. Nutr.* **2018**, *108*, 136–155. [CrossRef]
109. Graham, I.; Atar, D.; Borch-Johnsen, K.; Boysen, G.; Burell, G.; Cifkova, R.; Dallongeville, J.; De Backer, G.; Ebrahim, S.; Gjelsvik, B.; et al. European guidelines on cardiovascular disease prevention in clinical practice: Executive summary: Fourth Joint Task Force of the European Society of Cardiology and Other Societies on Cardiovascular Disease Prevention in Clinical Practice (Constituted by representatives of nine societies and by invited experts). *Eur. Heart J.* **2007**, *28*, 2375–2414. [CrossRef]
110. American Heart Association Nutrition Committee; Lichtenstein, A.H.; Appel, L.J.; Brands, M.; Carnethon, M.; Daniels, S.; Franch, H.A.; Franklin, B.; Kris-Etherton, P.; Harris, W.S.; et al. Diet and lifestyle recommendations revision 2006: A scientific statement from the American Heart Association Nutrition Committee. *Circulation* **2006**, *114*, 82–96. [CrossRef]

111. Corley, J.; Kyle, J.A.; Starr, J.M.; McNeill, G.; Deary, I.J. Dietary factors and biomarkers of systemic inflammation in older people: The Lothian Birth Cohort 1936. *Br. J. Nutr.* **2015**, *114*, 1088–1098. [CrossRef] [PubMed]
112. Holt, E.M.; Steffen, L.M.; Moran, A.; Basu, S.; Steinberger, J.; Ross, J.A.; Hong, C.P.; Sinaiko, A.R. Fruit and vegetable consumption and its relation to markers of inflammation and oxidative stressin adolescents. *J. Am. Diet Assoc.* **2009**, *109*, 414–421. [CrossRef] [PubMed]
113. Arouca, A.; Michels, N.; Moreno, L.A.; González-Gil, E.M.; Marcos, A.; Gómez, S.; Díaz, L.E.; Widhalm, K.; Molnár, D.; Manios, Y.; et al. Associations between a Mediterranean diet pattern and inflammatory biomarkers in Europeanadolescents. *Eur. J. Nutr.* **2018**, *57*, 1747–1760. [CrossRef] [PubMed]
114. Jiang, Y.; Wu, S.H.; Shu, X.O.; Xiang, Y.B.; Ji, B.T.; Milne, G.L.; Cai, Q.; Zhang, X.; Gao, Y.T.; Zheng, W.; et al. Cruciferous vegetable intake is inversely correlated with circulating levels of proinflammatory markers in women. *J. Acad. Nutr. Diet.* **2014**, *114*, 700–708. [CrossRef] [PubMed]
115. Wongwarawipat, T.; Papageorgiou, N.; Bertsias, D.; Siasos, G.; Tousoulis, D. Olive Oil-related Anti-inflammatory effects on atherosclerosis: Potential clinical implications. *Endocr. Metab. Immune Disord. Drug Targets* **2018**, *18*, 51–62. [CrossRef] [PubMed]
116. Schwingshackl, L.; Christoph, M.; Hoffmann, G. Effects of olive oil on markers of inflammation and endothelial function-A systematic review and meta-analysis. *Nutrients* **2015**, *7*, 7651–7675. [CrossRef] [PubMed]
117. Casas, R.; Estruch, R.; Sacanella, E. The protective effects of extra virgin olive oil on immune-mediated inflammatory responses. *Endocr. Metab. Immune Disord. Drug Targets* **2018**, *18*, 23–35. [CrossRef]
118. Schwingshackl, L.; Hoffmann, G. Monounsaturated fatty acids, olive oil and health status: A systematic review and meta-analysis of cohort studies. *Lipids Health Dis.* **2014**, *13*, 154. [CrossRef]
119. Fitó, M.; Estruch, R.; Salas-Salvadõ, J.; Martínez-Gonzalez, M.A.; Arós, F.; Vila, J.; Corella, D.; Díaz, O.; Sáez, G.; De La Torre, R.; et al. Effect of the mediterranean diet on heart failure biomarkers: A randomized sample from the PREDIMED trial. *Eur. J. Heart Fail.* **2014**, *16*, 543–550. [CrossRef]
120. Sala-Vila, A.; Romero-Mamani, E.S.; Gilabert, R.; Núñez, I.; De La Torre, R.; Corella, D.; Ruiz-Gutiérrez, V.; López-Sabater, M.C.; Pintó, X.; Rekondo, J.; et al. Changes in ultrasound-assessed carotid intima-media thickness and plaque with a mediterranean diet: A substudy of the PREDIMED trial. *Arterioscler. Thromb. Vasc. Biol.* **2014**, *34*, 439–445. [CrossRef]
121. Murie-Fernandez, M.; Irimia, P.; Toledo, E.; Martínez-Vila, E.; Buil-Cosiales, P.; Serrano-Martínez, M.; Ruiz-Gutiérrez, V.; Ros, E.; Estruch, R.; Martínez-González, M.A. Carotid intima-media thickness changes with mediterranean diet: A randomized trial (PREDIMED-Navarra). *Atherosclerosis* **2011**, *219*, 158–162. [CrossRef] [PubMed]
122. Moreno-Luna, R.; Muñoz-Hernandez, R.; Miranda, M.L.; Costa, A.F.; Jimenez-Jimenez, L.; Vallejo-Vaz, A.J.; Muriana, F.J.G.; Villar, J.; Stiefel, P. Olive oil polyphenols decrease blood pressure and improve endothelial function in young women with mild hypertension. *Am. J. Hypertens.* **2012**, *25*, 1299–1304. [CrossRef] [PubMed]
123. Storniolo, C.E.; Casillas, R.; Bulló, M.; Castañer, O.; Ros, E.; Sáez, G.T.; Toledo, E.; Estruch, R.; Ruiz-Gutiérrez, V.; Fitó, M.; et al. A mediterranean diet supplemented with extra virgin olive oil or nuts improves endothelial markers involved in blood pressure control in hypertensive women. *Eur. J. Nutr.* **2017**, *56*, 89–97. [CrossRef] [PubMed]
124. Murphy, K.J. A Mediterranean diet lowers blood pressure and improves endothelial function: Results from the medley randomized intervention trial. *Am. J. Clin. Nutr.* **2017**, *105*, 1305–1313. [CrossRef]
125. Camargo, A.; Delgado-Lista, J.; Garcia-Rios, A.; Cruz-Teno, C.; Yubero-Serrano, E.M.; Perez-Martinez, P.; Gutierrez-Mariscal, F.M.; Lora-Aguilar, P.; Rodriguez-Cantalejo, F.; Fuentes-Jimenez, F.; et al. Expression of proinflammatory; proatherogenic genes is reduced by the Mediterranean diet in elderly people. *Br. J. Nutr.* **2012**, *108*, 500–508. [CrossRef] [PubMed]
126. Widmer, R.J.; Freund, M.; Flamme, J.; Sexton, J.; Lennon, R.; Romani, A.; Mulinacci, N.; Vinceri, F.; Lerman, L.O.; Lerman, A. Beneficial effects of polyphenol-rich olive oil in patients with early atherosclerosis. *Eur. J. Nutr.* **2013**, *52*, 1223–1231. [CrossRef] [PubMed]
127. Oliveras-Lópeza, M.J.; Bernáab, G.; Jurado-Ruizab, E.; de la Serrana, L.G.; Martínab, F. Consumption of extra-virgin olive oil rich in phenolic compounds has beneficial antioxidant effects in healthy human adults. *J. Funct. Foods* **2014**, *10*, 475–484. [CrossRef]

128. Visioli, F.; Caruso, D.; Grande, S.; Bosisio, R.; Villa, M.; Galli, G.; Sirtori, C.; Galli, C. Virgin Olive Oil Study (VOLOS): Vasoprotective potential of extra virgin olive oil in mildly dyslipidemic patients. *Eur. J. Nutr.* **2005**, *44*, 121–127. [CrossRef]
129. Guasch-Ferré, M.; Liu, X.; Malik, V.S.; Sun, Q.; Willett, W.C.; Manson, J.E.; Rexrode, K.M.; Li, Y.; Hu, F.B.; Bhupathiraju, S.N. Nut Consumption and Risk of Cardiovascular Disease. *J. Am. Coll. Cardiol.* **2017**, *70*, 2519–2532. [CrossRef]
130. Aune, D.; Keum, N.; Giovannucci, E.; Fadnes, L.T.; Boffetta, P.; Greenwood, D.C.; Tonstad, S.; Vatten, L.J.; Riboli, E.; Norat, T. Nut consumption and risk of cardiovascular disease, total cancer, all-cause and cause-specific mortality: A systematic review and dose-response meta-analysis of prospective studies. *BMC Med.* **2016**, *14*, 207. [CrossRef]
131. Mente, A.; de Koning, L.; Shannon, H.S.; Anand, S.S. A systematic review of the evidence supporting a causal link between dietary factors and coronary heart disease. *Arch. Intern. Med.* **2009**, *169*, 659–669. [CrossRef] [PubMed]
132. Mozaffarian, D.; Hao, T.; Rimm, E.B.; Willett, W.C.; Hu, F.B. Changes in diet and lifestyle and long-term weight gain in women and men. *N. Engl. J. Med.* **2011**, *364*, 2392–2404. [CrossRef] [PubMed]
133. Del Gobbo, L.C.; Falk, M.C.; Feldman, R.; Lewis, K.; Mozaffarian, D. Effects of tree nuts on blood lipids, apolipoproteins, and blood pressure: Systematic review, meta-analysis, and dose-response of 61 controlled intervention trials. *Am. J. Clin. Nutr.* **2015**, *102*, 1347–1356. [CrossRef] [PubMed]
134. Banel, D.K.; Hu, F.B. Effects of walnut consumption on blood lipids and other cardiovascular risk factors: A meta-analysis and systematic review. *Am. J. Clin. Nutr.* **2009**, *90*, 56–63. [CrossRef] [PubMed]
135. Zhou, D.; Yu, H.; He, F.; Reilly, K.H.; Zhang, J.; Li, S.; Zhang, T.; Wang, B.; Ding, Y.; Xi, B. Nut consumption in relation to cardiovascular disease risk and type 2 diabetes: A systematic review and meta-analysis of prospective studies. *Am. J. Clin. Nutr.* **2014**, *100*, 270–277. [CrossRef] [PubMed]
136. Guo, K.; Zhou, Z.; Jiang, Y.; Li, W.; Li, Y. Meta-analysis of prospective studies on the effects of nut consumption on hypertension and type 2 diabetes mellitus. *J. Diabetes* **2015**, *7*, 202–212. [CrossRef] [PubMed]
137. Yu, Z.; Malik, V.S.; Keum, N.; Hu, F.B.; Giovannucci, E.L.; Stampfer, M.J.; Willett, W.C.; Fuchs, C.S.; Bao, Y. Associations between nut consumption and inflammatory biomarkers. *Am. J. Clin. Nutr.* **2016**, *104*, 722–728. [CrossRef] [PubMed]
138. Neale, E.P.; Tapsell, L.C.; Guan, V.; Batterham, M.J. The effect of nut consumption on markers of inflammation and endothelial function: A systematic review and meta-analysis of randomised controlled trials. *BMJ Open* **2017**, *7*, e016863. [CrossRef] [PubMed]
139. Xiao, Y.; Xia, J.; Ke, Y.; Cheng, J.; Yuan, J.; Wu, S.; Lv, Z.; Huang, S.; Kim, J.H.; Wong, S.Y.; et al. Effects of nut consumption on selected inflammatory markers: A systematic review and meta-analysis of randomized controlled trials. *Nutrition* **2018**, *54*, 129–143. [CrossRef] [PubMed]
140. Casas-Agustench, P.; López-Uriarte, P.; Bulló, M.; Ros, E.; Cabré-Vila, J.J.; Salas-Salvadó, J. Effects of one serving of mixed nuts on serum lipids, insulin resistance and inflammatory markersin patients with the metabolic syndrome. *Nutr. Metab. Cardiovasc. Dis.* **2011**, *21*, 126–135. [CrossRef] [PubMed]
141. Hernández-Alonso, P.; Salas-Salvadó, J.; Baldrich-Mora, M.; Juanola-Falgarona, M.; Bulló, M. Beneficial effect of pistachio consumption on glucose metabolism, insulin resistance, inflammation, and related metabolic risk markers: A randomized clinical trial. *Diabetes Care* **2014**, *37*, 3098–3105. [CrossRef] [PubMed]
142. Liu, J.F.; Liu, Y.H.; Chen, C.M.; Chang, W.H.; Chen, C.Y. The effect of almonds on inflammation and oxidative stress in Chinese patients with type 2 diabetes mellitus: A randomized crossover controlled feeding trial. *Eur. J. Nutr.* **2013**, *52*, 927–935. [CrossRef] [PubMed]
143. Chiva-Blanch, G.; Arranz, S.; Lamuela-Raventos, R.M.; Estruch, R. Effects of wine, alcohol and polyphenols on cardiovascular disease risk factors: Evidences from human studies. *Alcohol Alcohol.* **2013**, *48*, 270–277. [CrossRef] [PubMed]
144. Haseeb, S.; Alexander, B.; Baranchuk, A. Wine and cardiovascular health: A comprehensive review. *Circulation* **2017**, *136*, 1434–1448. [CrossRef] [PubMed]
145. Costanzo, S.; Di Castelnuovo, A.; Donati, M.B.; Iacoviello, L.; de Gaetano, G. Wine, beer or spirit drinking in relation to fatal and non-fatal cardiovascular events: A meta-analysis. *Eur. J. Epidemiol.* **2011**, *26*, 833–850. [CrossRef] [PubMed]
146. Haseeb, S.; Alexander, B.; Santi, R.L.; Liprandi, A.S.; Baranchuk, A. What's in wine? A clinician's perspective. *Trends Cardiovasc. Med.* **2018**, *S1050–S1738*. in press. [CrossRef] [PubMed]

147. Janssen, I.; Landay, A.L.; Ruppert, K.; Powell, L.H. Moderate wine consumption is associated with lower hemostatic and inflammatory risk factorsover 8 years: The study of women's health across the nation (SWAN). *Nutr. Aging* **2014**, *2*, 91–99. [CrossRef]
148. Estruch, R.; Sacanella, E.; Badia, E.; Antúnez, E.; Nicolás, J.M.; Fernández-Solá, J.; Rotilio, D.; de Gaetano, G.; Rubin, E.; Urbano-Márquez, A. Different effects of red wine and gin consumption on inflammatory biomarkers of atherosclerosis: A prospective randomized crossover trial. Effects of wine on inflammatory markers. *Atherosclerosis* **2004**, *175*, 117–123. [CrossRef]
149. Chiva-Blanch, G.; Urpi-Sarda, M.; Llorach, R.; Rotches-Ribalta, M.; Guillén, M.; Casas, R.; Arranz, S.; Valderas-Martinez, P.; Portoles, O.; Corella, D.; et al. Differential effects of polyphenols and alcohol of red wine on the expression of adhesion molecules and inflammatory cytokines related to atherosclerosis: A randomized clinical trial. *Am. J. Clin. Nutr.* **2012**, *95*, 326–334. [CrossRef]
150. Roth, I.; Casas, R.; Medina-Remón, A.; Lamuela-Raventós, R.M.; Estruch, R. Consumption of aged white wine modulates cardiovascular risk factors via circulating endothelial progenitor cells and inflammatory biomarkers. *Clin. Nutr.* **2018**, *S0261–S5614*, 30219-X. [CrossRef]
151. Estruch, R.; Sacanella, E.; Mota, F.; Chiva-Blanch, G.; Antúnez, E.; Casals, E.; Deulofeu, R.; Rotilio, D.; Andres-Lacueva, C.; Lamuela-Raventos, R.M.; et al. Moderate consumption of red wine, but not gin, decreases erythrocyte superoxide dismutase activity: A randomized cross-over trial. *Nutr. Metab. Cardiovasc. Dis.* **2011**, *21*, 46–53. [CrossRef] [PubMed]
152. De Gaetano, G.; Constanzo, S.; Castelnuovo, A.D.; Badimon, L.; Bejko, D.; Alkerwi, A.; Chiva-Blanch, G.; Estruch, R.; La Vecchia, C.; Panico, S. Effects of moderate beer consumption on health and disease: A consensus document. *Nutr. Metab. Cardiovasc. Dis.* **2016**, *26*, 443–467. [CrossRef] [PubMed]
153. Wannamethee, S.G.; Shaper, A.G. Type of alcoholic drink and risk of major coronary heart disease event and all-cause mortality. *Am. J. Public Health* **1999**, *89*, 685–690. [CrossRef] [PubMed]
154. Chiva-Blanch, G.; Magraner, E.; Condines, X.; Valderas-Martínez, P.; Roth, I.; Arranz, S.; Casas, R.; Navarro, M.; Hervas, A.; Sisó, A.; et al. Effects of alcohol and polyphenols from beer on atherosclerotic biomarkers in high cardiovascular risk men: A randomized feeding trial. *Nutr. Metab. Cardiovasc. Dis.* **2015**, *24*, 36–45. [CrossRef] [PubMed]
155. Sánchez-Muniz, F.J. Dietary fibre and cardiovascular health. *Nutr. Hosp.* **2012**, *27*, 31–45. [CrossRef] [PubMed]
156. Huang, T.; Xu, M.; Lee, A.; Cho, S.; Qi, L. Consumption of whole grains and cereal fiber and total and cause-specific mortality: Prospective analysis of 367,442 individuals. *BMC Med.* **2015**, *13*, 59. [CrossRef]
157. Yang, Y.; Zhao, L.G.; Wu, Q.J.; Ma, X.; Xiang, Y.B. Association between dietary fiber and lower risk of all-cause mortality: A meta-analysis of cohort studies. *Am. J. Epidemiol.* **2015**, *181*, 83–91. [CrossRef]
158. McRae, M.P. Dietary fiber is beneficial for the prevention of cardiovascular disease: An umbrella review of Meta-analyses. *J. Chiropr. Med.* **2017**, *16*, 289–299. [CrossRef]
159. Effects of Dietary Fiber Intake on Cardiovascular Risk Factors. Available online: https://www.intechopen.com/books/recent-advances-in-cardiovascular-risk-factors/effects-of-dietary-fiber-intake-on-cardiovascular-risk-factors (accessed on 26 October 2018).
160. Ma, Y.; Hébert, J.R.; Li, W.; Bertone-Johnson, E.R.; Olendzki, B.; Pagoto, S.L.; Tinker, L.; Rosal, M.C.; Ockene, I.S.; Ockene, J.K.; et al. Association between dietary fiber and markers of systemic inflammation in the Women's Health Initiative Observational Study. *Nutrition* **2008**, *24*, 941–949. [CrossRef]
161. Nguyen, N.T.; Magno, C.P.; Lane, K.T.; Hinojosa, M.W.; Lane, J.S. Definition of Metabolic Syndrome-Scott M. Grundy. Association of Hypertension, Diabetes, Dyslipidemia, and Metabolic Syndrome with Obesity: Findings from the National Health and Nutrition Examination Survey, 1999 to 2004. *J. Am. Coll. Surg.* **2008**, *207*, 928–934. [CrossRef]
162. Qi, L.; van Dam, R.M.; Liu, S.; Franz, M.; Mantzoros, C.; Hu, F.B. Whole-grain, bran, and cereal fiber intakes and markers of systemic inflammation in diabetic women. *Diabetes Care* **2006**, *29*, 207–211. [CrossRef]
163. Estruch, R.; Martínez-González, M.A.; Corella, D.; Basora-Gallisá, J.; Ruiz-Gutiérrez, V.; Covas, M.I.; Fiol, M.; Gómez-Gracia, E.; López-Sabater, M.C.; Escoda, R.; et al. Effects of dietary fibre intake on risk factors for cardiovascular disease in subjects at high risk. *J. Epidemiol. Community Health* **2009**, *63*, 582–588. [CrossRef]
164. Masters, R.C.; Liese, A.D.; Haffner, S.M.; Wagenknecht, L.E.; Hanley, A.J. Whole and refined grain intakes are related to inflammatory protein concentrations in human plasma. *J. Nutr.* **2010**, *140*, 587–594. [CrossRef] [PubMed]

165. North, C.J.; Venter, C.S.; Jerling, J.C. The effects of dietary fibre on C-reactive protein, an inflammation marker predicting cardiovascular disease. *Eur. J. Clin. Nutr.* **2009**, *63*, 921–933. [CrossRef] [PubMed]
166. Esposito, K.; Nappo, F.; Giugliano, F.; Di Palo, C.; Ciotola, M.; Barbieri, M.; Paolisso, G.; Giugliano, D. Meal modulation of circulating interleukin 18 and adiponectin concentrations in healthy subjects and in patients with type 2 diabetes mellitus. *Am. J. Clin. Nutr.* **2003**, *78*, 1135–1140. [CrossRef]
167. Kopf, J.C.; Suhr, M.J.; Clarke, J.; Eyun, S.I.; Riethoven, J.M.; Ramer-Tait, A.E.; Rose, D.J. Role of whole grains versus fruits and vegetables in reducing subclinical inflammation and promoting gastrointestinal health in individuals affected by overweight and obesity: A randomized controlled trial. *Nutr. J.* **2018**, *17*, 72. [CrossRef] [PubMed]
168. Toole, J.F.; Malinow, M.R.; Chambless, L.E.; Spence, J.D.; Pettigrew, L.C.; Howard, V.J.; Sides, E.G.; Wang, C.H.; Stampfer, M. Lowering homocysteine in patients with ischemic strole to prevent recurrent stroke, myocardial infarction and death: The Vitamin Intervention for Stroke Prevention (VISP) randomized controlled-trial. *JAMA* **2004**, *291*, 565–575. [CrossRef]
169. Spence, J.D.; Bang, H.; Chambles, L.E.; Stampfer, M.J. Vitamin Intervention for Stroke Prevention trial: An efficacy analysis. *Stroke* **2005**, *36*, 2404–2409. [CrossRef] [PubMed]
170. Spence, J.D. Homocysteine: Call off the funeral. *Stroke* **2006**, *37*, 282–283. [CrossRef] [PubMed]
171. Root, M.M.; McGinn, M.C.; Nieman, D.C.; Henson, D.A.; Heinz, S.A.; Shanely, R.A.; Knab, A.M.; Jin, F. Combined fruit and vegetable intake is correlated with improved inflammatory and oxidant status from a cross-sectional study in a community setting. *Nutrients* **2012**, *4*, 29–41. [CrossRef] [PubMed]
172. Helmersson, J.; Arnlöv, J.; Larsson, A.; Basu, S. Low dietary intake of alpha-carotene, beta-tocopherol and ascorbic acid is associated with increased inflammatory and oxidative stress status in a Swedish cohort. *Br. J. Nutr.* **2009**, *101*, 1775–1782. [CrossRef] [PubMed]
173. Wang, L.; Gaziano, J.M.; Norkus, E.P.; Buring, J.E.; Sesso, H.D. Associations of plasma carotenoids with risk factors and biomarkers related to cardiovascular disease in middle-aged and older women. *Am. J. Clin. Nutr.* **2008**, *88*, 747–754. [CrossRef] [PubMed]
174. Lee, H.; Lee, I.S.; Choue, R. Obesity, inflammation and diet. *Pediatr. Gastroenterol. Hepatol. Nutr.* **2013**, *16*, 143–152. [CrossRef] [PubMed]
175. Gammoh, N.Z.; Rink, L. Zinc in Infection and Inflammation. *Nutrients* **2017**, *9*, 624. [CrossRef] [PubMed]
176. Mazidi, M.; Rezaie, P.; Banach, M. Effect of magnesium supplements on serum C-reactive protein: A systematic review and meta-analysis. *Arch. Med. Sci.* **2018**, *14*, 707–716. [CrossRef] [PubMed]
177. Simental-Mendia, L.E.; Sahebkar, A.; Rodriguez-Moran, M.; Zambrano-Galvan, G.; Guerrero-Romero, F. Effect of magnesium supplementation on plasma C-reactive protein concentrations: A systematic review and Meta-analysis of randomized controlled trials. *Curr. Pharm. Des.* **2017**, *23*, 4678–4686. [CrossRef] [PubMed]
178. Rodriguez, A.J.; Mousa, A.; Ebeling, P.R.; Scott, D.; de Courten, B. Effects of vitamin D supplementation on inflammatory markers in heart failure: A systematic review and meta-analysis of randomized controlled trials. *Sci. Rep.* **2018**, *8*, 1169. [CrossRef]
179. Saboori, S.; Shab-Bidar, S.; Speakman, J.R.; Rad, E.Y.; Djafarian, K. Effect of vitamin E supplementation on serum C-reactive protein level: A meta-analysis of randomized controlled trials. *Eur. J. Clin. Nutr.* **2015**, *69*, 867–873. [CrossRef]
180. De Oliveira Otto, M.C.; Alonso, A.; Lee, D.H.; Delclos, G.L.; Jenny, N.S.; Jiang, R.; Lima, J.A.; Symanski, E.; Jacobs, D.R., Jr.; Nettleton, J.A. Dietary micronutrient intakes are associated with markers of inflammation but not with markers of subclinical atherosclerosis. *J. Nutr.* **2011**, *141*, 1508–1515. [CrossRef]
181. Wang, Q.; Zhu, Z.; Liu, Y.; Tu, X.; He, J. Relationship between serum vitamin D levels and inflammatory markers in acute stroke patients. *Brain Behav.* **2018**, *8*, e00885. [CrossRef]
182. Pilz, S.; Tomaschitz, A.; März, W.; Drechsler, C.; Ritz, E.; Zittermann, A.; Cavalier, E.; Pieber, T.R.; Lappe, J.M.; Grant, W.B.; et al. Vitamin D, cardiovascular disease and mortality. *Clin. Endocrinol.* **2011**, *75*, 575–584. [CrossRef] [PubMed]
183. Brewer, L.C.; Michos, E.D.; Reis, J.P. Vitamin D in atherosclerosis, vascular disease, and endothelial function. *Curr. Drug Targets* **2011**, *12*, 54–60. [CrossRef] [PubMed]
184. Oh, J.; Weng, S.; Felton, S.K.; Bhandare, S.; Riek, A.; Butler, B.; Proctor, B.M.; Petty, M.; Chen, Z.; Schechtman, K.B.; et al. 1,25(OH)2 vitamin d inhibits foam cell formation and suppresses macrophage cholesterol uptakein patients with type 2 diabetes mellitus. *Circulation* **2009**, *120*, 687–698. [CrossRef] [PubMed]

185. Tabesh, M.; Azadbakht, L.; Faghihimani, E.; Tabesh, M.; Esmaillzadeh, A. Calcium-Vitamin D cosupplementation influences circulating inflammatory biomarkers and adipocytokines in vitamin D-insufficient diabetics: A randomized controlled clinical trial. *J. Clin. Endocrinol. Metab.* **2014**, *99*, E2485–E2493. [CrossRef] [PubMed]
186. Shargorodsky, M.; Debby, O.; Matas, Z.; Zimlichman, R. Effect of long-term treatment with antioxidants (vitamin C, vitamin E, coenzyme Q10 and selenium) on arterial compliance, humoral factors and inflammatory markers in patients with multiple cardiovascular risk factors. *Nutr. Metab.* **2010**, *7*, 55. [CrossRef]
187. Ellulu, M.S.; Rahmat, A.; Patimah, I.; Khaza'ai, H.; Abed, Y. Effect of vitamin C on inflammation and metabolic markers in hypertensive and/or diabetic obese adults: A randomized controlled trial. *Drug Des. Dev. Ther.* **2015**, *9*, 3405–3412. [CrossRef]
188. Christen, W.G.; Cook, N.R.; Van Denburgh, M.; Zaharris, E.; Albert, C.M.; Manson, J.E. Effect of Combined Treatment with folic acid, Vitamin B6, and Vitamin B12 on plasmabiomarkers of inflammation and endothelial dysfunction in women. *J. Am. Heart Assoc.* **2018**, *7*, e008517. [CrossRef]
189. Massaro, M.; Scoditti, E.; Carluccio, M.A.; De Caterina, R. Nutraceuticals and prevention of atherosclerosis: Focus on omega-3 polyunsaturated fatty acids and Mediterranean diet polyphenols. *Cardiovasc. Ther.* **2010**, *28*, e13–e19. [CrossRef]
190. Hamer, M.; Steptoe, A. Influence of specific nutrients on progression of atherosclerosis, vascular function, haemostasis and inflammation in coronary heart disease patients: A systematic review. *Br. J. Nutr.* **2006**, *95*, 849–859. [CrossRef]
191. Burke, M.F.; Burke, F.M.; Soffer, D.E. Review of cardiometabolic effects of prescription Omega-3 fatty acids. *Curr. Atheroscler. Rep.* **2017**, *19*, 6. [CrossRef]
192. Calder, P.C. The role of marine omega-3 (n-3) fatty acids in inflammatory processes, atherosclerosis and plaque stability. *Mol. Nutr. Food Res.* **2012**, *56*, 1073–1080. [CrossRef] [PubMed]
193. Wang, Q.; Liang, X.; Wang, L.; Lu, X.; Huang, J.; Cao, J.; Li, H.; Gu, D. Effect of omega-3 fatty acids supplementation on endothelial function: A meta-analysis of randomized controlled trials. *Atherosclerosis* **2012**, *221*, 536–543. [CrossRef] [PubMed]
194. Leslie, M.A.; Cohen, D.J.A.; Liddle, D.M.; Robinson, L.E.; Ma, D.W.L. A review of the effect of omega-3 polyunsaturated fatty acids on blood triacylglycerol levels in normolipidemic and borderline hyperlipidemic individuals. *Lipids Health Dis.* **2015**, *14*, 53. [CrossRef] [PubMed]
195. Yagi, S.; Aihara, K.I.; Fukuda, D.; Takashima, A.; Hara, T.; Hotchi, J.; Ise, T.; Yamaguchi, K.; Tobiume, T.; Iwase, T.; et al. Effects of Docosahexaenoic Acid on the Endothelial Function in Patients with Coronary Artery Disease. *J. Atheroscler. Thromb.* **2015**, *22*, 447–454. [CrossRef] [PubMed]
196. Kelley, D.S.; Adkins, Y. Similarities and differences between the effects of EPA and DHA on markers of atherosclerosis in human subjects. *Proc. Nutr. Soc.* **2012**, *71*, 322–331. [CrossRef] [PubMed]
197. Cawood, A.L.; Ding, R.; Napper, F.L.; Young, R.H.; Williams, J.A.; Ward, M.J.; Gudmundsen, O.; Vige, R.; Payne, S.P.; Ye, S.; et al. Eicosapentaenoic acid (EPA) from highly concentrated n-3 fatty acid ethyl esters is incorporated into advanced atherosclerotic plaques and higher plaque EPA is associated with decreasedplaque inflammation and increased stability. *Atherosclerosis* **2010**, *212*, 252–259. [CrossRef] [PubMed]
198. Thies, F.; Garry, J.M.C.; Yaqoob, P.; Rerkasem, K.; Williams, J.; Shearman, C.P.; Gallagher, P.J.; Calder, P.C.; Grimble, R.F. Association of n-3 polyunsaturated fatty acids with stability of atherosclerotic plaques: A randomised controlled trial. *Lancet* **2003**, *361*, 477–485. [CrossRef]
199. Robinson, J.G.; Stone, N.J. Antiatherosclerotic and antithrombotic effects of omega-3 fatty acids. *Am. J. Cardiol.* **2006**, *98*, 39i–49i. [CrossRef]
200. Kaliora, A.C.; Dedoussis, G.V. Natural antioxidant compounds in risk factors for CVD. *Pharmacol. Res.* **2007**, *56*, 99–109. [CrossRef]
201. Valderas-Martinez, P.; Chiva-Blanch, G.; Casas, R.; Arranz, S.; Martínez-Huélamo, M.; Urpi-Sarda, M.; Torrado, X.; Corella, D.; Lamuela-Raventós, R.M.; Estruch, R. Tomato sauce enriched with olive oil exerts greater effects on cardiovascular disease risk factors than raw tomato and tomato sauce: A randomized trial. *Nutrients* **2016**, *8*, 170. [CrossRef]
202. Mozos, I.; Stoian, D.; Caraba, A.; Malainer, C.; Horbańczuk, J.O.; Atanasov, A.G. Lycopene and Vascular Health. *Front. Pharmacol.* **2018**, *9*, 521. [CrossRef]

203. Costa-Rodrigues, J.; Pinho, O.; Monteiro, P.R.R. Can lycopene be considered an effective protection against cardiovascular disease? *Food Chem.* **2018**, *245*, 1148–1153. [CrossRef] [PubMed]
204. Cheng, H.M.; Koutsidis, G.; Lodge, J.K.; Ashor, A.; Siervo, M.; Lara, J. Tomato and lycopene supplementation and cardiovascular risk factors: A systematic review and meta-analysis. *Atherosclerosis* **2017**, *257*, 100–108. [CrossRef] [PubMed]
205. Biddle, M.J.; Lennie, T.R.; Bricker, G.V.; Kopec, R.E.; Schwartz, S.J.; Moser, D.K. Lycopene dietary intervention: A pilot study in patients with heart failure. *Cardiovasc. Nurs.* **2016**, *30*, 205–212. [CrossRef] [PubMed]
206. Wang, Y.; Chung, S.J.; McCullough, M.L.; Song, W.O.; Fernandez, M.L.; Koo, S.I.; Chun, O.K. Dietary carotenoids are associated with cardiovascular disease risk biomarkers mediated by serum carotenoid concentrations. *J. Nutr.* **2014**, *144*, 1067–1074. [CrossRef] [PubMed]
207. Xu, X.R.; Zou, Z.Y.; Huang, Y.M.; Xiao, X.; Ma, L.; Lin, X.M. Serum carotenoids in relation to risk factors for development of atherosclerosis. *Clin. Biochem.* **2012**, *45*, 1357–1361. [CrossRef]
208. Thies, F.; Masson, L.F.; Rudd, A.; Vaughan, N.; Tsang, C.; Brittenden, J.; Simpson, W.G.; Duthie, S.; Horgan, G.W.; Duthie, G. Effect of a tomato-rich diet on markers of cardiovascular disease risk in moderately overweight, disease-free, middle-aged adults: A randomized controlled trial. *Am. J. Clin. Nutr.* **2012**, *95*, 1013–1022. [CrossRef]
209. Ras, R.T.; Geleijnse, J.M.; Trautwein, E.A. LDL-cholesterol-lowering effect of plant sterols and stanols across different dose ranges: A meta-analysis of randomised controlled studies. *Br. J. Nutr.* **2014**, *112*, 214–219. [CrossRef]
210. Cabra, C.E.; Simas-TorresKlein, M.R. Phytosterols in the Treatment of Hypercholesterolemia and Prevention of Cardiovascular Diseases. *Arq. Brasil. Cardiol.* **2017**, *109*, 475–482. [CrossRef]
211. Demonty, I.; Ras, R.T.; van der Knaap, H.C.; Duchateau, G.S.; Meijer, L.; Zock, P.L.; Geleijnse, J.M.; Trautwein, E.A. Continuous dose-response relationship of the LDL-cholesterol-lowering effect of phytosterol intake. *J. Nutr.* **2009**, *139*, 271–284. [CrossRef]
212. Rocha, V.Z.; Ras, R.T.; Gagliardi, A.C.; Mangili, L.C.; Trautwein, E.A.; Santos, R.D. Effects of phytosterols on markers of inflammation: A systematic review and meta-analysis. *Atherosclerosis* **2016**, *48*, 76–83. [CrossRef] [PubMed]
213. Ras, R.T.; Fuchs, D.; Koppenol, W.P.; Schalkwijk, C.G.; Otten-Hofman, A.; Garczarek, U.; Greyling, A.; Wagner, F.; Trautwein, E.A. Effect of a plant sterol-enriched spread on biomarkers of endothelial dysfunction and low grade inflammation in hypercholesterolaemic subjects. *J. Nutr. Sci.* **2016**, *5*, e44. [CrossRef] [PubMed]
214. Devaraj, S.; Jialal, I.; Rockwood, J.; Zak, D. Effect of orange juice and beverage with phytosterols on cytokines and PAI1 activity. *Clin. Nutr.* **2011**, *30*, 668–671. [CrossRef] [PubMed]
215. Heggen, E.; Kirkhus, B.; Pedersen, J.I.; Tonstad, S. Effects of margarine enriched with plant sterol esters from rapeseed and tall oils on markers of endothelial function, inflammation and hemostasis. *Scand. J. Clin. Lab. Investig.* **2015**, *75*, 189–192. [CrossRef] [PubMed]
216. Mozaffarian, D.; Wu, J.H.Y. Flavonoids, Dairy Foods and Cardiovascular and Metabolic Health: A review of emerging biologic pathways. *Circ. Res.* **2018**, *122*, 369–384. [CrossRef] [PubMed]
217. Tressera-Rimbau, A.; Arranz, S.; Eder, M.; Vallverdú-Queralt, A. Dietary Polyphenols in the Prevention of Stroke. *Oxid. Med. Cell. Longev.* **2017**, *2017*, 7467962. [CrossRef] [PubMed]
218. González-Gallego, J.; García-Mediavilla, M.V.; Sánchez-Campos, S.; Tuñón, M.J. Fruit polyphenols immunity and inflammation. *Br. J. Nutr.* **2010**, *104*, S15–S27. [CrossRef]
219. Bahramsoltani, R.; Ebrahimi, F.; Farzaei, M.H.; Baratpourmoghaddam, A.; Ahmadi, P.; Rostamiasrabadi, P.; Rasouli Amirabadi, A.H.; Rahimi, R. Dietary polyphenols for atherosclerosis: A comprehensive review and future perspectives. *Crit. Rev. Food Sci. Nutr.* **2017**, 1–19. [CrossRef]
220. Witkowska, A.M.; Waśkiewicz, A.; Zujko, M.E.; Szcześniewska, D.; Pająk, A.; Stepaniak, U.; Drygas, W. Dietary polyphenol intake but not the dietary total antioxidant capacity is inversely related to cardiovascular disease in postmenopausal polish women: Results of WOBASZ and WOBASZ II Studies. *Oxid. Med. Cell. Longev.* **2017**, *2017*, 5982809. [CrossRef]
221. Chiva-Blanch, G.; Badimon, L. Effects of polyphenol intake on metabolic syndrome: Current Evidences from Human Trials. *Oxid. Med. Cell. Longev.* **2017**, *2017*, 5812401. [CrossRef]
222. Miranda, A.M.; Steluti, J.; Fisberg, R.M.; Marchioni, D.M. Association between Coffee Consumption and Its Polyphenols with Cardiovascular Risk Factors: A Population-Based Study. *Nutrients* **2017**, *9*, 276. [CrossRef]

223. Ding, M.; Bhupathiraju, S.N.; Satija, A.; van Dam, R.M.; Hu, F.B. Long-term coffee consumption and risk of cardiovascular disease: A systematic review and a dose-response meta-analysis of prospective cohort studies. *Circulation* **2014**, *129*, 643–659. [CrossRef] [PubMed]
224. Larsson, S.C.; Orsini, N. Coffee consumption and risk of stroke: A dose-response meta-analysis of prospective studies. *Am. J. Epidemiol.* **2011**, *174*, 993–1001. [CrossRef] [PubMed]
225. Shen, L.; Song, L.G.; Ma, H.; Jin, C.N.; Wang, J.A.; Xiang, M.X. Tea consumption and risk of stroke: A dose-response meta-analysis of prospective studies. *J. Zhejiang Univ. Sci. B* **2012**, *13*, 652–662. [CrossRef] [PubMed]
226. Manach, C.; Mazur, A.; Scalbert, A. Polyphenols and Prevention of cardiovascular diseases. *Curr. Opin. Lipidol.* **2005**, *16*, 77–84. [CrossRef] [PubMed]
227. Hooper, L.; Kroon, P.A.; Rimm, E.B.; Cohn, J.S.; Harvey, I.; Le Cornu, K.A.; Ryder, J.J.; Hall, W.L.; Cassidy, A. Flavonoids, flavonoid-rich foods, and cardiovascular risk: A meta-analysis of randomized controlled trials. *Am. J. Clin. Nutr.* **2008**, *88*, 38–50. [CrossRef]
228. Van Bussel, B.C.T.; Henry, R.M.A.; Schalkwijk, C.G.; Dekker, J.M.; Nijpels, G.; Feskens, E.J.M.; Stehouwer, C.D.A. Alcohol and red wine consumption but not fruit vegetables fish or dairy products are associated with less endothelial dysfunction and less low-grade inflammation: The Hoorn Study. *Eur. J. Nutr.* **2018**, *57*, 1409–1419. [CrossRef] [PubMed]
229. Huang, H.; Chen, G.; Liao, D.; Zhu, Y.; Xue, X. Effects of Berries Consumption on Cardiovascular Risk Factors: A Meta-analysis with Trial Sequential Analysis of Randomized Controlled Trials. *Sci. Rep.* **2016**, *6*, 23625. [CrossRef]
230. Luís, Â.; Domingues, F.; Pereira, L. Association between berries intake and cardiovascular diseases risk factors: A systematic review with meta-analysis and trial sequential analysis of randomized controlled trials. *Food Funct.* **2018**, *9*, 740–757. [CrossRef]
231. De Bacquer, D.; Clays, E.; Delanghe, J.; De Backer, G. Epidemiological evidence for an association between habitual tea consumption and markers of chronic inflammation. *Atherosclerosis* **2006**, *189*, 428–435. [CrossRef]
232. Vazquez-Agell, M.; Urpi-Sarda, M.; Sacanella, E.; Camino-Lopez, S.; Chiva-Blanch, G.; Llorente-Cortes, V.; Tobias, E.; Roura, E.; Andres-Lacueva, C.; Lamuela-Raventos, R.M.; et al. Cocoa consumption reduces NF-kB activation in peripheral blood mononuclear cells in humans. *Nutr. Metab. Cardiovasc. Dis.* **2013**, *23*, 257–263. [CrossRef] [PubMed]
233. Monagas, M.; Khan, N.; Andres-Lacueva, C.; Casas, R.; Urpí-Sardà, M.; Llorach, R.; Lamuela-Raventós, R.M.; Estruch, R. Effect of cocoa powder on the modulation of inflammatory biomarkers in patients at high risk of cardiovascular disease. *Am. J. Clin. Nutr.* **2009**, *90*, 1144–1150. [CrossRef] [PubMed]
234. Basu, A.; Du, M.; Sanchez, K.; Leyva, M.J.; Betts, N.M.; Blevins, S.; Wu, M.; Aston, C.E.; Lyons, T.J. Green tea minimally affects biomarkers of inflammation in obese subjects with metabolicsyndrome. *Nutrition* **2011**, *27*, 206–213. [CrossRef] [PubMed]
235. Zhang, X.; Zhu, Y.; Song, F.; Yao, Y.; Ya, F.; Li, D.; Ling, W.; Yang, Y. Effects of purified anthocyanin supplementation on platelet chemokines in hypocholesterolemic individuals: A randomized controlled trial. *Nutr. Metab.* **2016**, *13*, 86. [CrossRef] [PubMed]
236. Song, F.; Zhu, Y.; Shi, Z.; Tian, J.; Deng, X.; Ren, J.; Andrews, M.C.; Ni, H.; Ling, W.; Yang, Y. Plant food anthocyanins inhibit platelet granule secretion in hypercholesterolaemia: Involving the signaling pathway of PI3K–Akt. *Thromb. Haemost.* **2014**, *112*, 981–991. [CrossRef] [PubMed]
237. Davinelli, S.; Bertoglio, J.C.; Zarrelli, A.; Pina, R.; Scapagnini, G. A Randomized clinical trial evaluating the efficacy of an anthocyanin-maqui berry extract (Delphinol®) on oxidative stress biomarkers. *J. Am. Coll. Nutr.* **2015**, *34*, 28–33. [CrossRef] [PubMed]
238. Hall, W.L.; Vafeiadou, K.; Hallund, J.; Bügel, S.; Koebnick, C.; Reimann, M.; Ferrari, M.; Branca, F.; Talbot, D.; Dadd, T.; et al. Soy-isoflavone-enriched foods and inflammatory biomarkers of cardiovascular disease risk in postmenopausal women: Interactions with genotype and equol production. *Am. J. Clin. Nutr.* **2005**, *82*, 1260–1268. [CrossRef] [PubMed]
239. Hodis, H.N.; Mack, W.J.; Kono, N.; Azen, S.P.; Shoupe, D.; Hwang-Levine, J.; Petitti, D.; Whitfield-Maxwell, L.; Yan, M.; Franke, A.A.; et al. Isoflavone soy protein supplementation and atherosclerosis progression in healthy postmenopausal women: A randomized controlled trial. *Stroke* **2011**, *42*, 3168–3175. [CrossRef] [PubMed]

240. Tomé-Carneiro, J.; Gonzálvez, M.; Larrosa, M.; García-Almagro, F.J.; Avilés-Plaza, F.; Parra, S.; Yáñez-Gascón, M.J.; Ruiz-Ros, J.A.; García-Conesa, M.T.; Tomás-Barberán, F.A.; et al. Consumption of a grape extract supplement containing resveratrol decreases oxidized LDL and ApoB in patients undergoing primary prevention of cardiovascular disease: A triple-blind, 6-month follow-up, placebo-controlled, randomized trial. *Mol. Nutr. Food Res.* **2012**, *56*, 810–821. [CrossRef] [PubMed]
241. Agarwal, B.; Campen, M.J.; Channell, M.M.; Wherry, S.J.; Varamini, B.; Davis, J.G.; Baur, J.A.; Smoliga, J.M. Resveratrol for primary prevention of atherosclerosis: Clinical trial evidence for improved gene expression in vascular endothelium. *Int. J. Cardiol.* **2013**, *166*, 246–248. [CrossRef] [PubMed]
242. Seyyedebrahimi, S.; Khodabandehloo, H.; Nasli Esfahani, E.; Meshkani, R. The effects of resveratrol on markers of oxidative stress in patients with type 2 diabetes: A randomized, double-blind, placebo-controlled clinical trial. *Acta Diabetol.* **2018**, *55*, 341–353. [CrossRef] [PubMed]

Permissions

All chapters in this book were first published by MDPI; hereby published with permission under the Creative Commons Attribution License or equivalent. Every chapter published in this book has been scrutinized by our experts. Their significance has been extensively debated. The topics covered herein carry significant findings which will fuel the growth of the discipline. They may even be implemented as practical applications or may be referred to as a beginning point for another development.

The contributors of this book come from diverse backgrounds, making this book a truly international effort. This book will bring forth new frontiers with its revolutionizing research information and detailed analysis of the nascent developments around the world.

We would like to thank all the contributing authors for lending their expertise to make the book truly unique. They have played a crucial role in the development of this book. Without their invaluable contributions this book wouldn't have been possible. They have made vital efforts to compile up to date information on the varied aspects of this subject to make this book a valuable addition to the collection of many professionals and students.

This book was conceptualized with the vision of imparting up-to-date information and advanced data in this field. To ensure the same, a matchless editorial board was set up. Every individual on the board went through rigorous rounds of assessment to prove their worth. After which they invested a large part of their time researching and compiling the most relevant data for our readers.

The editorial board has been involved in producing this book since its inception. They have spent rigorous hours researching and exploring the diverse topics which have resulted in the successful publishing of this book. They have passed on their knowledge of decades through this book. To expedite this challenging task, the publisher supported the team at every step. A small team of assistant editors was also appointed to further simplify the editing procedure and attain best results for the readers.

Apart from the editorial board, the designing team has also invested a significant amount of their time in understanding the subject and creating the most relevant covers. They scrutinized every image to scout for the most suitable representation of the subject and create an appropriate cover for the book.

The publishing team has been an ardent support to the editorial, designing and production team. Their endless efforts to recruit the best for this project, has resulted in the accomplishment of this book. They are a veteran in the field of academics and their pool of knowledge is as vast as their experience in printing. Their expertise and guidance has proved useful at every step. Their uncompromising quality standards have made this book an exceptional effort. Their encouragement from time to time has been an inspiration for everyone.

The publisher and the editorial board hope that this book will prove to be a valuable piece of knowledge for researchers, students, practitioners and scholars across the globe.

List of Contributors

Rosa Lombardi and Anna Ludovica Fracanzani
Department of Pathophysiology and Transplantation, University of Milan, 20122 Milan, Italy
Ca' Granda IRCCS Foundation, Policlinico Hospital of Milan, 20122 Milan, Italy

Federica Iuculano, Giada Pallini and Silvia Fargion
Department of Pathophysiology and Transplantation, University of Milan, 20122 Milan, Italy

Susan Hewlings
Department of Nutrition and Dietetics, Central Michigan University, Mount Pleasant, MI 48859, USA
GRAS Associates/Nutrasource, Guelph, ON N1G 0B, Canada

Areej Ali Alkhaldy, Reem Saleh Alamri, Rozana Khalid Magadmi and Nrvana Yasser Elshini
Clinical Nutrition Department, Faculty of Applied Medical Sciences, King Abdulaziz University, Jeddah 21589, Saudi Arabia

Rania Abd El Hamid Hussein
Clinical Nutrition Department, Faculty of Applied Medical Sciences, King Abdulaziz University, Jeddah 21589, Saudi Arabia
Internal Medicine Department, Gamal Abd El Nasser Hospital, Health Insurance Authority, Alexandria 21516, Egypt

Kamal Waheeb Alghalayini
Department of Medicine, Faculty of Medicine, King Abdulaziz University, Jeddah 21589, Saudi Arabia

Krasimir Kostov
Department of Pathophysiology, Medical University-Pleven, 1 Kliment Ohridski Str., 5800 Pleven, Bulgaria

Lyudmila Halacheva
Department of Physiology, Medical University-Pleven, 1 Kliment Ohridski Str., 5800 Pleven, Bulgaria

Daniel N. Roffe-Vazquez, Anna S. Huerta-Delgado, José R. Villarreal-Calderón and Adrian M. Gonzalez-Gil
Tecnologico de Monterrey, Center for Research in Clinical Nutrition, Escuela de Medicina, Monterrey 64710, N.L., Mexico

Elena C. Castillo and Cecilio Enriquez
Tecnologico de Monterrey, Centro de Investigacion Biomedica, Hospital Zambrano Hellion, San Pedro Garza-Garcia 66278, N.L., Mexico

Gerardo Garcia-Rivas
Tecnologico de Monterrey, Centro de Investigacion Biomedica, Hospital Zambrano Hellion, San Pedro Garza-Garcia 66278, N.L., Mexico
Tecnologico de Monterrey, Cardiovascular and Metabolomics Research Group, Escuela de Medicina, San Pedro Garza-Garcia 66278, N.L., Mexico

Leticia Elizondo-Montemayor
Tecnologico de Monterrey, Center for Research in Clinical Nutrition, Escuela de Medicina, Monterrey 64710, N.L., Mexico
Tecnologico de Monterrey, Cardiovascular and Metabolomics Research Group, Escuela de Medicina, San Pedro Garza-Garcia 66278, N.L., Mexico

Jacqueline K. Innes
School of Human Development and Health, Faculty of Medicine, University of Southampton, Southampton SO16 6YD, UK

Philip C. Calder
School of Human Development and Health, Faculty of Medicine, University of Southampton, Southampton SO16 6YD, UK
National Institute for Health Research Southampton Biomedical Research Centre, University Hospital Southampton NHS Foundation Trust and University of Southampton, Southampton SO16 6YD, UK

Fatou Balla Wade, Marie Parsine Sall, Fatimata Mbaye and Mbacké Sembene
Genetics and Population Management Team, Department of Animal Biology, Faculty of Sciences and Techniques, Cheikh Anta Diop University, Dakar 5005, Senegal

Juan M. Castro, Victoria García-Espinosa, Agustina Zinoveev, Mariana Marin, Daniel Bia and Yanina Zócalo
Departamento de Fisiología, Facultad de Medicina, Centro Universitario de Investigación, Innovación y Diagnóstico Arterial, Universidad de la República, General Flores 2125, 11800 Montevideo, Uruguay

Cecilia Severi
Departamento de Medicina Preventiva y Social, Instituto de Higiene, Facultad de Medicina, Universidad de la República, Alfredo Navarro 3051, 11600 Montevideo, Uruguay

Pedro Chiesa
Servicio de Cardiología Pediátrica, Centro Hospitalario Pereira-Rossell, ASSE-Facultad de Medicina, Universidad de la República, Bulevar Artigas 1550, 11600 Montevideo, Uruguay

Akshay Goel, Naga Venkata Pothineni, Hakan Paydak, Tom Saldeen and Jawahar L. Mehta
Division of Cardiology, University of Arkansas for Medical Sciences and Central Arkansas Veterans Healthcare System, Little Rock, AR 72205, USA

Mayank Singhal
Cape Fear Valley Hospital, Fayetteville, NC 28304, USA

Ali Salami
Rammal Hassan Rammal Research Laboratory, Physio-toxicity (PhyTox) Research Group, Lebanese University, Faculty of Sciences (V), Nabatieh 1700, Lebanon

Christy Costanian
Faculty of Medicine, University of Ottawa, Ottawa 61350, ON K1G 5Z3, Canada
School of Medicine, Lebanese American University, Beirut 1102 2801, Lebanon

Said El Shamieh
Department of Medical Laboratory Technology, Faculty of Health Sciences, Beirut Arab University, Beirut 115020, Lebanon

Natasa Cvetinovic
Department of Cardiology, University Clinical Hospital Center "Dr. Dragisa Misovic—Dedinje", 11000 Belgrade, Serbia

Goran Loncar
Institute for Cardiovascular Diseases Dedinje, 11000 Belgrade, Serbia
School of Medicine, University of Belgrade, 11000 Belgrade, Serbia

Andjelka M. Isakovic
School of Medicine, University of Belgrade, 11000 Belgrade, Serbia

Stephan von Haehling
Department of Cardiology and Pneumology, University of Goettingen Medical Center, DE-37075 Goettingen, Germany
German Center for Cardiovascular Research (DZHK), partner site Goettingen, DE-37099 Goettingen, Germany

Wolfram Doehner
Berlin Institute of Health Center for Regenerative Therapies (BCRT) and Department of Cardiology (Virchow Klinikum), German Centre for Cardiovascular Research (DZHK) partner site Berlin, Charité Universitätsmedizin Berlin, DE-13353 Berlin, Germany

Mitja Lainscak
Division of Cardiology, General Hospital Murska Sobota, SI-9000 Murska Sobota, Slovenia
Faculty of Medicine, University of Ljubljana, SI-1000 Ljubljana, Slovenia

Jerneja Farkas
Research Unit, General Hospital Murska Sobota, SI-9000 Murska Sobota, Slovenia
National Institute of Public Health, SI-1000 Ljubljana, Slovenia

Rosa Casas, Ramon Estruch and Emilio Sacanella
Department of Internal Medicine, Hospital Clinic, Institut d'Investigació Biomèdica August Pi I Sunyer (IDIBAPS), University of Barcelona, Villarroel, 170, 08036 Barcelona, Spain
CIBER 06/03: Fisiopatología de la Obesidad y la Nutrición, Instituto de Salud Carlos III, 28029 Madrid, Spain

Sara Castro-Barquero
Department of Internal Medicine, Hospital Clinic, Institut d'Investigació Biomèdica August Pi I Sunyer (IDIBAPS), University of Barcelona, Villarroel, 170, 08036 Barcelona, Spain

Index

www.ingramcontent.com/pod-product-compliance
Lightning Source LLC
LaVergne TN
LVHW060543210926
848485LV00005B/1249